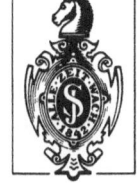

Clinical Practice in Urology
Series Editor: Geoffrey D. Chisholm

Titles in the series already published

Urinary Diversion
Edited by Michael Handley Ashken

Chemotherapy and Urological Malignancy
Edited by A. S. D. Spiers

Urodynamics
Paul Abrams, Roger Feneley and Michael Torrens

The Pharmacology of the Urinary Tract
Edited by M. Caine

Bladder Cancer
Edited by E. J. Zingg and D. M. A. Wallace

Percutaneous and Interventional Urology and Radiology
Edited by Erich K. Lang

Adenocarcinoma of the Prostate
Edited by Andrew W. Bruce and John Trachtenberg

Controversies and Innovations in Urological Surgery
Edited by Clive Gingell and Paul Abrams

Forthcoming titles in the series

Ultrasound in Urology
Edited by W. B. Peeling and D. Rickards

Practical Management of the Urinary Tract in Spinal Cord Damaged Man
Edited by Keith Parsons and John M. Fitzpatrick

Urological Prostheses, Appliances and Catheters
Edited by J. P. Pryor

Male Infertility (Second Edition)
Edited by T. B. Hargreave

Combination Therapy in Urological Malignancy

Edited by
Philip H. Smith

With 28 Figures

Springer-Verlag
London Berlin Heidelberg New York
Paris Tokyo

Philip H. Smith, MB, FRCS
Consultant Urologist, St James's University Hospital, Beckett Street,
Leeds LS9 7TF, UK

Series Editor

Geoffrey D. Chisholm, ChM, FRCS, FRCSEd
Professor of Surgery, University of Edinburgh; and Consultant
Urological Surgeon, Western General Hospital, Edinburgh, Scotland

ISBN-13:978-1-4471-1657-8   e-ISBN-13:978-1-4471-1655-4
DOI: 10.1007/978-1-4471-1655-4

British Library Cataloguing in Publication Data
Combination therapy in urological malignancy.
1. Man. Urogenital System. Cancer. Therapy
I. Smith, P.H. (Philip Henry), *1934–*
II. Series
616.99'4606
ISBN-13:978-1-4471-1657-8

Library of Congress Cataloging-in-Publication Data
Combination therapy in urological malignancy/edited by P.H. Smith
p. cm.— (Clinical practice in urology)
Includes bibliographies and index.
ISBN-13:978-1-4471-1657-8 (Berlin)
1. Genitourinary organs—Cancer—Treatment. 2. Genitourinary organs—Cancer—
Adjuvant treatment.   I. Smith, P.H. (Philip Henry)   II. Series.
[DNLM: 1. Combined Modality Therapy. 2. Urologic Neoplasms—therapy. WJ
160 C731]   RC280.U74C65 1989   616.99'4606—dc19   DNLM/DLC

© Springer-Verlag Berlin Heidelberg 1989
Softcover reprint of the hardcover 1st edition 1989

Filmset by Wilmaset, Birkenhead, Merseyside

2128/3916–543210   Printed on acid-free paper

Series Editor's Foreword

Any discussion of the present success in management of urological cancers evokes a mixed response. Oncologists and urologists can enjoy the success with chemotherapy for testicular cancers but cannot forget the dismal results with any form of treatment, other than surgery, for renal carcinoma. But these are the less frequent urological tumours: what are the attitudes to the more common prostate and bladder cancers. Intensive study, many clinical trials and much debate lead us to the conclusion that we understand them better, we can tailor the treatment more appropriately to the individual patient but there remains some uncertainty as to the overall success that we have achieved. There have been no striking changes in the 5-year survival data.

Clinicians tend to see their success in terms of their special interest. Radiotherapists point to their success in stage-reduction but what are we to do with the many patients whose tumour is unaltered by radiotherapy. Urological surgeons, and especially those who are still influenced by the shadow of Halsted, point to their success in excising the cancer but apart from that highly selected group, what are we to do for the very large number of patients for whom surgery is inappropriate. Bystanders can only watch and listen to the arguments for and against these views.

Could one conclusion be that we have reached the limits for each of these methods of attack on cancer?

An earlier volume in this series concentrated on chemotherapy and urological malignancy. It is a measure of the change in emphasis in the attack on cancer that this book now considers combination therapy and urological malignancy. Mr Philip Smith has gathered together a most impressive group of contributors from no less than 10 different countries. The experience of these contributors gives an authority to the chapters that will be readily appreciated. The contributors analyse the facts and the reader will quickly find a state-of-the-art opinion. Controversial topics such as the value of clinical trials, the quality of

life and the cost of treatment are included in this volume. These and
the chapters by other contributors have created an important addition
to the aim of this Series which is to bring to the reader the best possible
opinions in the clinical practice of urology.

Edinburgh   Geoffrey D. Chisholm
January 1989

Preface

Any new volume must justify its existence. This contribution is based upon the premise that chemotherapy, radiotherapy or surgery alone is inadequate to control the majority of urological tumours.

For many years surgeons and radiotherapists have explored the possibilities of combination therapy and within the last decade the medical oncologist has played an increasing role as treatment by cytotoxic chemotherapy has been shown to be of major importance in at least some urological tumours.

Whilst surgery may be adequate to control the localised lesion it is still often difficult to be certain that a tumour which is clinically localised within its organ of origin is not, microscopically at least, already invading lymph nodes or spreading elsewhere. The recognition of this fact justifies the increasingly determined search for effective cytotoxic drugs which must eventually play a primary role in the management of all tumours.

Once control of the local lesion, distant metastases and micro-metastases has been accomplished the surgeon may still have a role in excising residual tumour and in some cases in reconstruction of the urinary tract.

Within the last ten years many of those interested in urological oncology have been invited to visit Erice in Sicily for informal and in-depth workshops organised most expertly by Professor Michele Pavone-Macaluso. These courses have provided an unrivalled milieu in which exchanges of views and cross fertilisation of opinion could occur.

At least one of the authors of each chapter in this book has visited Erice; all have responded warmly to the view that combination treatment must be the aim, to the need for such a volume and to the concept that it should appear without delay and with acknowledgement of the indebtedness of the authors to the effort, commitment and insight shown by Professor Pavone-Macaluso, to whom this volume is dedicated – without his permission or his knowledge. His co-authors hope that he will not be offended and thank him for his unstinting and continuing efforts to assist the development of urological oncology.

This volume outlines the current possibilities for combination therapy in the battle against urological cancer and highlights some of the problems which remain to be solved, including the place of surveillance in patients with Stage 1 tumours of the testis and the problems of administering effective chemotherapy to patients with invasive bladder cancer many of whom are in poor general health. It also explores the increasing possibilities offered by reconstructive surgical techniques and attempts to assess both the cost of treatment and the quality of life for the patient.

If it encourages those interested in these conditions to think regularly beyond the confines of their own speciality its main aim will have been achieved.

Leeds   Philip H. Smith
June 1988

Contents

Contributors

N. K. Aaronson, PhD
The Netherlands Cancer Institute, Plesmanlaan 121, 1066 CX
Amsterdam, The Netherlands

R. Ackermann, MD
Department of Urology, University of Dusseldorf Medical School,
Moorenstrasse 5, D-4000 Dusseldorf, FRG

W. W. Bonney, MD
Department of Urology, University of Iowa Hospital, Iowa City, Iowa
52240, USA

S. A. Brosman, MD
Kaiser-Permanante, 4900 Sunset Boulevard, Los Angeles, California
90027, USA

F. Calais da Silva, MD
Consultant Urologist, Hospital Desterro, Lisbon, Portugal

T. Ebert, MD
Department of Urology, University of Dusseldorf Medical School,
Moorenstrasse 5, D-4000 Dusseldorf, FRG

Sophie D. Fosså, MD, PhD
Consultant, the Norwegian Radium Hospital, Department of Medical
Oncology and Radiotherapy, 0310 Oslo 3, Norway

F. S. Freiha, MD, FACS
Stanford University School of Medicine, Division of Urology, Stanford University Medical Center, Stanford, California 94305, USA

B. Goldwasser, MD
Acting Chairman, Department of Urology, Chaim Sheba Medical
Center and Senior Lecturer, Sackler School of Medicine, Tel-Aviv
University, Department of Urology, Chaim Sheba Medical Center,
Tel-Hashomer 52621, Israel

A. Horwich, PhD, MRCP, FRCP
The Royal Marsden Hospital and Institute of Cancer Research,
Academic Unit of Radiotherapy and Oncology, The Royal Marsden
Hospital, Downs Road, Sutton SM2 5PT, UK

J. Hutton, BSc, BPhil
Senior Research Fellow, Centre for Health Economics, University of
York, Heslington, York YO1 5DD, UK

W. G. Jones, MB, ChB, FRCR, DMRT
Senior Lecturer in Radiotherapy and Honorary Consultant, Univer-
sity Department of Radiotherapy, Tunbridge Building, Cookridge
Hospital, Leeds LS16 6QB, UK

O. Nativ, MD
Consultant, Department of Urology, Chaim Sheba Medical Center,
Tel-Hashomer 52621, Israel

D. W. W. Newling, MB, BChir, FRCS
Consultant Urological Surgeon, Department of Urology, Princess
Royal Hospital, Salthouse Road, Hull HU8 9HE, UK

M. Pavone-Macaluso, MD
University of Palermo, Institute of Urology, Polyclinico P. Giaccone,
Via Del Vespro 129, 90127 Palerma, Italy

D. Raghavan, MB, BS, PhD, FRACP
Research Director, Urological Cancer Research Unit and Oncologist,
Royal Prince Alfred Hospital, Missenden Road, Camperdown, New
South Wales 2050, Australia

J. Ramon, MD
Resident in Urology, Department of Urology, Chaim Sheba Medical
Center, Tel-Hashomer 52621, Israel

C. J. Rodenburg, MD, PhD
Department of Medical Oncology, Rotterdam Cancer Institute,
Groene Hilledijk 301, 3075 EA Rotterdam. The Netherlands

H. I. Scher, MD
Assistant Attending Physician, Memorial Sloan-Kettering Cancer
Center and Assistant Professor of Medicine, Cornell University
Medical College, Memorial Sloan-Kettering Cancer Center, 1275
York Avenue, New York, New York 10021, USA

W. U. Shipley, MD
Harvard Medical School and Massachusetts General Hospital Cancer
Center, Department of Radiation Medicine, Massachusetts General
Hospital Cancer Center, Boston, Massachusetts, USA

Cora N. Sternberg, MD
Clinical Assistant Attending Memorial Sloan-Kettering Cancer
Center and Clinical Instructor, Department of Medicine, Cornell
University Medical College, Memorial Sloan-Kettering Cancer
Center, 1275 York Avenue, New York, New York 10021, USA

G. Stoter, MD
Medical Oncologist, Rotterdam Cancer Institute, Groene Hilledijk
301, 3075 EA Rotterdam, The Netherlands

I. F. Tannock, MD, PhD
Princess Margaret Hospital and University of Toronto, 500 Sher-
bourne Street, Toronto, Ontario M4X 1K9, Canada

Radiation Therapy: its Integration with Surgery and Chemotherapy in the Management of Patients with Urological Malignancy

W.U. Shipley

The combination of radiation therapy with surgery and/or chemotherapy in the treatment of urological malignancy varies widely in this heterogeneous group of tumours, both in usefulness in the curative management of the primary tumour as well as in palliation (and cure in testis cancer) of patients with metastatic disease. Thus, these combinations – radiation and surgery, radiation and chemotherapy – will be dealt with separately and by tumour site.

Radiation Therapy Combined with Surgery

Bladder Cancer

Radiation therapy has its main potential usefulness in patients with invasive (of muscle) bladder cancer. Thus, in patients with superficial tumours, only specialised techniques of brachytherapy or electron beam intraoperative radiation therapy will be addressed.

The Selection of Patients with Tumours that Respond Well to Irradiation

If the patient is to be treated well with radiation therapy for an invasive bladder

Table 1.1.   Local control following external beam irradiation

	Number of patients	Clinical stage	Total dose (cGy)	Maintained local control (%)
Miller and Johnson (1973)	428	T1–T4	5800–6500	27
Parsons et al. (1981)	31	T3, T4	6300–6500	48
Shipley et al. (1985)	37	T2, T3	6400–6840	49
Timmer et al. (1985)	76	T2, T3	6000–6500	41
Quilty and Duncan (1986)	333	T3	5000–5750	24
Blandy et al. (1988)	138	T2, T3	6000	40

tumour, there must be close coordination and combination with the urological oncologist. This urologist is responsible for the initial thorough evaluation of the patient and thus plays a major role in the selection process as to whether the patient should be considered for initial cystectomy, with or without adjuvant chemotherapy or radiation, or for an initial attempt at bladder preservation by incorporating radiation and often chemotherapy in the treatment. In the absence of any positive selection, patients with invasive tumours who have been treated with full-dose radiation alone have had a 50% to 75% local tumour persistence or recurrence rate (Table 1.1). Thus, it is best to select subgroups that are relatively more likely to have the radiation succeed. Blandy was the first to report a favourable and significant correlation between achieving a complete local response following radiation therapy and patient survival (Blandy et al. 1980). He has recently updated the London Hospital experience with homogeneous radiation treatment using the radiation beam from a linear accelerator (Blandy et al. 1988). Between 1979 and 1985, 138 patients, all having clinical stage T2 or T3 invasive tumours, were treated. Cystoscopic evaluation 3 and 6 months after radiotherapy resulted in a complete response in 64 patients (47%). To date, all these patients are alive with intervals up to 5 years. Although 11 patients have had a local relapse none has developed distant metastases. Local recurrences were treated in 10 patients by radical salvage cystectomy and in one by chemotherapy. Of the 74 patients, 41 (53%) who showed incomplete regression of the tumour at the completion of radiation therapy have died of bladder cancer. Only 17 of this group were judged fit to undergo radical cystectomy (the remainder were either medically unfit or developed distant metastases). All 17 patients tolerated cystectomy well but only two have been longterm survivors. Blandy's conclusions are:

1. Compared to his prior results, patients needing salvage cystectomy have been able to tolerate that operation much better, perhaps because of improvements in both radiation therapy and perioperative care
2. The response to radiation therapy identifies those for whom cystectomy is likely to confer benefit. Those who have an excellent response to radiation may benefit from cystectomy if local relapse occurs. When radiation produces only incomplete regression, subsequent cystectomy is unlikely to be associated with prolonged survival
3. Cystectomy may be safely deferred in the complete responders, most of whom will not require this operation
4. The radiation response rate has not improved significantly compared to the prior series, and thus further progress with conventional radiation therapy alone and prompt salvage cystectomy seems unlikely

Unfavourable prognostic factors in patients irradiated for clinical stage T2 and T3 disease include ureteral obstruction on excretory urography (Shipley et al. 1985; Greiner et al. 1977), the absence of papillary surface histological character- istics (Shipley et al. 1985; Timmer et al. 1985), and the absence of a visibly complete transurethral resection prior to radiation (Shipley et al. 1987b). Thus, in patients with only solid surface histological characteristics and/or with ureteral obstruction, and/or in whom a transurethral resection resulting in substantial tumour debulking is not possible, additional therapy to radiation alone should be considered.

Transurethral Surgical Resection and Radiation Therapy

In 1973 the M. D. Anderson Hospital first reported a favourable subset of 43 patients with clinical stage T2 and T3 tumours who had undergone complete resection of their tumours prior to full-dose radiation therapy (Miller and Johnson 1973). Resection was either transurethral or by open fulguration. The 5-year survival was 45% in this group of patients – significantly better than in those patients with similar stage tumours who were either incompletely resected or biopsied only (26% for stage T2 patients and 20% for stage T3 patients). In addition, the permanent local control rate was higher in the completely resected subgroup – 65% compared to 27%. In the Massachusetts General Hospital series (Shipley et al. 1985), we noted a favourable outcome for permanent local control, patient survival and freedom from distant metastases in those patients in whom the urologist was able to carry out a "visibly complete" transurethral resection prior to radiation therapy (Fig. 1.1). The 5-year survival from bladder cancer in the group who underwent a "complete" resection was 54% versus 17% in the group who did not ($P = 0.009$). The extent of transurethral surgery was, on multivariate analysis, an independent and the most significant variable predicting permanent local control. Thus, combining transurethral techniques which will safely provide maximum tumour debulking prior to radiation therapy seems clinically important. A thorough transurethral resection substantially reduces the number of remaining tumour cells that must be inactivated by radiation but is frequently only done in tumours of small initial size or of exophytic type. By waiting 3 to 4 weeks following completion of a conventionally thorough transurethral resection, treating with 180-cGy fractions for 5 sessions a week, and boosting high dose (6840 cGy) only for the bladder tumour volume and not the whole bladder, patients have usually been able to tolerate full-dose radiation therapy without significant reduction in bladder capacity (Shipley et al. 1985).

Intraoperative Radiation Therapy of Bladder Cancer (IORT)

In appropriate patients open surgery can provide the ability to deliver more radiation safely and selectively directly to the tumour and less to the uninvolved portion of the bladder. The flagship experience over the last 25 years is with brachytherapy using radium-226 implants (van der Werf-Messing et al. 1983a,b; 1988). Intraoperatively the radium needles were inserted into and immediately adjacent to the tumour through an open cystotomy. Recently, the radioactive source has been changed to caesium-137. Sutures are attached to needles and

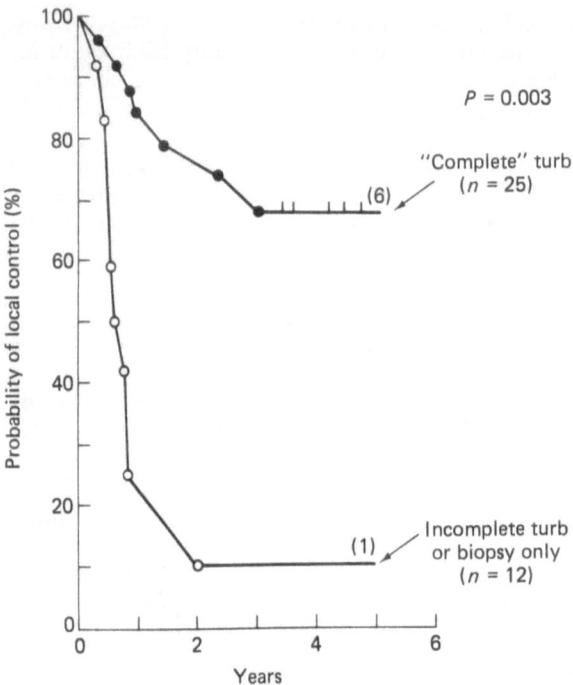

Fig. 1.1. The probability of local control by full-dose radiation therapy in patients with stage T2 and T3 bladder cancer in whom a "visibly complete" transurethral resection of the bladder tumour (*TURB*) was possible, and in patients in whom only an incomplete resection or biopsy was done. The numbers in parentheses indicate the number of patients followed beyond 5 years. (Reproduced from WU Shipley, GR Prout Jr., SD Kaufman et al. (1987) *Cancer* 60: 511–520).

brought out through a separate tract or from the incision and are used to remove the needles following the delivery of from 3250 to 6500 cGy of radiation over 3 to 6 days. Problems with wound seeding resulting from the open cystotomy have been solved by the use of preoperative radiation therapy with doses of 1050 cGy over 3 elapsed days. Selection criteria include that the tumour is usually solitary and always less than 5 cm in diameter. In 196 patients with Ta and T1 tumours, only 12% had a recurrence in their bladder in 5 years (van der Werf-Messing et al. 1988). In 328 stage T2 patients, but not all with proven muscle invasion, who were implanted, 77% have remained free of recurrence for at least 5 years (van der Werf-Messing et al. 1983a). With this treatment T2 tumours with non-papillary histology or poor differentiation have a significantly poorer result, but a recent treatment modification of 40 Gy preoperatively and only 50% dose by implant seems to give better results (van der Werf-Messing et al. 1988). For patients with stage T3 tumours less than 5 cm in diameter, a 3500-cGy tumour implant was preceded by 1050 cGy of preoperative radiation therapy and followed by an additional 3000 cGy in 15 fractions of external beam treatment to the bladder as well as to the pelvic lymph nodes. In 41 patients, the overall 5-year survival was 57%, and the local recurrence rate 18% (van der Werf-Messing et al. 1983b). A similar good experience has been reported by Batterman and Tierie (1986) from Amsterdam. A slightly different brachytherapy approach has recently been reported by Mazeron et al. (1985) using a single-plane afterloading iridium-192 implant, combined with complete gross tumour removal (usually by limited partial cystectomy) and an external lymph node dissection. The results are also very good (Table 1.2) but a limitation of this technique is that only 1-cm thickness can be irradiated by the single-plane afterloading implant. This precludes treatment of patients with clinical or pathological stage T3b tumours.

Table 1.2. Intraoperative radiation therapy: clinical stage T2 bladder cancer

	Number of patients	Treatment[a]	5-year local control (%)	5-year survival (%)
van der Werf-Messing et al. 1983a	328	XRT, Ra–226	77	56
Batterman and Tierie 1986	85	XRT, Ra–226	74	55
Mazeron et al. 1985	24	Resection, Ir–192, XRT	92	58
Matsumoto et al. 1981	28	IORT, XRT	82	62

[a] XRT, External beam irradiation.
Ra–226, brachytherapy by radium needles.
IR–192, brachytherapy by afterloading iridium in catheters.
IORT, single dose electron beam irradiation.

In Japan, intraoperative radiation therapy has been given by electron beam irradiation with single 2500 to 3000 cGy doses to the bladder tumour volume at the time of open cystotomy. Most patients have been given an additional 3000 to 4000 cGy postoperatively in 15 or 20 daily treatments. The procedure has been well tolerated and the freedom from local recurrence rates were: 94% for stage Ta, 88% for stage T1, and 82% for stage T2 (Matsumoto et al. 1981). Of the 57 patients who have been followed for at least 5 years, 81% are without evidence of recurrence.

While such retrospective reports may include some unclear patient selection factors, they all indicate that intraoperative radiation therapy either by electron beam or by temporary interstitially implanted radioactivity is effective against superficial and minimally invasive tumours. The Radiation Therapy Oncology Group (RTOG) is now planning a prospective evaluation of combining intraoperative electron beam radiation therapy following initial treatment with multiple-drug chemotherapy for patients with invasive bladder tumours that are less than 5 cm and in or adjacent to the trigone. External beam radiation therapy will be given as a short preoperative course to prevent the possibility of tumour seeding but any additional pelvic external beam radiation therapy will be reserved only for those patients who have biopsy-proven residual disease, i.e. who do not have a surgically confirmed complete response following the initial debulking trans-urethral surgery and the neoadjuvant chemotherapy. By a combination of selection of the appropriate electron beam energy, lateral angulation of the beam and the use of a temporary thin lead shield posterior to the tumour during IORT, significant doses of radiation to the rectum can be avoided.

Radiation Therapy as an Adjuvant to Cystectomy

Over the last two decades preoperative radiation therapy followed by total or radical cystectomy has been the standard treatment. While there are still questions as to the value of such adjuvant radiation treatment, the patients in each reported series who reached a post-irradiation pathological stage of pTO, pTis, or pT1 experienced marked improvement in survival when compared to historical or control populations (van der Werf-Messing 1982; Prout 1984; Bloom et al. 1982). A retrospective review of all published series by clinical stage with and without preoperative radiation therapy indicates a 10% or more survival advantage to those patients treated by preoperative radiation therapy rather than by radical cystectomy alone. However, despite good local control with preoperative radiation therapy (Table 1.3), in at least 85% to 90% of patients, these series also revealed a significant incidence of distant metastases. Thus, since it is currently hoped that multi-drug cisplatin-containing chemotherapy may be effective against distant metastases that are undetected by the physician at the time of diagnosis, precystectomy chemotherapy (sometimes with radiation therapy) is now undergoing extensive phase I/II and soon, phase III evaluation. At our institution we have reserved precystectomy radiation therapy only for those patients with clinical T3b or larger tumours who present with sufficient upper urinary tract compromise to preclude the use of methotrexate, cisplatin, and vinblastine neoadjuvant chemotherapy combined with 4000-cGy preoperative radiation therapy (*vida infra*, page 17). Usually percutaneous upper tract drainage during the $4\frac{1}{2}$ weeks of preoperative radiation therapy is adequate and a pretreatment urinary diversion can be avoided.

Table 1.3. Local-regional control following adjuvant pre-operative external beam irradiation and cystectomy

	Number of patients	Clinical stage	Total dose (cGy)	Surgery[a]	Maintained pelvic control
Miller and Johnson 1973	101	T3	5000	RC alone	87%
Batata et al. 1981	133	T3, T4	2000	RC and PL	88%
van der Werf-Messing 1982	183	T3 (>5 cm)	4000	RC alone	100%
Shipley et al. 1986	175	T2–T4a	4000	RC and PL	92%

[a] RC, Radical cystectomy.
PL, Pelvic lymphadenectomy.

Prostate Cancer

For patients with prostatic adenocarcinoma of comparable clinical stage – T2A or the B1 nodular tumours – the 15-year overall survival following either radical prostatectomy (Jewett 1980; Jewett and Walsh 1982; Gibbons et al. 1984) or radiation therapy (Bagshaw 1985) is similar and ranges from 51% to 57% (Fig. 1.2). While some differences may exist in these series, the overall efficacy of either radiation therapy or surgery is high and similar. An earlier American Veterans' Administration study for patients with stage T2 (B) tumours treated either by radical surgery or by observation showed no clear benefit from surgery on overall survival (Byar and Corle 1981). However, these patients were not staged with present techniques that use radionuclide bone scans and the number

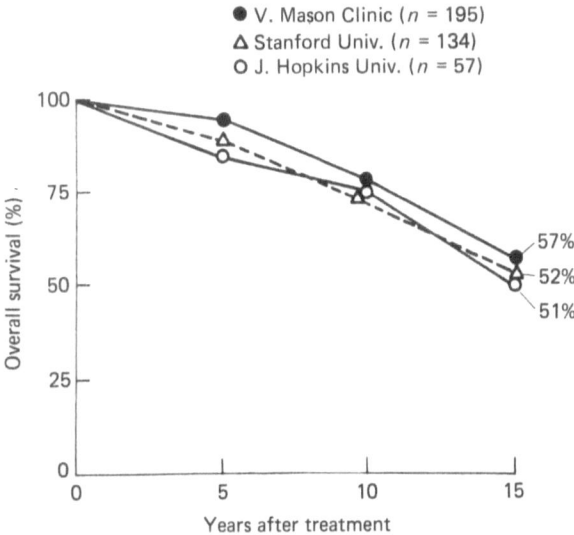

Fig. 1.2. The reported overall survival following treatment for patients with stage T2a (B1) prostatic carcinoma following radical prostatectomy at either Johns Hopkins University (Jewett 1980; Jewett and Walsh 1982) or the Virginia Mason Clinic (Gibbons et al. 1984), or following external beam radiation therapy at Stanford University (Bagshaw 1985).

of patients in each group was small and accessioned from a large number of institutions.

Based on present-day information, a US National Institutes of Health Consensus Development Conference (15–17 June 1987) judged that patients with stage T1b (A2) or stage T2 (B) tumours with substantial expected longevity should be offered treatment either by radical surgery or by radiation therapy, and that the patient should decide himself which treatment he would prefer after being fully informed of possible treatment complications (Livingston et al. 1987). In his introductory remarks to the conference, Dr. Willet F. Whitmore, Jr. emphasised some of the important dilemmas facing clinicians caring for patients with prostatic adenocarcinoma – a disease so heterogeneous and unpredictable that it may well be that the biology of the tumour is more important with regard to outcome than is the treatment. He defined three subgroups – patients whose tumours are such that they will do well regardless of treatment, those in whom the treatment efficacy determines the outcome, and those whose tumours are such that they will do poorly regardless of treatment. He pointed out that it is not possible to know into which of these three subgroups an individual patient belongs at diagnosis. In all the series presented to the NIH panel, the initial tumour size or stage at diagnosis was the dominant significant factor in predicting outcome (survival, survival without evidence of tumour progression, or without evidence of local tumour recurrence) whether the treatment was radical surgery or radiation therapy. These series revealed that when a palpable primary tumour was limited to the prostate (stage T2, or B) only 10% or so of the patients would have local recurrence, and only 20% to 25% would have progression with distant metastasis after treatment with either surgery or radiation therapy. In contrast, in patients who presented with a palpable tumour extending outside the prostate (stage T3 and T4, or stage C) the local recurrence rates were 25% to 40% and the probability of progression with distant metastases was 50% to 75%. The implications of these observations are that earlier diagnosis will be of enormous benefit to patients. Unfortunately, the majority of patients who present with localised prostatic adenocarcinoma do so with the more locally advanced stage T3, or C tumours, and in those patients progression with distant metastases is *the* major clinical problem. The solution awaits the development of effective, tolerable adjuvant systemic therapies, or of the medical ability to diagnose these tumours sooner.

Pelvic Lymph Node Excision Prior to External Beam Radiation Therapy

Staging pelvic lymphadenectomy prior to radiation therapy is used infrequently and the indications for it are not clear. Between 1978 and 1983, the Radiation Therapy Oncology Group (RTOG) found that only 26% of 445 patients with stage T1b (A2) or T2 (B) tumours were evaluated by lymph nodal staging prior to entrance into their studies (Asbell et al. 1987). A figure of about 25% is also the one cited in many single institutions' retrospective analyses reported in the last few years (Bagshaw 1985; Perez 1983; Pilepich et al. 1987; Zagars et al. 1987; Shipley et al. 1988b). In the multi-institutional RTOG study, the incidence of significant complications was not affected by previous pelvic lymph nodal staging. However, those patients found surgically to be without evidence of lymph nodal metastases had a lower probability of progressing with distant metastases than did those patients whose lymph nodes were staged only by a "negative" lymphangio-gram (Asbell et al. 1987). The rationale for carrying out this invasive pre-irradiation staging procedure is to select for radiation therapy only those patients who do not have metastasising tumours. While this is an eminently reasonable rationale, the reason it is clinically not judged either wise or practical is that the majority of men treated by external beam radiation therapy are over 70 years old and thus may tolerate the surgical procedure with more difficulty than they would the radiation. Persistent radiation-related morbidity following external beam radiation therapy is now less than 10% (Shipley et al. 1988b; Pilepich 1988; Hanks 1988) and in most cases only requires the persistent use of medication to decrease bowel hyperactivity. Only in fewer than 2% of patients is open surgery necessary for control or correction of a urological or gastrointestinal complication. However, erectile impotence in previously potent patients is reported following irradiation in from one-third to one-half of patients (Shipley et al. 1988b; Pilepich 1988).

In summary, the major enthusiasm for the use of pre-irradiation staging pelvic lymphadenectomy seems to be in patients who are entering carefully controlled clinical trials and for men who present with localised prostatic cancer and are under 60 years old. In the former group, the information is of great value in multivariate analysis with regard to treatment outcome. In the latter group, radiation treatment, which may cause a substantial decrease in the quality of life by causing erectile impotency, can be avoided in patients with numerous pelvic lymph nodal metastases, as their chance of cure from any local treatment is very low indeed (Bagshaw 1985; Scardino et al. 1986; Scardino 1988; Thayer et al. 1987).

Transurethral Surgery or Biopsy Before or After Radiation Therapy

Based on careful multivariate analysis of the American Patterns of Care Study, Hanks and colleagues (Hanks 1988) identified a clear association between transurethral surgery prior to radiation therapy and subsequent progression with distant metastases. However, this relationship has *only* been found in irradiated patients with stage T3 (C) tumours that are of *poor* histological differentiation. Recently, in a large group of patients treated by combined external beam radiation therapy and gold-198 interstitial therapy, Scardino and colleagues (Scardino 1988) found a statistical association between the need for a transurethral resection and tumour size, as well as the incidence of pelvic lymph node metastases. Thus, while the earlier observations suggested a causal relationship between transurethral surgery and the subsequent development of distant metastases, recent work suggests that it may be only a reflection of a more virulent biology of the tumour at diagnosis. No study has resolved this issue. At this institution we favour a transurethral prostatectomy prior to radiation therapy in patients judged to have significant urinary outflow obstruction. Such patients have a 10%–15% incidence of developing a bladder neck or prostatic urethral stricture subsequent to radiation therapy, but these are usually easily managed by a single minor transurethral procedure (Shipley et al. 1988b). While the incidence of benign bladder neck or prostatic urethral stricture is less in patients not having prior transurethral surgery (1.7%), healing from a "significant" transurethral resection following high-dose irradiation is compromised and may result in incontinence.

The clinical value or importance of post-irradiation prostatic biopsy as a routine method of evaluating patients is not clear. Several investigators have shown that the incidence of clinically undetected microscopic cancer in patients irradiated for stage T2b (B2) or T3 (C) tumour ranges from 20% to 60%. Further, there is a correlation between a positive post-irradiation biopsy and the subsequent development of distant metastases (Scardino 1988; Freiha and Bagshaw 1984). However, since no clear benefit has been shown from the use of adjuvant systemic hormone or chemotherapy, the "early" prediction of the subsequent development of distant metastases may be of no benefit to the individual patient. In addition, the correlation between the positive post-irradiation biopsy and the development of distant metastases is likely to result from the fact that both events are strongly influenced by the initial tumour volume rather than as a consequence of a microscopic volume of tumour cells persisting at the primary tumour site. Only when a large series of patients with similar sized tumours of similar differentiation are analysed for the relationship between positive tumour biopsy following irradiation and progression with distant metastases could a causal relationship be identified. We recommend the routine use of post-irradiation biopsy *only* in those patients who are participating in a rigorous clinical trial testing the efficacy of one form of local radiation therapy against another. Further, in the absence of symptoms or of a progressing local prostatic tumour, we do not recommend any treatment for patients with biopsy-persistent tumour cells two or more years following radiation therapy. Serial transrectal ultrasonic studies as an improved method of following gross prostatic cancer response to radiation therapy warrants evaluation. Transrectal ultrasound may well be a better approach to monitoring local tumour response following radiation therapy than prostatic-specific antigen which may rise on serial evaluations due either to local tumour regrowth or to progression of distant metastases.

Interstitial Radiation Therapy

For patients with stage T2 (B) tumours as well as those with some minimal stage T3 tumours, the Memorial Sloan–Kettering Cancer Center Group (Grossman et al. 1982) and others (Peschel et al. 1985; DeLaney et al. 1986) report that the iodine-125 retropubic implant yields an overall 5-year survival from 83% to 87%. The initial impression that the iodine-125 implant gave less radiation-related morbidity and preserved erectile potency better than external beam irradiation, has not subsequently been borne out (Shipley et al. 1988b; Hanks 1988; Peschel et al. 1985; DeLaney et al. 1986). In addition, when the initial tumour size has been large and/or when the radiation implant has yielded inhomogeneous doses of radiation across the tumour (Thayer et al. 1987), the local control rate has been less than seen following radical prostatectomy (Gibbons et al. 1984) or external beam radiation therapy (Bagshaw 1985). However, when tumour size has been small and iodine-125 doses have been homogeneous the local recurrence rate appears to be very similar to that achieved with external beam irradiation (Fig. 1.3). A combination of external beam irradiation (4000–5000 cGy), lymphade-

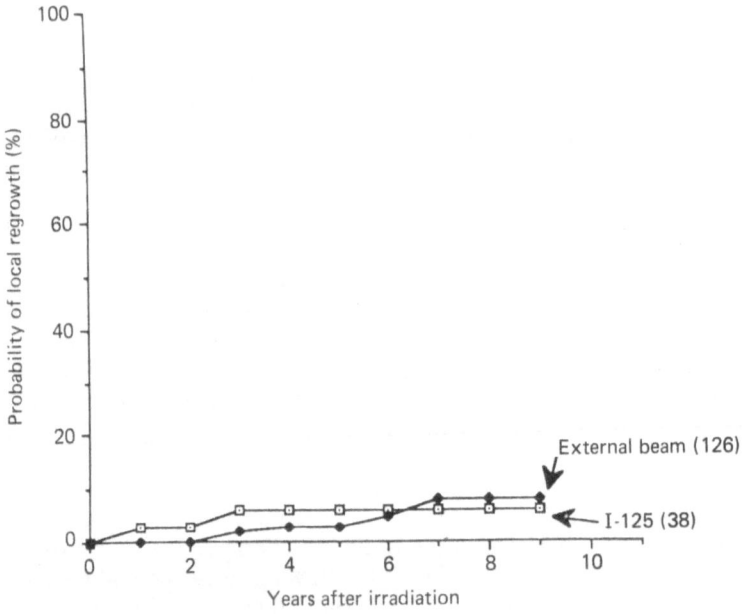

Fig. 1.3. The cumulative incidence for local tumour regrowth for patients with stage T2 tumours treated either by external beam radiation therapy or iodine-125 implantation.

nectomy and retropubic implantation with gold-198 (2500–3500 cGy to the tumour nodule) has been used by the Baylor Group (Scardino et al. 1986) yielding very satisfactory 5- (90%) and 10- (68%) year survivals in 232 patients, with minimal radiation-related morbidity. However, this group showed a clear correlation between a positive post-radiation biopsy and the development of distant metastases, which suggests some possible ineffectiveness of the radiation therapy. The high actuarial local recurrence rate at 10 years (49%) may be due to this fact or, since no patient was given hormonal treatment, to the lack of this possible additional therapy (Scardino et al. 1986; Scardino 1988).

Radiation Therapy Following Radical Prostatectomy

Patients who are found to have microscopic invasion of the seminal vesicles or positive resection margins following radical prostatectomy have an impaired local control and overall survival (Jewett 1980; Gibbons et al. 1986). Local radiation therapy in such patients with unfavourable pathology leads to a reduction in local recurrence (Gibbons et al. 1986; Anscher and Prosnitz 1987; Forman et al. 1986; Ray et al. 1984). The impact on survival remains controversial (Paulson et al. 1986; Bosch et al. 1987) even though two retrospective series suggest important benefit (Gibbons et al. 1986; Anscher and Prosnitz 1987). While such controversy is likely to persist until, and possibly after, a definitive randomised trial is completed, one relatively clear fact has emerged. The dose of radiation therapy needed in the adjuvant setting is likely to be *less* than when given without radical surgery. A dose in the range of 5500–6100 cGy with conventional fractionation is probably adequate as fewer tumour cells need to be eradicated and the patient's tolerance for radiation therapy following radical surgery may be less (Ray et al. 1984) due to some reduction in the blood supply to the lower urinary tract and the rectum from surgery. Our institutional policy has been to offer adjuvant postoperative radiation therapy to patients with positive resection margins, with microscopic involvement of the seminal vesicles, and to those with a few unsuspected (microscopic) metastases in the pelvic lymph nodes. We have found this approach well tolerated and one that has so far, prevented local recurrence of tumour.

Palliation of Patients Presenting With Spinal Cord Compression By Metastatic Tumour

In patients presenting with paraplegia at diagnosis and who have an expected longevity of more than 12 months, we have used initial decompression by laminectomy followed by postoperative radiation therapy. With this approach, 50% of our patients have become ambulatory compared to only 20% when radiation is used alone (D. Flynn, personal communication). However, in patients who present with pain but are ambulatory and whose radiographic studies (myelogram or MRI) show spinal cord compression by metastatic prostatic cancer, over 75% are ambulatory following treatment, whether by radiation therapy alone or by laminectomy followed by radiation therapy. In 53 patients analysed retrospectively following spinal cord compression from metastatic prostatic cancer, the rates of ambulation post-treatment were highest when the neurological damage at diagnosis was the least, i.e. 82% in those patients who were ambulatory at presentation, 52% for those who were para-paretic at diagnosis, and only 32% for those patients who were paraplegic at presentation. Thus, if patients are advised to come immediately for evaluation and treatment if severe back pain and/or leg weaknesses should develop, they are likely to maximise the benefit we can offer with palliative treatment. Further, if they do present with paralysis and have an expected longevity of greater than 12 months, laminectomy with prompt decompression should be strongly considered prior to attempted palliation with local radiation therapy.

Testis Cancer

Seminoma

Seminoma is exquisitely sensitive to radiation therapy and usually presents at an early stage. Postorchidectomy external beam radiation therapy to the retroperitoneal lymph nodes achieves a very high cure rate for patients presenting with early stage tumours (Table 1.4). When the orchidectomy has been done through a radical inguinal incision, a dose to the retroperitoneal lymph nodes of 2500–3000 cGy can be given with satisfactory shielding; the other testicle is very likely to maintain fertility (Kubo and Shipley 1982). Supradiaphragmatic radiation therapy is not given for stage I or stage IIA patients because prophylactic mediastinal radiation has been judged of no additional benefit (Peckham 1981; Thomas et al. 1982).

Table 1.4. Results of postorchidectomy radiation therapy in Stage I seminoma testis

Treatment centre	Total number of patients	5-year survival (%)
Walter Reed Army Hosp. (Maier and Sulak 1973)	284	97
Royal Marsden Hosp. (Hamilton et al. 1986)	232	98
M. D. Anderson Hosp. (Zagars and Babaian 1987a)	161	95
Stanford University Hosp. (Earle et al. 1973)	71	100
Massachusetts General Hosp. (Dosoretz et al. 1981)	135	98
US Patterns of Care Study (Hanks et al. 1981)	229	98
Cross Cancer Institute (Willan and McGowan 1985)	139	98
Total	1251	98

Non-seminomatous Germ Cell Tumours

Because of the very high success rate with chemotherapeutic regimens and the very satisfactory results using surgical resection for residual disease, many clinicians do not appreciate the marked radiation sensitivity of embryonal and teratocarcinoma to local radiation. These histologies are about as sensitive to radiation therapy as are Hodgkin's disease and the other lymphomas. Nevertheless, radiation is non-seminomatous germ-cell tumours is reserved for those patients whose metastases are shown radiographically to respond incompletely to maximal chemotherapy regimens and which are not amenable to postchemotherapy surgical resection. Such metastatic sites include the central mediastinum, the bone, and the brain. Radiation therapy is also indicated when surgical resection of residual disease has been incomplete. Doses with conventional fractionations are used for radiation in this setting, usually in the range of 3600 cGy over 4 weeks. In sites in which the heart and the central nervous system can be completely excluded, higher doses should be considered.

Cancer of the Kidney and Ureter

Radiation Therapy as Adjuvant to Nephrectomy for Renal Cell Carcinoma

Because patients with renal cell carcinoma have a variable and protracted natural history it has been difficult to demonstrate survival benefit from any therapy adjunctive to nephrectomy. Studies of the possible benefit of irradiation combined with nephrectomy are inconclusive. Benefit has been reported from only one non-randomised trial (Rafia 1973). Two randomised trials of postoperative radiation therapy showed no benefit in survival, although in both series significant radiation complications may have masked that benefit (Finney 1973; Kjaer et al. 1987). For instance, in the recent Danish series, the radiation dose per fraction was 250 cGy given to a total dose of 5000 cGy over approximately 4 weeks (Kjaer et al. 1987). These investigators reported severe complications, mainly gastrointestinal in 44%, of which 19% were fatal. Two studies of radiation therapy prior to nephrectomy showed no benefit (van der Werf-Messing 1973; Juusela et al. 1977). However, in both trials the radiation dose was low and in many instances the pathological stage was also low and thus very unlikely to benefit from adjuvant therapy.

Patients who may benefit from postoperative adjunctive radiation therapy include those with pathological evidence of invasion of tumour into Gerota's fascia, to adjacent organs, or with proven metastasis to regional lymph nodes, but without known distant metastatic disease. Radiation therapy is probably best given in 180–200-cGy fractions daily with 10 to 25 MV beams from linear accelerators to the renal fossa and tumour bed, as well as to the para-aortic and para-caval lymph nodes. For right-sided tumours field reduction at 3600–4000 cGy is often necessary in order not to treat more than 30% of the liver parenchyma to the tumour-bed dose of 4500 cGy. Unless there is clear evidence of wound contamination by spill at the time of nephrectomy, no effort is usually made to include, the entire surgical incision in the treatment field.

Adjuvant Radiation Therapy for Transitional Cell Carcinoma of the Renal Pelvis or Ureter

Therapy adjuvant to surgery is unnecessary for low-stage upper tract transitional cell tumours because fewer than 20% of the patients will fail following the primary surgical procedure (Heney et al. 1981; Johannson et al. 1976). A recent retrospective review of patients with poor risk (high tumour stage and/or high histological grade) transitional cell carcinoma of the renal pelvis and ureter suggested benefit from adjuvant radiation therapy (Brookland and Richter 1985). Patients treated with postoperative irradiation of 4000–5000 cGy had a lower incidence of local recurrence (11% against 46%) and a higher 5-year survival (27% against 17%) when compared with patients treated with surgery alone. However, these authors also reported that 45% of the patients in the poor-prognosis group developed distant metastases – the main cancer-related cause of death.

We consider patients with locally advanced disease as possible candidates for postoperative radiation therapy. The dose is in the range of 4500 cGy in 180-cGy fractions over 5 weeks to the tumour bed, and to the regional pelvic lymph nodes with a boost to the tumour bed, if safely possible, to 5000 cGy. However, based on the high incidence of distant metastases, we have recently embarked on a pilot study combining local radiation therapy with adjuvant cisplatin-based chemotherapy. In this instance, when adjuvant chemotherapy is given, doses of radiation therapy are decreased by 10%–15%.

Palliation of Metastatic Renal Cell Carcinoma

The major sites of haematogeneous metastasis from renal cell carcinoma are to bone, lung, and brain. Treatment in virtually all instances is non-curative and the role of the radiation therapist and surgeon in the local management of these metastases is nearly always palliative. Nevertheless, approximately 30% of patients presenting with an initial solitary metastatic lesion will survive 5 years. Therefore, a goal of assuring a durable palliative response in this setting is appropriate. For patients presenting with a "solitary" lung metastasis, spinal metastasis or brain metastasis, initial surgical resection should be considered, usually followed by postoperative radiation therapy. For "solitary" metastasis to the spine, vertebral body resection by the anterior approach has been successful in some carefully selected patients (Sundaresan et al. 1984).

External beam radiation therapy alone is the usual initial palliative approach for patients presenting with symptomatic metastases. A subjective or at times objective response occurs in between one-half and two-thirds of the patients (Fosså et al. 1982; Onufrey and Mohiuddin 1985; Halperin and Harisiadis 1983). To achieve a durable palliative response, doses equivalent to at least 5000 cGy in $5\frac{1}{2}$ weeks would seem necessary (Onufrey and Mohiuddin 1985). The delivery of such high doses often demands the use of multiple field techniques.

Radiation Combined with Systemic Chemotherapy

Bladder Cancer

A randomised phase III trial by Richards et al. (1983) failed to show improvement in patient survival for local control when conventional external beam radiation was combined with post-irradiation 5-fluorouracil (5FU) and adriamycin. However, a decade ago Yagoda and colleagues at the Memorial Sloan–

Table 1.5. Local complete response rates

	Agents[a]	Number of patients	Local complete response rate (%)
Full-dose XRT alone			
London Hospital (1979–85) (Blandy et al. 1988)	XRT	138	47
Institute of Urology (Bloom et al. 1982)	XRT	85	40
Yorkshire Urology Group (Richards et al. 1983)	XRT	55	51
Full-dose XRT and drug			
Yorkshire Urology Group (Richards et al. 1983)	XRT, 5FU, ADR	55	51
National Bladder Cancer Group (Shipley et al. 1987a)	DDP, XRT	57	77
University of Innsbruck (Jakse et al. 1985)	DDP, XRT, ± ADR	44	75
Norwegian Radium Hospital (Shipley et al. 1988a)	DDP, MTX, XRT	19	74
Erlangen, West Germany (Sauer et al. 1987)	DDP, XRT	25	80

[a] XRT, external beam irradiation.
5FU, 5-fluorouracil.
ADR, doxorubicin hydrochloride (adriamycin).
DDP, cisplatin.
MTX, methotrexate.

Kettering Cancer Center showed good activity with systemic cisplatin against metastatic transitional cell carcinoma. This stimulated interest in the possibility of combining cisplatin chemotherapy with radiation therapy in the treatment of patients with locally advanced bladder cancer (Yagoda et al. 1976). To date, the "evidence" for increased efficacy of cisplatin plus radiation is based on reports of high local complete response rates using cisplatin plus radiation therapy when compared (historically, or in non-randomised series) to radiation therapy alone (Table 1.5). Two series have follow-up of from 4 to 5 years. The National Bladder Cancer Group treated patients with stage T2–T4b bladder cancer (all with muscle invasion) who were *not* candidates for cystectomy (Shipley et al. 1987a). Cisplatin (70 mg/m^2) plus external beam radiation therapy (6480 cGy) were used to treat 57 patients who had gross residual disease and who were re-evaluated cystoscopically following treatment. The initial complete response rate was 77%, although 23% of these completely responding tumours recurred. The actuarial 4-year survival rate for the entire group, whether or not they completed the planned treatment, was 35%, significantly better for patients with clinical stage T2 tumours (64%) than for those with clinical stage T3 and T4 tumours (24%, Fig. 1.4). Jakse and colleagues from Innsbruck report a progressive experience in 44 patients with an updated complete response rate of 75% but with local relapse in only 15% of the completely responding group (Jakse et al. 1985; Shipley et al. 1988a). The actuarial 5-year survival for all patients in this series is 46% and 66% for the completely responding patients. Using non-randomised historical comparisons (Table 1.5) the response rate for full-dose external beam irradiation

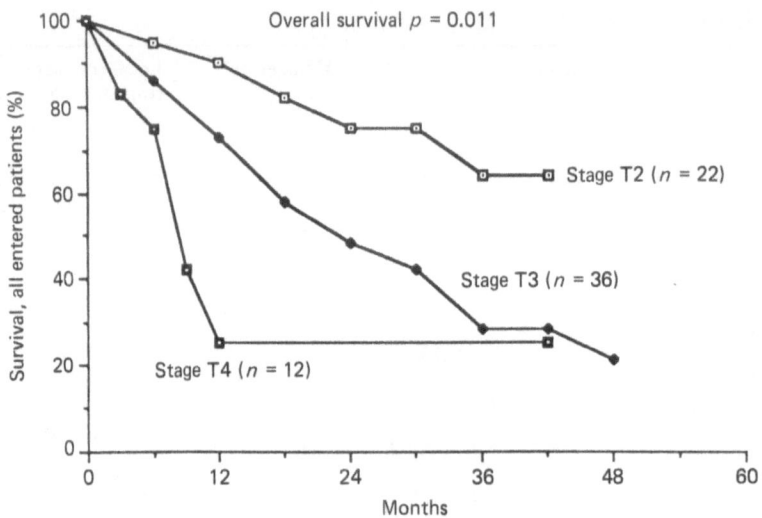

Fig. 1.4. The actuarial survival by clinical stage for all 70 patients entered on the National Bladder Cancer Group protocol of cisplatin and full-dose radiation therapy (Shipley et al. 1987a).

alone ranges from 40% to 51% while the complete response rates using cisplatin plus full-dose radiation, alone or in combination with one other drug, range from 74% to 80%. This gives substantial encouragement for the use of the combination of cisplatin plus radiation therapy *but* this has not yet been demonstrated to be better by a phase III trial evaluating either complete response rate or long-term

Table 1.6. Local complete response rates following chemotherapy alone

	Agents[a]	Number of patients	Local complete response rate (%)
Institute of Urology (Oliver et al. 1984)	MTX	32	9
National Bladder Cancer Group (Soloway et al. 1983)	DDP ± CTX	30	7
Memorial Hospital (Sternberg et al. 1988)	MTX, VLB, ADR, DDP	22	27[b]
M. D. Anderson Hospital (Logothetis et al. 1985)	DDP, CTX, ADR	28	46
NCOG (Meyers et al. 1985)	DDP, MTX, VLB	12	50
Cleveland Clinic (Batman et al. 1986)	DDP, CTX, ADR	24	25
Mass. General Hospital (Prout et al. 1988)	MTX, DDP, VLB	27	39[b]

[a] MTX, methotrexate.
DDP, cisplatin.
CTX, cyclophosphoramide.
VLB, vinblastine.
ADR, doxorubicin hydrochloride (adriamycin).
[b] includes a urine cytology that is not positive.

survival. However, cisplatin plus full-dose radiation therapy seems substantially better than single- and multi-drug chemotherapy without radiation therapy (Table 1.6).

Currently, many institutions and multi-institutional groups are doing phase I/II pilot studies with combinations of chemotherapy and radiation therapy, both together and alone, as "upfront" or neoadjuvant treatment in patients with invasive bladder carcinoma, to evaluate the possibility of selecting for treatment with bladder preservation only patients who have had a complete response to this regimen and who thus have a high probability of having had, without cystectomy, local cure of their bladder cancer (Prout et al. 1988). Therefore, the number of patients having to undergo a salvage cystectomy for recurrence will be substantially minimised. However, it is too soon yet to be certain that any of these specific programmes will increase either bladder preservation or patient survival. Randomised phase III trials are now being initiated, both within the EORTC and within several American institutions and groups, to study this important question.

Prostate Cancer

There are no data to support the use of systemic chemotherapy or hormonal therapy adjuvant to radiation therapy in the treatment of patients with locally advanced prostatic cancer. Two reports of the use of hormonal therapy *after* radiation therapy for patients irradiated in the decade 1965–1975 have shown no benefit (Neglia et al. 1977; van der Werf et al. 1976). However, two more recent series have suggested improved local control of bulky prostatic carcinoma treated with hormonal therapy before radiation therapy (Greene et al. 1984; Pilepich et al. 1987). This has led the Radiation Therapy Oncology Group to initiate a phase III study of combination of Zoladex and Flutamide (2-methyl-N-[4-nitro-3-(trifluoromethyl) phenyl] propanamide) to be used as cyto-reductive agents *prior to and during* definitive radiation therapy in patients with locally advanced carcinoma of the prostate.

Testis Cancer

Treatment of Advanced Seminoma

Prior to the recognition of effective, usually cisplatin-based, chemotherapy, radiation therapy was the treatment of choice for patients with stage IIB, III, or IV seminoma. The cure rate with radiation therapy alone for stage IIB was 60% and the cure rate for stages III and IV ranged from 20% to 60% (Dosoretz et al. 1981; Peckham 1981). Extended field radiation therapy to nodal sites above and below the diaphragm often precludes the administration of doses of chemotherapy effective to control sites of failure following radiation therapy (Loehrer et al. 1987). The cure rate when effective chemotherapy (either PVB or VAB-6) leads to a complete response (which happens in about three-quarters of the patients) is very high, and may be over 90% (Loehrer et al. 1987).

The medical oncologists judge seminoma to be as chemosensitive to cisplatin-based chemotherapy as any other germ cell tumour type. Cisplatin, even as a

single agent, has produced excellent results at the Institute of Urology in London
(Oliver 1984). Cisplatin given at 50 mg/m^2 on days 1 and 2 every 3 weeks for 4
courses resulted in a complete response in 13 of 14 patients. Patients with
disseminated seminoma had high response rates to cisplatin-based chemotherapy
whether given as the first treatment with no prior radiation therapy (Table 1.7) or
when used as salvage treatment for patients relapsing after initial radiation
therapy (Table 1.8). The Southeastern Cancer Study Group has recently
published its large experience in the treatment of patients with advanced
seminoma, both with and without prior radiation therapy (Loehrer et al. 1987).
They report 43 of 62 patients, or 69% of patients treated, achieving and
maintaining a complete response. However, in 13 of these 43 patients the
complete response was "consolidated" by surgery and/or radiation therapy at the
site of the original tumour bulk. They reported 6 drug-related fatalities and 12
patients dying of progressive disease, 11 of whom were never disease-free.

Only about 50% of patients treated with the platinum-containing chemotherapeutic regimens will have a radiographically complete response. To date, it is still

Table 1.7. Results of postorchidectomy chemotherapy in stages IIB, III, and IV seminoma testis:
chemotherapy as initial treatment[a]

Treatment centre	Chemotherapy schedule	Number of patients	Maintained complete response
London Institute of Urology (Oliver 1984)	cisplatin	10	9
M. D. Anderson Hosp. (Zagars and Babaian 1987b)	cisplatin ± cytoxan	10	8
University of Munich (Clemm et al. 1986)	VIP[b]	6	5
Southeastern Cancer Study Group (Loehrer et al. 1987)	PVB[b] ± doxorubicin, etoposide	27	21
Total		53	43 (81%)

[a] Includes some "consolidation" by surgery or radiation.
[b] VIP, vinblastine, Ifosfamide, cisplatin.
PVB, cisplatin, vinblastine, bleomycin.

Table 1.8. Results of chemotherapy following orchidectomy and radiation therapy for relapse of
disseminated seminoma testis: chemotherapy as salvage treatment[a]

Treatment centre	Chemotherapy schedule	Number of patients	Maintained complete response
London Inst. Urology (Oliver 1984)	cisplatin, etoposide	4	4
University of Munich (Clemm et al. 1986)	VIP[b]	7	5
Southeastern Cancer Study Group (Loehrer et al. 1987)	PVB[b] ± doxorubicin, etoposide	33	20
Total		44	29 (66%)

[a] Includes some "consolidation" by surgery.
[b] VIP, vinblastine, Ifosfamide, cisplatin.
PVB, cisplatin, vinblastine, bleomycin.

unclear whether the incompletely responding patients need further treatment or only close observation. The recent Memorial Sloan–Kettering Cancer Center review of patients with bulky stage II or III seminoma reported that residual viable seminoma was found only in those patients whose residual mass, radiographically, was 3 cm or more (Motzer et al. 1987).

In summary, advanced seminoma is a rare and curable disease but its treatment remains controversial. One reasonable approach, shared by many major treatment centres, is the use of multi-drug platinum-based chemotherapy. If there is radiographical evidence of a complete response, no further treatment is given. However, in those with a residual mass or masses, either careful close observation or "consolidation" by local radiotherapy or surgery is appropriate.

Non-seminomatous Germ Cell Tumours

Many clinicians do not appreciate the marked radiation sensitivity of embryonal and teratocarcinoma to local radiation therapy, similar to that of non-Hodgkin's lymphoma. The Royal Marsden Hospital experience documents that only 2 of 84 patients irradiated with clinical stage I tumours developed a retroperitoneal recurrence – one in 44 patients with primary teratocarcinoma and one in 40 patients with primary embryonal carcinoma (Tyrrell and Peckham 1976). When the retroperitoneal lymph nodal metastases were 2 cm or less by lymphangiographic evaluation, radiation therapy sterilised these deposits in 93% of the patients. However, radiation therapy was only effective in permanently sterilising retroperitoneal lymph nodes in 31% of the patients who were irradiated for bulky (5 cm in diameter or greater) metastatic deposits. This result is inferior to that which can be achieved with first-line multiple drug chemotherapy, which will completely sterilise retroperitoneal disease in over 50% of such patients. Thus, radiation therapy is used only in special circumstances in patients with this disease, being reserved for those with radiographic evidence of incompletely responding metastases that are not amenable to surgical "consolidation". The sites of such metastatic deposits include the central mediastinum, the bone, and the brain. With conventional fractionation doses that are commonly used in this setting are in the range of 3600 cGy over 4 weeks. In sites in which the heart and the central nervous system can be completely excluded, boosts to higher doses should be considered.

Acknowledgement. I warmly thank both Ms. Anne Macaulay for her assistance in the preparation of this chapter and my clinical colleagues, especially Dr. G. R. Prout, Jr. and Dr. S. D. Kaufman, for sharing their wisdom and judgement in the management of patients with urological tumours. Supported in part by a grant from the National Cancer Institute (USA) CA2661 to the Radiation Therapy Oncology Group.

References

Anscher MS, Prosnitz LR (1987) Postoperative radiotherapy for patients with carcinoma of the prostate undergoing radical prostatectomy with positive surgical margins: seminal vesicle involvement and/or penetration through the capsule. J Urol 138: 1407–1412

Asbell SO, Martz KL, Pilepich MV et al. (1987) Impact of surgical staging in evaluating the radiotherapeutic outcome in RTOG phase III study for stage A_2 and B prostatic carcinoma. Int J Radiat Oncol Biol Phys 13: suppl. 1: 2

Bagshaw MA (1985) Potential for radiation therapy alone in cancer of the prostate. Cancer 55: 2079–2085

Batata MA, Chu FC, Hilaris BS et al. (1981) Preoperative whole pelvis versus true pelvis irradiation and/or cystectomy for bladder cancer. Int J Radiat Oncol Biol Phys 7: 1349–1354

Batman TJ, Montie JE, Bukowski RN et al. (1986) Intra-arterial chemotherapy as an adjuvant to surgery in transitional cell carcinoma of the bladder. J Urol 135: 256–260

Battermann JJ, Tierie AH (1986) Results of implantation for T1 and T2 bladder tumors. Radiother Oncol 1986: 5: 85–90

Blandy JP, England HR, Evans SJW et al. (1980) T3 bladder cancer – the case for salvage cystectomy. Br J Urol 52: 506–510

Blandy JP, Jenkins BJ, Fowler CG et al. (1988) Radical radiotherapy and salvage cystectomy for T2 and T3 cancer of the bladder. In: Smith PH, Pavone-Macaluso MM (eds) The treatment of advanced prostate and bladder cancer. A. R. Liss, Inc, New York, 447–452

Bloom HCG, Hendry WR, Wallace DM et al. (1983) Treatment of T3 bladder cancer: a controlled trial of preoperative radiotherapy and radical cystectomy versus radical radiotherapy, second report and review. Br J Urol 54: 136–151

Bosch RJ, Kurth KH, Schroeder FH (1987) Surgical treatment of locally advanced (T3) prostatic carcinoma: early results. J Urol 138: 816–822

Brookland RK, Richter MP (1985) Postoperative irradiation of transitional cell carcinoma of the renal pelvis and ureter. J Urol 133: 952–955

Byar DP, Corle DK (1981) VACURG randomized trial of radical prostatectomy for stages I and II prostate cancer. Veterans Administration Cooperative Urological Research Group. Urology [suppl. 4] 17: 7–13

Clemm C, Hartenstein R, Willich N et al. (1986) Vinblastine-ifosfamide-cisplatin treatment of bulky seminoma. Cancer 58: 2203–2207

DeLaney TF, Shipley WU, O'Leary MP, Biggs PJ, Prout GR Jr (1986) Preoperative irradiation, lymphadenectomy, and Iodine-125 implantation for patients with localized carcinoma of the prostate. Int J Radiat Oncol Biol Phys 12: 1779–1785

Dosoretz DE, Shipley WU, Blitzer PH et al. (1981) Megavoltage irradiation for pure testicular seminoma: results and patterns of failure. Cancer 48: 2184–2190

Earle JD, Bagshaw MA, Kaplan HS (1973) Supervoltage radiation therapy of testicular tumors. A JR 117: 653–661

Finney R (1973) Radiotherapy in the treatment of hypernephroma: a clinical trial. Br J Urol 45: 258–269

Forman JD, Wharam MD, Lee DJ, Zinreich ES, Order SE (1986) Definitive radiotherapy following prostatectomy: results and complications. Int J Radiat Oncol Biol Phys 12: 185–188

Fosså SD, Kjolseth I, Lund G (1982) Radiotherapy of metastasis from renal cancer. Eur Urol 8: 340–342

Freiha SF, Bagshaw MA (1984) Carcinoma of the prostate: results of post-irradiation biopsy. Prostate 5: 19–24

Gibbons RP, Cole BS, Richardson RB, Correa GJ Jr, Brannen GE, Mason JT, Taylor WJ, Hafermann MD (1986) Adjuvant radiotherapy following radical prostatectomy: results and complications. J Urol 135: 65–71

Gibbons RP, Correa RJ, Brannen GE (1984) Total prostatectomy for localized prostatic cancer. J Urol 131: 73–76

Greene N, Bodner H, Broth E et al. (1984) Improved control of bulky prostatic carcinoma with sequential estrogen and radiation therapy. Int J Radiat Oncol Biol Phys 10: 971–976

Greiner R, Skaleric C, Veraguth P (1977) The prognostic significance of ureteral obstruction in carcinoma of the bladder. Int J Radiat Oncol Biol Phys 2: 1095–1102

Grossman HB, Whitmore WF Jr, Hilaris B et al. (1982) Iodine-125 implantation for carcinoma of the prostate: further follow-up of the first 100 cases. Urol 20: 591–598

Halperin EC, Harisiadis L (1983) The role of radiation therapy in the management of metastatic renal cell carcinoma. Cancer 51: 614–617

Hamilton C, Horwich A, Peckham MJ et al. (1986) Radiotherapy for stage I testis seminoma: results of treatment and complications. Radiat Ther Oncol 6: 115–120

Hanks GE (1988) National practiced results of external beam radiation therapy for clinically localized prostatic cancer. NIH Consensus Development Conference, Bethesda, Maryland, June 15–17, 1987 NCI Monographs 7: 75–84

Hanks GE, Herring DF, Kramer S (1981) Patterns of care outcome studies results of the national practice in seminoma of the testis. Int J Radiat Oncol Biol Phys 7: 1413–1417

Heney NM, Nocks BN, Daly JJ et al. (1981) Prognostic factors in carcinoma of the ureter. J Urol 125: 632–636

Jakse G, Frommhold H, Nedden DZ (1985) Combined radiation and chemotherapy for locally advanced transitional cell carcinoma of the urinary bladder. Cancer 55: 1659–1664

Jewett HJ (1980) Radical perineal prostatectomy for palpable, clinically localized, non-obstructive cancer: experience at the Johns Hopkins Hospital: 1909–1963. J Urol 124: 492–497

Jewett HJ, Walsh PC (1982) Radical perineal prostatectomy for clinical stage T2 carcinoma of the prostate. J Urol 127: 704–709

Johansson A, Angerval L, Bengtsson U et al. (1976) A clinicopathologic and prognostic study of epithelial tumors of the renal pelvis. Cancer 37: 1376–1381

Juusela H, Malmio K, Alfthan D et al. (1977) Preoperative irradiation in the treatment of renal adenocarcinoma. Scand J Urol Nephrol 11: 277–281

Kjar M, Frederiksen PL, Engelholm SA (1987) Postoperative radiotherapy in stages II and III renal adenocarcinoma: a randomized trial by the Copenhagen renal cancer study group. Int J Radiat Oncol Biol Phys 13: 665–672

Kubo HD, Shipley WU (1982) Reduction of the scatter dose to the testicle outside the radiation treatment fields. Int J Radiat Oncol Biol Phys 8: 1741–1745

Lange PH et al. (1988) Adjuvant postoperative radiation therapy following radical prostatectomy. NIH Consensus Development Conference, Bethesda, Maryland, June 15–17, 1987. NCI Monographs 7: 141–150

Livingston RB et al. (1987) The management of clinically localized prostatic cancer: NIH concensus development conference. JAMA 258: 727–730

Loehrer PJ, Birch R, Williams SD et al. (1987) Chemotherapy of metastatic seminoma: the Southeastern Cancer Study Group experience. J Clin Oncol 5: 1212–1220

Logothetis CJ, Samuels ML, Ogden S et al. (1985) Cyclophosphamide, adriamycin, and cisplatin chemotherapy for patients with locally advanced urothelial tumors with or without nodal metastases. J Urol 134: 460–464

Maier JG, Sulak MH (1973) Radiation therapy in malignant testis tumors: Part I: seminoma. Cancer 32: 1212–1216

Matsumoto L, Kakizoe T, Mikuriya S et al. (1981) Clinical evaluation of intraoperative radiotherapy for carcinoma of the urinary bladder. Cancer 47: 509–513

Mazeron JJ, Marinello G, Pierquin B et al. (1985) Treatment of bladder tumors by iridium-192 implantation: the Creteil technique. Radiother Oncol 4:111–119

Meyers FJ, Palmer JM, Freiha FS et al. (1985) The fate of the bladder in patients with metastatic bladder cancer treated with cisplatin, methotrexate, and vinblastine: a Northern California Oncology Group Study. J Urol 134: 1118–1121

Miller LS, Johnson DE (1973) Megavoltage radiation for bladder carcinoma: alone, postoperative, or preoperative. Seventh National Cancer Conference Proceedings 771–782

Motzer R, Bosl G, Heelan R et al. (1987) Residual mass: an indication for surgery in patients with advanced seminoma following systemic chemotherapy. J Clin Oncol 5: 1064–1070

Neglia WJ, Hussey DH, Johnson DE (1977) Megavoltage radiation therapy for carcinoma of the prostate. Int J Radiat Oncol Biol Phys 2: 873–882

Oliver RTD (1984) Single-agent cisplatin for metastatic seminoma. Proc Am Soc Clin Oncol [abstr.] 3: 162

Oliver RTD, England HR, Risdon RA et al. (1984) Methotrexate in the treatment of metastatic and recurrent primary transitional cell carcinoma. J Urol 131: 483–485

Onufrey V, Mohiuddin M (1985) Radiation therapy in the treatment of metastatic renal cell carcinoma. Int J Radiat Oncol Biol Phys 11: 2007–2009

Parsons JJ, Thar TL, Bova FS et al. (1981) An evaluation of split-course irradiation for pelvic malignancies. Int J Radiat Oncol Biol Phys 6: 175–181

Paulson DF, Stone AR, Walther PH, Tucker JA, Cox EB (1986) Radical prostatectomy: anatomical predictors of success or failure. J Urol 136: 1041–1044

Peckham MJ (1981) Testicular tumors: investigation and staging. In: Peckham MJ (ed) The management of testicular tumors. Edwin Arnold, Ltd, London. pp 89–101

Perez CA (1983) Carcinoma of the prostate. Int J Radiat Oncol Biol Phys 9: 1427–1438

Peschel RE, Fogel T, Kazinski B et al. (1985) Iodine-125 implants for carcinoma of the prostate. Int J Radiat Oncol Biol Phys 11: 1777–1782

Pilepich MV (1988) Radiation therapy in patients with localized prostatic carcinoma: RTOG data. NIH Consensus Development Conference, Bethesda, Maryland, June 15–17, 1987. NCI

Monographs 7: 61–66

Pilepich MV, Krall JM, John MJ et al. (1987) Hormonal cytoreduction in locally advanced carcinoma of the prostate treated with definitive radiotherapy. Int J Radiat Oncol Biol Phys [suppl. 1] 13: 104–105

Pilepich MV, Krall JM, Sause WT et al. (1987) Prognostic factor in carcinoma of the prostate – analysis of RTOG study 75–06. Int J Radiat Oncol Biol Phys 13: 339–349

Prout GR Jr. (1984) Radiation therapy and cystectomy. Urol [suppl 4] 23: 104–118

Prout GR Jr, Kaufman SD, Shipley WU et al. (1988) Combined therapies in the treatment of patients with muscle-invading bladder carcinoma: a preliminary report of a bladder-sparing effort. Abstract submitted to the American Urologic Association Meeting, June 1988, Boston, Massachusetts

Quilty PM, Duncan W (1986) Primary radical radiotherapy for T3 transitional cell cancer of the bladder: an analysis of survival and control. Int J Radiat Oncol Biol Phys 12: 853–860

Rafla S (1970) Renal cell carcinoma. Cancer 25: 26–40

Ray GR, Bagshaw MA, Freiha F (1984) External beam radiation salvage for residual or recurrent local tumor following radical prostatectomy. J Urol 132: 926–929

Richards B, Bastable JRG, Freedman L et al. (1983) Adjuvant chemotherapy with adriamycin and 5-Fluorouracil in T3, Nx, MO bladder cancer treated with radiotherapy. Br J Urol 55: 386–391

Sauer R, Schrott KM, Dunst J et al. (1987) Improved response rate of T3/T4 carcinomas of the urinary bladder treated by radiotherapy under cisplatin-sensitization. Int J Radiat Oncol Biol Phys [Suppl. 1] 13:101–102

Scardino PT, Wheeler TM (1988) Local control of prostatic cancer with radiation therapy: frequency and significance of positive post-irradiation prostatic biopsy results. NIH Consensus Development Conference, Bethesda, Maryland, June 15–17, 1987. NCI Monographs 7: 95–106

Scardino PT, Franel JM, Weiler TM (1986) The prognostic significance of post-irradiation biopsy results in patients with prostatic cancer. J Urol 135: 510–515

Shipley WU, Rose MA, Perrone TL, Mannix CM, Heney NM, Prout GR Jr (1985) Full-dose irradiation for patients with invasive bladder carcinoma: clinical and histological factors prognostic of improved survival. J Urol 134: 679–683

Shipley WU, Coombs LJ, Prout GR Jr (1986) Preoperative irradiation and radical cystectomy for invasive cancer – patterns of failure and prognostic factors associated with patient survival and disease progression. J Urol 135: 222A.

Shipley WU, Prout GR Jr, Einstein AB et al. (1987a) Treatment of invasive bladder cancer by cisplatin and radiation in patients unsuited for surgery. JAMA 258: 931–935

Shipley WU, Prout GR Jr, Kaufman SD, Perrone TL (1987b) Invasive bladder carcinoma: the importance of initial transurethral surgery and other significant prognostic factors for improved survival with full-dose irradiation. Cancer 60: 514–520

Shipley WU, Kitagawa P, Jones W et al. (1988a) Guidelines in 1987 for multi-center radiation therapy protocols for clinical research on bladder cancer. In Niijima T, Denis L, Koontz, W (eds) Guidelines for clinical research on bladder cancer. A. R. Liss, Inc, New York

Shipley WU, Prout GR Jr, Coachman NM et al. (1988b) The Massachusetts General Hospital experience in patients irradiated for localized prostatic carcinoma: presented at NIH Consensus Development Conference on the Management of Clinically Localized Prostatic Cancer, Bethesda, Maryland, June 15–17, 1987. NCI Monographs 7: 67–74

Solway MS, Einstein AB, Corder MP et al. (1983) A comparison of cisplatin and the combination of cisplatin and cyclophosphamide in advanced urothelial cancer: a National Bladder Cancer Group study. Cancer 52: 767–771

Sternberg CN, Yagoda A, Scher HI et al. (1988) M-VAC (methotrexate, vinblastine, adriamycin, and cisplatin) for advanced transitional cell carcinoma of the urothelium. J Urol 139: 461–469

Sundaresan N, Galicich JH, Baines MS et al. (1984) Vertebral body resection in the treatment of cancer involving the spine. Cancer 53: 1393–1396

Thayer WR, Hilaris B, Herr HW et al. (1987) Interstitial irradiation in prostatic cancer: report of 10 year results. Abstract, American Urological Association Meeting, May 1987. J Urol 37: 200A

Thomas GM, Rider WD, Dembo AJ, Cummings BJ, Gospodarowicz M, Hawkins NV, Herman JG, Keen CW (1982) Seminoma of the testis: results of treatment and patterns of failure after radiation therapy. Int J Radiat Oncol 8: 165–174

Timmer PR, Hartlief HA, Hoojikaas JA (1985) Bladder cancer: pattern of recurrence in 142 patients. Int J Radiat Oncol Biol Phys 11: 899–905

Tyrrell CJ, Peckham MJ (1976) The response of lymph node metastases of testicular teratoma to radiation therapy. Br J Urol 48: 363–370

van der Werf-Messing B (1973) Carcinoma of the kidney. Cancer 32: 1056–1062
van der Werf-Messing B (1982) Carcinoma of the urinary bladder T3 NX MO treated by preoperative radiation followed by simple cystectomy. Int J Radiat Oncol Phys 8: 1849–1855
van der Werf-Messing B, Menon RS, Hop WL (1983a) Cancer of the urinary bladder T2, T3 (NXMO) treated by interstitial radium implant: second report. Int J Radiat Oncol Biol Phys 7: 481–485
van der Werf-Messing B, Menon RS, Hop WL (1983b) Carcinoma of the urinary bladder T3 NXMO treated by combination radium implant and external beam radiation: second report. Int J Radiat Oncol Biol Phys 9: 177–180
van der Werf-Messing B, Menon RS, Hop WCJ (1988) Carcinoma of the urinary bladder category T2, T3, Nx, MO, treated by interstitial radium implant. In Smith PH, Pavone-Macaluso MM (eds) The treatment of advanced prostate and bladder cancer. A. R. Liss, Inc, New York, 511–524
van der Werf-Messing B, Sourek-Zikova V, Blonk DI (1976) Localized advanced carcinoma of the prostate. Radiation therapy vs. hormonal therapy. Int J Radiat Oncol Biol Phys 1: 1043–1048
Willan BD, McGowan DG (1985) Seminoma of the testis: a 22-year experience with radiation therapy. Int J Radiat Oncol Biol Phys 11: 1769–1775
Yagoda A, Watson RC, Gonzales JC, Grabstald H, Whitmore WF Jr (1976) Cis-dichlorodiammineplatinum II in advanced bladder cancer. Cancer Treat Rep 60: 917–923
Zagars GK, Babaian RJ (1987a) Stage I testicular seminoma: rationale for postorchiectomy radiation therapy. Int J Radiat Oncol Biol Phys 13: 155–162
Zagars GK, Babaian RJ (1987b) The role of radiation therapy in stage II testicular seminoma. Int J Radiat Oncol Biol Phys 13: 163–170
Zagars GK, Von Eschenback AC, Johnson DE (1987) The management of stage C adenocarcinoma of the prostate with external beam radiation therapy. Abstract, American Urologic Association Meeting, May 1987. J Urol 37: 199A

Chapter 2

Chemotherapy

G. Stoter and C.J. Rodenburg

The history of cancer chemotherapy started with the incidental discovery that nitrogen mustard was cytotoxic to lymphoid malignancies. The initial enthusiasm was soon tempered by the observation that most responses were short-lived due to the development of drug resistance.

With the development of new cytotoxic agents the concept of combination chemotherapy was introduced to circumvent acquired (secondary) drug resistance, and eventually the combination of drugs with different mechanisms of action led to the curative potential of combination chemotherapy in Hodgkin's disease in 1964 (Longo et al. 1986).

In the 1970s the development of new drugs and the use of combination treatment led to the development of effective treatment for disseminated non-seminomatous testicular cancer. Before the era of chemotherapy this was a rapidly lethal disease. Initial attempts with single agents showed that this malignancy is responsive to a variety of drugs but will progress after short periods of remission. In the early 1960s a triple-drug combination of actinomycin-D, methotrexate and chlorambucil improved the results and resulted in a few cures (Li et al. 1960).

Other drugs were needed to improve these encouraging results. The next step forward was made with the combination of vinblastine and bleomycin (Samuels et al. 1975), but the real cure for disseminated testicular cancer did not appear before the discovery of cisplatin, the first inorganic compound in the history of cancer chemotherapy (Einhorn and Donohue 1977). At present, about 70% of patients can be cured with combination chemotherapy consisting of cisplatin, VP16–213, and bleomycin. It has been noted that patients with few and small metastases have a much better prognosis than their counterparts (Stoter et al. 1987a).

Today, disseminated tumours originating from head and neck, breast, lung, stomach, ovary, uterus and bladder can all be treated effectively in terms of response rates and limited periods of palliation of symptoms; but cures will hardly ever be achieved, as combination chemotherapy has not proved to be the answer to secondary drug resistance in these solid tumours. It appears that curative treatment of the vast majority of the one hundred or so existing tumour types will require the development of new and more effective cytotoxic agents, either chemotherapeutic drugs, hormones, biological response modifiers or combinations of these.

Apart from germ cell tumours of the testis and the ovary, and choriocarcinoma of the uterus, chemotherapy has no curative potential in the treatment of genitourinary tumours. Renal cell cancer is primarily resistant to any known form of hormonal and chemotherapy, and chemotherapy is, as yet, of little benefit in prostate cancer patients. Progress has, however, been made in the treatment of disseminated transitional cell cancer of the urothelial tract. In the early 1970s doxorubicin was the most widely used agent, yielding a response rate of about 20% for a median duration of 3 months, whether or not in combination with other drugs. The introduction of cisplatin improved these results but complete responses were usually seen in fewer than 10% of cases, and no survival advantage could be demonstrated. Recent trials combining cisplatin and methotrexate with or without doxorubicin and vinblastine have demonstrated an increase of complete response rates varying from 25% to 40%, including a suggestion of improved duration of response and survival in complete responders (Stoter et al. 1987b).

Although the early work led to progress in Phase II studies by showing evidence of temporary response in patients with advanced disease, the hope has always been that it may be possible to give the cytotoxic agents in the adjuvant situation, i.e. after excision of the apparently non-metatastic primary lesion, or in association with such treatment, i.e. as neoadjuvant therapy.

Preclinical experiments have shown that chemotherapy is more effective in microscopic disease in animal models. The theoretical explanation for this is better vascularisation and drug access, a higher proportion of cells in cycle which makes them more vulnerable to chemotherapy, and a lower probability of the development of drug-resistant cell mutations, which are estimated to occur at a frequency of one per million cells in the human (Goldie and Coldman 1984). However, the clinical usefulness of adjuvant chemotherapy, in addition to radical treatment of the primary tumour with surgery and radiotherapy, appears to be much more limited than could be expected on the basis of preclinical observations. In the predominant tumour types such as gastrointestinal and lung tumours no disease-free and overall survival benefit has yet been achieved, and the benefit in certain categories of breast-cancer patients is so far only marginal (NIH 1986).

With the notable exception of testicular cancer, adjuvant chemotherapy has not been shown to be beneficial in the management of genitourinary tumours. In addition, it is often difficult to administer toxic chemotherapy to these patients, who are usually elderly, once they have undergone major local treatment procedures such as are used in head and neck cancer and in bladder cancer. These difficulties and the desirability of attacking micrometastases even earlier, i.e. before or concurrent with local therapies, has led to the introduction of neoadjuvant chemotherapy. At present, a series of neoadjuvant clinical studies are under way in invasive stage T3–4 bladder cancer with the use of cisplatin and methotrexate-based chemotherapy concurrent with radiotherapy or prior to cystectomy. No conclusive data are available yet, but it seems that only patients who achieve a complete pathological response of the primary tumour are likely to benefit from the combined modality treatment (Scher et al. 1988). Large cooperative study groups are now at the start of randomised controlled clinical trials.

A major impediment to the administration of chemotherapy is the side-effect of granulocytopenia which renders the patient more susceptible to infections and sepsis. This problem frequently leads to dose reductions and delays. For instance, in an EORTC study of cisplatin and methotrexate in disseminated bladder cancer and in a MSKCC (Memorial Sloan–Kettering Center) study of these drugs with doxorubicin and vinblastine, 70%–80% of the patients were subject to dose and interval modifications. Very recently, haematopoietic growth factors have been introduced into clinical use (Nienhuis et al. 1987; Groopman et al. 1987). The first reports show that minute amounts of granulocyte-macrophage colony stimulating factor (GM–CSF), in the order of 3–10 µg/kg per day intravenously or subcutaneously, will prevent granulocytopenia completely and reduce infectious complications accordingly, thus not only facilitating the correct dose-interval application of chemotherapy, but also opening possibilities of intensification of treatment which, in turn, may yield better antitumour effect. Side effects of the above-mentioned doses are unremarkable. Interleukin-3 (IL3), which prevents thrombocytopenia, is shortly expected to be available and will further aid to serve these goals.

Finally, a few words about adoptive immunotherapy in urological malignancies are appropriate. Renal cell cancer, which is a notoriously chemotherapy-resistant disease, appeared to be sensitive to treatment with lymphokine-activated-killer (LAK) cells (Rosenberg et al. 1987; West et al. 1987). The therapeutic procedure consists of a priming phase with intravenous administration of interleukin-2 (IL2). Thereafter, lymphocytes are obtained from the patient's blood by leukopheresis and are activated ex vivo with IL2; they are then infused with IL2 into the patient's circulation. So far, wide variations in schedules are being tested. Response rates vary from 30%–50% and little information is, as yet, available about the durability of responses. Another open question is whether the ex vivo activation of lymphocytes is better than the in vivo administration of IL2 alone. Although it is clear that the key to the fine-tuning of the immunotherapeutic mechanisms has not yet been found, the present results open an exciting prospect of effective therapy in renal cell cancer, as well as in other tumours and indications, including intralesional treatment of superficial bladder tumours. It is most likely that adoptive immunotherapy and the application of haematopoietic growth factors will become the fourth modality in the armoury of anti-cancer treatment.

References

Einhorn LH, Donohue JP (1977) Cisdiamminedichloroplatinum, vinblastine and bleomycin combination chemotherapy in disseminated testicular cancer. Ann Intern Med 87: 293–298

Goldie JH, Coldman AJ (1984) The genetic origin of drug resistance in neoplasms: implications for systemic therapy. Cancer Res 44: 3643–3653

Groopman JE et al. (1987) Effect of recombinant human granulocyte-macrophage colony-stimulating factor on myelopoiesis in the Acquired Immunodeficiency Syndrome. N Engl J Med 317: 593–598

Li MC, Whitmore Jr WF, Golbey R, Grabstald H (1960) Effects of combined drug therapy on metastatic cancer of the testis. JAMA 174: 145–153

Longo DL, Young RC, Wesley M, Hubbard SM, Duffey PL, Jaffe ES, De Vita Jr, VT (1986) Twenty years of MOPP therapy for Hodgkin's disease. J Clin Oncol 9: 1295–1306

National Institutes of Health (1986) Consensus development panel on adjuvant chemotherapy and endocrine therapy for breast cancer. Introduction and conclusions. NCI Monographs 1: 1–17

Nienhuis AW et al. (1987) Recombinant human GM-CSF shortens the period of neutropenia after autologous bone marrow transplantation in a primate model. J Clin Invest 80: 573–577

Rosenberg SA, Lotze MT, Muul LM et al. (1987) A progress report on the treatment of 157 patients with advanced cancer using lymphokine-activated killer cells and interleukin-2 or high-dose interleukin-2 alone. N Engl J Med 316: 889–897

Samuels ML, Holoye PY, Johnson DE (1975) Bleomycin combination chemotherapy in the management of testicular neoplasia. Cancer 36: 318–326

Scher H, Yagoda A, Herr H et al. (1988) Neoadjuvant M-VAC (methotrexate, vinblastine, adriamycin and cisplatin): effect on the primary bladder lesion. J Urol 139: 470–474

Stoter G, Sylvester R, Sleijfer DT, ten Bokkel Huinink WW, Kaye SB, Jones WG, van Oosterom AT, Vendrik CPJ, Spaander P, de Pauw M (1987a) Multivariate analysis of prognostic factors in patients with disseminated nonseminomatous testicular cancer: results from a European Organization for Research on Cancer Multiinstitutional Phase III Study. Cancer Res 47: 2714–2718

Stoter G, Splinter TAW, Child JA, Fosså SD, Denis L, van Oosterom AT, de Pauw M, Sylvester R for the European Organization for Research on Treatment of Cancer Genito-urinary Group (1987b) Combination chemotherapy with cisplatin and methotrexate in advanced transitional cell cancer of the bladder. J Urol 137: 663–667

West WH, Tauer KW, Yannelli JR et al. (1987) Constant-infusion recombinant interleukin-2 in adoptive immunotherapy of advanced cancer. N Engl J Med 316: 898–905

Chapter 3

Immunotherapy

S.A. Brosman

The manipulation of the immune system as a means of cancer therapy has held the interest of researchers and clinicians for many years. Rapidly developing knowledge in molecular biology, recombinant DNA technology and hybridoma technology has allowed a more sophisticated approach to the understanding of the immune system and its role in tumour immunology.

The immune system plays a key role in host recognition and control of cellular transformation. This natural defence and regulatory system functions through an intricate network which requires the recognition of novel or foreign proteins. The basis of immunotherapy is the presence of an immunogenic tumour in a host which can recognise and respond appropriately to transformed cells. In order for the host to respond to a malignant cell, there must be alterations in that cell which confer immunogenicity. If the tumour has no or very little immunogenicity, there will be no effective host response even if there is activation of the immune system. It is thought that those clones of tumour cells which are highly immunogenetic are destroyed early in the development of the malignancy, leaving behind cells with no immunogenicity or with the ability to inactivate the host's response. Cancer cells can create a protective environment by producing substances which mask their immunogenicity and prevent certain segments of the immune response from functioning. In order for immunotherapy to be effective, the tumour should be altered to become highly immunogenic and the immune system activated in such a way as to stimulate the appropriate immunocytes, in the proper sequence, to respond to the cancer antigens.

Past efforts to achieve beneficial results with immunotherapy failed because of the inability to satisfy these criteria. Animal model systems demonstrated dramatic successes largely because the tumours were immunogenic, the number of tumour cells could be controlled and the immune system activated by specific and non-specific methods.

The Immune Response and Tumour Immunology

In order to understand recent developments in immunotherapy, it is necessary to review the basic steps in the immune response and learn where and under what circumstances the immune system can be modulated to function as an anti-cancer device.

In order for the immune system to respond to the presence of a transformed cell, it must respond to circulating antigen, or bring its forces to the site where transformation is occurring, either at a primary or a metastatic site. There are elaborate mechanisms which guide circulating antigens to sites where there is maximum opportunity for exposure to lymphoctyes. There is a heterogeneous group of immune cells consisting of monocytes and macrophages, fixed tissue histocytes, dendritic cells, Langerhan's cells, and others which can be identified at the site of a neoplasm. These cells comprise the reticuloendothelial system and are known as antigen capturing cells and accessory cells. The macrophage has been the most extensively studied cell in this group and is a cornerstone of the immune response. Macrophages can capture soluble antigen molecules and interact directly with tumour associated antigens expressed on the cell surface: they possess a great deal of motility and respond to chemotactic products emanating from the cancer site.

Tumour associated antigens (TAA) are broken down or processed into smaller molecular fragments which are expressed on the cell surface and react with receptors on the surface of T lymphocytes (Fig 3.1). These antigenic fragments are known as epitopes. The epitopes can be carried on the cell surface of a macrophage, where they are accessible to passing lympocytes, for an extended period of time. The macrophage carries specialised glycoproteins on its cell surface which are known as histocompatibility proteins. These combine with the epitopes in forming a complex which is important for immune activation. This complex or restriction element allows a distinction to be made between an antigenic and a non-antigenic protein and prevents the host from initiating an immune response against its own tissues and proteins.

Since immunity is specific, molecular mechanisms of recognition exist such as the histocompatibility-epitope complex. Both the antigen-specific receptors on lymphocytes and the antibody molecules that are formed must recognise and unite with particular antigenic molecules or molecular fragments. The immune system does not know in advance what it will be asked to recognise and must possess the capability of responding to any conceivable antigen. One difference between T-cell and B-cell receptors is that T cells will recognise only those antigens displayed with the appropriate restriction element. Restriction elements are slightly homologous to immunoglobulins and are coded for by the major histocompatibility complex (MHC). In humans this is known as the HLA complex, and in mice it is H-2. MHC molecules consist of two classes based on

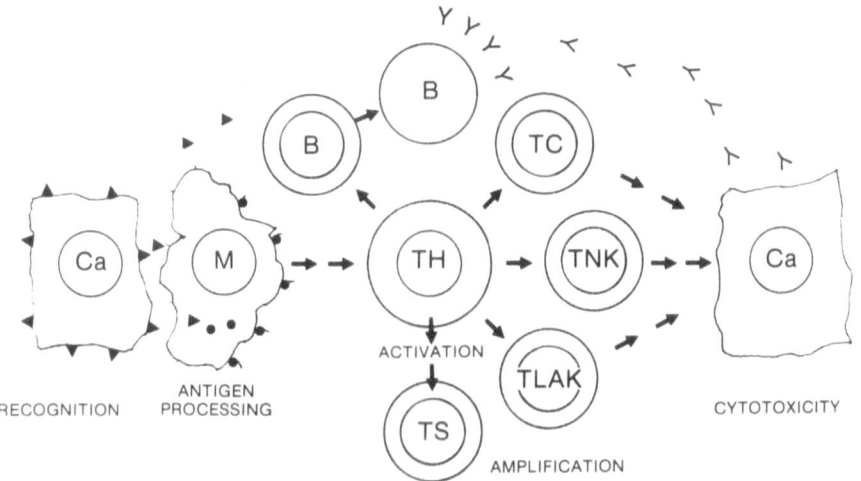

Fig. 3.1. Immune response to cancer antigens. The immune response can be divided into four components. Tumour-associated antigens displayed on the surface or shed into the circulation by cancer cells are recognised by macrophages (*M*) and some B cells. Macrophages process tumour antigens and display these peptides in a complex formed with histocompatibility antigens. T lymphocyte helper cells are activated when they come in contact with this complex and begin the effector cell response. This involves the recruitment of effector cells which develop tumour specificity. Amplification is the mechanism whereby the numbers of effector cells are increased. A cytotoxic response is generated by direct cell killing or indirectly by the production of cytotoxic lymphokines and cytokines.

their tissue distribution, the structure of the expressed antigens, and their functions. Class I molecules are the serologically defined histocompatibility markers on which tissue typing was originally based. They are present on all nucleated cells and are composed of a 45 kd (kilodalton) heavy chain associated with a B_2 microgobulin. They serve as restriction elements for a subset of T cells known as CD8 or T8 suppressor/cytotoxic lymphocytes.

T-cell receptors do not recognise or respond to antigen itself but only when the antigen has been processed into a peptide which is associated with HLA molecules. Class II antigens have a more limited tissue distribution. They are found on macrophages, B cells and activated T cells in humans. They serve as restriction elements for the CD4 or T4-positive helper/inducer T-lymphocyte subset. When macrophages process tumour antigens, they display the epitopes on their surfaces in combination with the Class II molecules. The helper T cells recognise this complex.

Both T-cell and B-cell receptors arise as a result of random somatic translocations in immunocyte precursor cells. This creates the characteristic diversity inherent in T- and B-cell recognition. Each cell has a single, unique combining specificity which creates clones of specific immunocytes when there is selective stimulation of properly presented antigen.

This activation of lymphocytes respresents the next step in the host response to cancer antigens. The typical immune response to cancer antigens involves a complex cascade of intercellular interactions. A B cell does not begin making antibodies just because a cancer antigen is in the vicinity. These responses require the collaborative help of accessory cells (macrophages) and the CD4/T4-positive helper/inducer T cell. The function of these markers which are recognisable by monoclonal antibodies is unclear, but T cells carry either CD4 or CD8 and never carry both. CD4-positive cells always use Class II-positive MHC molecules as restrictive elements and CD8 positive cells use Class I. It is thought that these markers act to stabilise or strengthen the bond between the T-cell receptor and the antigen-restriction element complex.

The antigen-MHC complex on the accessory cell surface engages the receptors of an appropriate T4 helper cell that migrates past, or is at the site of tumour development. Engagement and aggregation of the T-cell receptors occur. The macrophage secretes interleukin-1 (IL-1), a coactivating molecule which stimulates cell growth. IL-1 is produced by many different cell types and participates in multiple activities. Some of these include inflammation, fibroblast proliferation, fever, sleep, interleukin 2 (IL-2) release, T cell activation, B cell activation, collagenase and prostaglandin induction and osteoclast activation. In the presence of IL-1, the T4 helper cell enlarges, begins to secrete a group of various lymphokines (soluble protein mediators of various biological events) and divides to form a clone. These lymphokines stimulate additional T cell, B cell and macrophage growth and consist of some substances used for immunotherapy. As a group, they are known as biological response moderators (BRMs) which are non-specific agents acting as modulators of the immune system by enhancing, suppressing and restoring immune activity. They consist of the interferons (alpha, beta, and gamma), the interleukins (IL-1, IL-2, IL-3, IL-4), a variety of colony stimulating factors (CSF) which mobilise bone marrow precursors of granulocytes, macrophages, etc., and are involved in cellular growth and differentiation and additional substances such as tumour necrosis factor (TNF) which is produced by macrophages and seems to be identical to cachetin (Fig. 3.2).

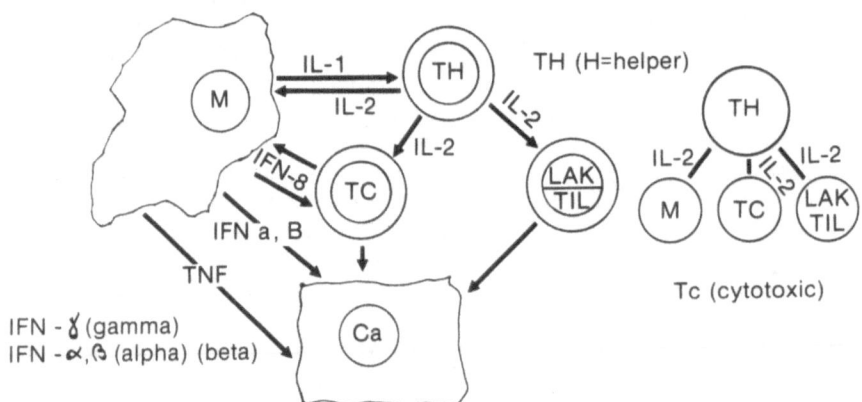

Fig. 3.2. Cytokines are substances released by cells in the immune system which regulate their function. Many of these are referred to as biological response modifiers. Macrophages (*M*) release interleukin-1 (*IL-1*) which activates T helper cells (*TH*). These in turn produce interleukin-2 (*IL-2*) which stimulates cytotoxic T cells, lymphokine activated killer cells (*LAK*) and tumour infiltrating lymphocytes (*TIL*). IL-2 also acts on macrophages which produce tumour necrosis factor (*TNF*) and interferon alpha and beta (*IFN-a, IFN-B*) which have a direct cytotoxic effect on cancer cells.

When the T cell and B cell have receptors for different epitopes of the same antigen, the antigen serves as a molecular bridge uniting the two cells. This allows for the targeting delivery of B cell growth and differentiation factors from the T cell. Since B cells possess Class II MHC molecules on their surface, they can present antigen to T cells in a manner similar to that used by macrophages. The B cell is activated by a combination of biological signals delivered in a certain sequence. These signals are produced as a result of antigen binding and T-cell stimulation. The B cell enlarges, divides, and differentiates to antibody secreting status. Some T-cell products encourage a switch in production from IgM, the first formed antibody type, to other isotypes such as IgG, IgA or IgE.

A similar process activates the CD8 positive/cytotoxic lymphocyte which can produce lytic damage to targeted cancer cells. Another CD8 positive cell is the suppressor T lymphocyte which cannot yet be separated from the cytotoxic T lymphocyte on the basis of cell surface markers. These cells seem to be responsible for down-regulating and immune response. Their function has been shown to be abnormally activated in cancer patients as a part of the protective mechanism exerted by the neoplasm.

T helper cells manufacture gamma interferon which stimulates macrophage growth and reproduction and increases Class II-MHC expression and macrophages and B cells. Recognition and lymphocyte activation involve immunological specificity, but there are many non-specific events that are initiated and which mediate many of the effector functions of these cells. This linkage between specific and non-specific segments of the immune response serves to amplify and deploy the immunological message.

Interleukin 2 (IL-2) is one of the lymphokines which is produced only by T cells. Although IL-2 mediates some macrophage and B cell functions, its major effects are on other T cells. Resting T cells are not responsive to IL-2 because they do not express the IL-2 receptor. When T cells are stimulated by the antigen-MHA complex in the presence of IL-1, they begin to express the IL-2 receptor and manufacture IL-2. IL-2 stimulates T cell and macrophage proliferation, the production of gamma interferon and enhances the cytotoxicity of T cells, macrophages and natural killer (NK) cells. T cells also produce IL-3 and IL-4. IL-3 regulates haemopoiesis and cellular proliferation and differentiation. IL-4 is a very potent T- and B-cell activator.

Natural killer (NK) cells are named for their ability to exhibit cytotoxicity without prior sensitisation. NK activity was first recognised while studying cell-mediated responses against tumour cells in cancer patients and in healthy individuals. Not only was a subclass of cytotoxic lymphocytes found in normal individuals, but the targets of NK activity were not restricted to a particular histological tumour type.

There are multiple subpopulations of NK cells, all of which are responsive to IL-2. Their tumour specificity is not dependent on the presence of MHC antigens. The role of NK cells in controlling primary tumours is not clearly established. There is a low incidence of spontaneous or carcinogenic-induced tumours in animals with high NK activity, a high incidence of lymphoproliferative disease in humans and animals with low NK activity. Retinoic acid, a substance active during embryogenesis, slows tumour growth by causing the cells to differentiate toward normal and enhances NK activity. NK cells may serve as an early first defence mechanism against cellular transformation. Tumour cells that are successful in their growth are able to resist NK cells.

Another aid to deployment is the high mobility of lymphocytes. In patients with advanced cancer, it has been shown that this mobility is suppressed. Once a T cell or a B cell has been activated, these cells can leave the lymph node, spleen, other lymphoid tissue or the tumour site and join the recirculating pool of lymphocytes, thereby activating additional cells specifically against the cancer cells. These cells may also re-enter the lymph nodes by penetrating specially adapted venules. Some lymphocytes are deployed to sites of tumour metastasis, as well as to the primary tumour.

With this background in mind, we can begin to understand some of the current efforts taking place in immunotherapy and realise why therapeutic efforts failed in the past. Although attempts to modulate the immune system go back many years, it was not until the development of inbred strains of mice that the host–tumour relationship could be studied apart from allograft rejection reactions. Animal experiments in the 1960s demonstrated that stimulation of the immune system with both specific and non-specific substances could prevent the establishment of a neoplasm, deter the growth of an established cancer and reverse the process of metastases. Attempts to duplicate the laboratory successes in the clinical setting met with failure. Some of the reasons for these failures were the attempts to "cure" patients with large tumour burdens by the use of a therapy which was poorly understood and did not adhere to the biological principles which had been learned in the laboratory.

Immunotherapy

In order for any immunological manipulation to be effective in managing cancer, a number of criteria must be satisfied (Table 3.1). The tumour must be immunogenic and there need to be proper assays to evaluate tumour antigenicity and relate antigenicity to immunotherapy. Patients whose cancers lack or have poor immunogenicity are not suitable candidates for non-specific immunotherapy unless the cancer cells can be altered to induce an immunological response. Stimulating the immune system per se will have little benefit if the effector cells cannot recognise the appropriate target. Thus, one approach would involve altering the cancer cells in some way to cause the expression of novel antigens on their surface or strip away some of the cell surface substances and expose new recognition sites.

Table 3.1. Criteria for successful immunotherapy

1. Immunogenic tumour
2. Immunocompetent host
3. Ability to stimulate immunocompetency
4. Combination with other tumour reductive measures
5. Small tumour burden
6. The use of agents which have been proved to be of benefit in appropriate animal models
7. Adequate dosage
8. Proper delivery to tumour site
9. Maintenance of immunotherapeutic effect
10. Ability to overcome tumour heterogeneity

Another obstacle to overcome is the heterogeneity of the tumour cell population. As genetic and phenotypic diversity increases, the cancer cells experience a type of Darwinian selection process in which only those cells will survive which have the ability to exist within the host environment. A variety of immunotherapeutic strategies utilised in appropriate sequences will be necessary to solve this problem. These include not only the use of measures to augment host immunocompetence and cytotoxicity, but altering the tumour environment to induce cellular differentiation and reversal of the transformation process. Other methods of reducing the tumour cell population remain important, and immunotherapy combined with surgery, radiation and chemotherapy will optimise the chances for a successful outcome.

The tumour burden needs to be small enough to allow the limited number of cellular components in the immune system to be effective. Although antibodies can be generated and given in enormous doses, agents which act indirectly on the cancer by activating immunocytes or inducing them to produce cytotoxic substances have a limitation in their dosage because there seems to be an endpoint in what these cells can accomplish and what the host will tolerate. Adequate but non-toxic doses of the various agents have to be determined for each type of cancer and each individual. Early diagnosis remains important and will be aided by a variety of sophisticated and sensitive immunodiagnostic techniques.

The host must be immunocompetent or some means must be employed to augment immunocompetence. The manipulation of the immune response should involve the enhancement of the effector cell population and its products, while inhibiting the emergence of cells and factors that suppress a beneficial response.

Human trials should be restricted to agents and techniques which demonstrate at least 3 logs of tumour cell kill in appropriate animal models.

It is important to consider the means of delivery of the immunotherapeutic agent to the cancer site, as well as how to maintain its activity once it is there. Intravenous infusion may be adequate for some agents, while intraarterial administration is necessary for others. Repetitive dosing is necessary for many of these agents, since their effectiveness may be of brief duration. To prevent a premature breakdown of many of the immunotherapeutic molecules, they must be administered with some type of protection until they get to the tumour site. Liposome encapsulation has been one solution to this problem.

Immunotherapy can be classified into two categories: non-specific and specific. The non-specific group includes agents which alter the immune system in some manner and induce an anti-cancer effect (Table 3.2). These substances are not targeted to a specific tumour. They include bacteria, bacterial products, exogenous agents and biological response modifiers. All of these substances act indirectly on the tumour by stimulating immunocytes to become cytotoxic or produce chemicals which are selectively toxic to cancer cells.

Some of the earlier agents which were found to be effective include bacillus Calmette–Guerin and *Corynebacterium parvum*. Bacterial products, such as endotoxins, lipopolysaccharides, and synthetic products represented by muramyl dipeptide and the trehalose esters, have demonstrated a marked ability to stimulate the immune system, particularly through macrophage activation. Exogenous substances, such as Levamisole (2, 3, 5, 6-tetrahydro-6-phenylimidazo-[2, 1-b] thiazole) and viral antigens, have been shown to have anti-cancer effects as a result of their influence on the immune system.

Table 3.2.   Non-specific immunotherapy

Bacteria
  Intact microbial organisms
    BCG
    Corynebacterium parvum

Bacterial products – natural and synthetic
  Lipopolysaccharide (endotoxin)
  Staph phage lysate
  Methanol extraction residue of BCG (MER)
  Peptidoglycans (muramyl dipeptide)
  Glycolipids (trehalose dimycolate)
  Cell wall fractions of various organisms
  Cell wall skeleton fractions
  Glucans and other polysaccharides
  OK 432 (streptococcus)

Synthetic macrophage activators and interferon inducers
  Pyran copolymer
  MVE series
  Poly IC, poly ICLC, poly IC with mismatched bases
  Poly AU
  Pyrimidinoles
  Lysolecithin analogues
  Lipoidal amines

Chemical modulators
  Levamisole
  Thiazobenzimidazole (Wy 40453)
  Diethyldithiocàrbamate (DTC)
  Keyhole limpet haemocyanin (KLH)
  2-Mercapto-2-methylpropanoyl-L-cysteine (SA 96)
  Isoprinosine
  Inosine analogues
  Bestatin
  Cyclomunine
  NED 137
  BAY; 7433
  Azimexon
  Imexon
  Indomethacin and other PGE synthetase inhibitors
  Cimetidine
  Lynestrenol

Biological Response Modifiers/Cytokines
  Interferons
  Interleukins
  Transfer factor
  Tumour necrosis factor
  Transforming Growth Factor B
  Colony Stimulating Factors (CSF)
    Granulocyte-macrophage CSF (GM-CSF)
    Macrophage-CSF (M-CSF)
    Granulocyte-CSF (G-CSF)
  Thymic hormones: Thymosin F5, Thymosin a1, Thymic human factor, thymopoietin, thymostimulin

Non-specific tumour reductive procedures and measures to improve host immunocompetence
  Plasmapheresis
  Plasma exchange
  Vitamin A and conjugates
  Vitamin C
  Hyperalimentation
  Psychological factors

Specific immunotherapy implies that preparations are utilised which can provoke an immunocyte attack on cancer cells without inducing a generalised immune response (Table 3.3). Autologous tumour cells which have been altered to make them immunogenic can be given to the host with the expectation that the suppressed immunocytes will become active. Monoclonal antibodies which can target cancer cells can be used to direct cytotoxic agents and radioactive sources to the tumour cells.

Table 3.3.   Specific immunotherapy

Tumour cell vaccine, altered autologous tumour cells
Immune RNA
Transfer factor
Immune leukocyte infusions
MAB anti-tumour antibody
MAB conjugated with radioisotopes, drugs, toxins
Combination of BRMs and specific immunotherapy

Specific immunotherapy offers some hope of treating tumours with low immunogenicity by identifying a group of cell receptors which are inimicable to the tumour but are not shared by normal cells. These receptors can be targeted by a battery of specific antibodies which would not damage normal cells, nor would they induce an autoantibody response which would render them ineffective.

In recent years there has been a great deal of attention devoted to the biological response modifiers (BRM). These are natural biological products produced by cells in the immune system which regulate their own function by serving as cellular messengers. These monokines and lymphokines activate and deactivate the immune response. They include the interleukins and interferons.

The number of substances which have been used, and those which are currently undergoing investigation as immunotherapeutic agents, are too numerous to discuss. A brief description of some of these agents is given in the next section, and tables provide a listing of more of them. They represent a variety of ways in which the immune system can be affected.

Immunotherapy with Bacteria

Regression of neoplastic disease in patients with acute bacterial infections suggests that some bacteria produce substances which affect the growth of cancer cells. In 1893, W. B. Coley reported on the treatment of cancer patients with bacterial products and noted that tumour regressions were produced. The therapy was most effective when the substances were injected directly into the tumours. Despite these early reports, very little research was done in this area until 1965 when Villasor reported on the use of bacillus Calmette–Guerin (BCG) in combination with chemotherapy in patients with advanced cancer. Since that time, we are familiar with the many clinical trials using this agent and the place it has taken in the management of patients with Stage T_a, T_1 transitional cell carcinoma of the bladder, and carcinoma in situ.

BCG is an attenuated strain of *Mycobacterium bovis* that Calmette and Guerin developed from a virulent culture in 1908 by the addition of bile to the medium.

Although all cultures of BCG have originated from this strain, various vaccines are not identical as a result of differences in preparation, culture methods, and genetic drift.

The efficacy of BCG in treating neoplasia is related to its ability to stimulate the immune system through the inflammatory response, as well as inducing macrophage activation. The portion of the organism which is responsible for these actions has not been discovered. It is clear that live organisms are necessary for the anti-neoplastic effect, and that there must be direct contact made with the cancer. Other factors which govern the effectiveness of BCG include the immunocompetency of the host, a relatively small tumour burden, and a dose which is adequate to induce a response, but not enough to overwhelm the immune system and enhance tumour growth.

Macrophage activation by BCG initiates both an immune and an inflammatory reaction. The stimulated macrophages produce interleukin-1, which is necessary for T-cell activation, and tumour necrosis factor, which is responsible for direct cancer cell cytotoxicity. They also activate T helper/cytotoxic lymphocytes which in turn produce a number of lymphokines, including interferon, which also have an anti-cancer effect. Interleukin-1 has a number of biological effects (Table 3.4).

Table 3.4. Properties and effects of interleukin-1

Made by many cells

Multiple biological functions
Inflammation
Fibroblast proliferation
Fever
Sleep
IL-2 release
T cell activation
B cell activation
Collagenase, prostaglandin induction
Osteoclast activation

Corynebacterium parvum is a killed preparation of one of a number of anaerobic coryneforms with biological activity. The immunological effects of *C. parvum* include antibody production, delayed hypersensitivity, and anti-tumour immunity which may be stimulatory in some situations and suppressive in others.

Bacterial Products (muramyl dipeptides, trehalose diesters, methanol extracted residue)

Because of the sometimes unpredictable and untoward effects associated with the administration of live or dead organisms, attention has been devoted to an identification of those substances which are primarily responsible for immune cell activation. Studies of the chemical structure of mycobacterial cell walls and their hydrolysis products led to the isolation of water-soluble adjuvants and the identification of the peptidoglycans of which the muramyl dipeptides (MDP) are an example. These possess the minimal structure capable of replacing whole killed mycobacteria in complete Freund's adjuvant. The peptide moiety of these molecules is responsible for the immunologic activities. The peptidoglycan derivatives containing an L-alanine-D-glutamic acid sequence are those which are the most active and are recognised by macrophages. These substances are extremely potent macrophage activators. To enhance cell-mediated immunity and produce an anti-cancer effect, MDP must be given by inclusion in liposomes or as a fatty acid derivative.

The glycolipids as represented by the trehalose diesters (TD) are another group of bacterial cell wall substances that can be made synthetically. They induce a strong antibody response and stimulate immunity to tuberculous infections. The anti-tumour effect is also mediated by the macrophage. The combination of TD and MDP has a more potent anti-tumour effect than either used alone.

Another agent obtained from the mycobacterium cell wall which shows anti-cancer activity is the methanol-extracted residue (MER). Although it is very potent as a macrophage activator and is associated with tumour regression in some animal models, its toxicity has precluded its use in clinical trials. All of the bacterial products have demonstrated anti-cancer activity. When their toxicity can be reduced, they will play an important role as immunostimulants.

Chemical Modulators (Immunorestoratives)

These agents either augment or suppress various T-cell mediated and other immune responses, depending on the status of activity of the immune system at a given time, and the balance between suppressor and helper T cells. Most of the work in this area has been done with Levamisole. No careful dose–response studies have been conducted, but there are indications that the remission rate and duration can be extended in immunocompetent patients with minimal tumour burdens. Keyhole limpet haemocyanin (KLH) is a substance extracted from a mollusc. It has been used to prevent recurrences of bladder tumours by intravesical instillation. Its mechanism of action is uncertain.

Biologic Response Modifiers and Cytokines

Interleukin-2

In 1976, Morgan, Ruscetti and Gallo described a factor produced by phytohae-magglutinin activated human T cells that was capable of mediating the expansion of human cells in vitro. This factor, originally called T-cell growth factor, is now referred to as interleukin-2 (IL-2). It is a glycoprotein with a molecular weight of approximately 15 000 kd and is a potent modulator of the immune system in vitro (Table 3.5).

In experimental animals, the systemic injection of IL-2 has been shown to mediate a number of immunological effects. These include the induction of specific T helper cells, cytotoxic cells and antibody production.

In a variety of mouse models, including immunogenic and non-immunogenic sarcomas and colon adenocarcinomas, the administration of high doses of IL-2 alone can mediate the regression of pulmonary and hepatic metastases. Based upon a variety of animal studies, IL-2 has been administered to patients with

Table 3.5. Properties and effects of interleukin-2

Released by T cells
Effects are limited to lymphocytes and macrophages
Resting T cell does not express IL-2 receptor
T cells require antigen stimulation and IL-1 to express IL-2 receptor
Stimulates T cell and macrophage proliferation
Stimulates production of interferon gamma
Enhances cytotoxicity of T cells, macrophages, NK cells, LAK cells, TIL cells

advanced cancer. Doses of 100 000 u per kilogram given every 8 hours for 2 days and repeated at various intervals produced regression in a few patients. Patients with a variety of tumours have been treated, but those with renal adenocarcinomas and pulmonary metastases have demonstrated the best response. Some have obtained stabilisation and tumour regression, but only for a short term. The amount of IL-2 that can be administered is limited by serious toxic side effects. These include increased vascular permeability, pulmonary oedema, febrile reponses, skin rashes, nausea, vomiting, and diarrhoea.

Attempts are being made to find methods which would increase the potency of this immunotherapeutic approach and diminish the toxicity of IL-2. The increased vascular permeability can be substantially reduced by the concurrent administration of cyclophosphamide (CTX). Treatment with CTX enhances specific adoptive immunotherapy, presumably by eliminating tumour-induced suppressor cells and/or by direct tumoricidal activity. The combined administration of CTX plus IL-2 is far more effective in the treatment of mice with advanced pulmonary metastases than is therapy with either agent given alone. Using doses of IL-2 and CTX that produce no cures in mice, more than half of the mice with advanced pulmonary metastases can be cured with the combined administration of these agents.

Nakano et al. (1985) studied the effect of IL-2 on the cytotoxicity of peripheral blood lymphocytes (PBL) in a small group of patients with renal carcinoma. The cytotoxic activity of the PBL was impaired in all the patients. Attempts to enhance cytotoxicity by sensitising the effector cells with mitomycin C-treated tumour cells were futile. Adding IL-2 to this system produced tumour cell lysis in the effector cells from several patients, but IL-2 used alone accomplished the same result. Thus the cytotoxicity of PBL grown in culture with IL-2 was restored and enhanced without the need for prior sensitisation of the effector cells.

Similar experience has been shown in other tumour systems. Hershey et al. (1981) demonstrated cytotoxicity in 5 of 9 melanoma patients. Lotze et al. (1981) reported tumour cell lysis in 5 of 7 patients whose PBLs were grown in IL-2. Kedar et al. (1983) studied patients with lung cancer and found that IL-2 would increase cytotoxicity of cultured PBLs, but cytotoxicity could be enhanced even further if tumour cells were added to the medium. Although PBL treated with IL-2 can lyse their own tumours, this does not always occur. This failure may be due to defective host immunocompetence or differences in tumour immunogenicity.

One mechanism for the anti-tumour effect of IL-2 is the augmentation of natural killer cell (NK) activity. IL-2 stimulates the production of gamma interferon by T cells, which stimulates NK activity. Ordinarily, NK cells do not require the presence of IL-2 or IFN, but the presence of these mediators improves the cytotoxic response. Tumour cells that are resistant to NK cytolysis can be lysed by PBLs cultured in IL-2, suggesting that cytotoxic T cells can be generated independently from NK cells.

The use of IL-2 alone as a form of immunotherapy has not been demonstrated to be useful. Even though lower doses can be administered with minimal side effects and have an anti-tumour cell response in vitro, there are no significant in vivo effects.

Interleukin-2 plus LAK cells

This represents a combination of a BRM and adoptive specific immunotherapy. There is a subset of lymphocytes which become highly cytotoxic when they are cultured in vitro in the presence of IL-2. They are referred to as lymphokine activated killer cells (LAK). These cells are capable of killing autologous and allogeneic tumour cells but not normal cells. In animal models, these LAK cells are capable of causing dramatic regression of established tumours. The experience with LAK in humans indicates that human LAK cells are also capable of killing autologous and allogeneic tumour cells. Studies performed at the National Cancer Institute indicate that the adoptive transfer of LAK in conjunction with recombinant IL-2 is effective in eliminating pulmonary and hepatic metastases from a variety of murine tumours. The administration of autologous LAK cells and IL-2 to patients with advanced cancer can mediate the regression of metastatic disease in selected situations.

IL-2 administered in high doses can result in the endogenous generation of LAK cells in vivo. Regression of pulmonary and hepatic metastases in mice has occurred following the repetitive injection of large doses of IL-2. The severe toxicity produced by the large amount of IL-2 needed to achieve these beneficial effects limits the usefulness of this therapy.

Morita and colleagues (Morita et al. 1987) addressed the issue of whether or not LAK cells administered in vivo would reach tumour tissues and remain functional. They obtained peripheral blood lymphocytes from three patients with renal cancer who had no sign of metastasis. The lymphocytes were cultured with IL-2, radiolabelled with ^{111}In-oxine and infused into the renal artery. The authors learned that there was a selectivity for the accumulation of infused LAK cells into tumour tissue.

This form of adoptive immunotherapy, the introduction of externally activated effector cells, is not only maintained at the tumour site but exerts cytotoxic effects as well. Kinetic studies indicate that LAK cell activity can be generated in the presence of IL-2 within 3 days and the activity persists for 20 days.

Lotze reported that IL-2 activated LAK cells given intravenously would tend to localise primarily in the liver and spleen. Mazumder and Rosenberg (1984) observed that PHA-activated PBL administered intravenously migrated preferentially to the spleen and liver after transient localisation in the lungs. Repeat infusion increased the migration to tumour sites and lungs.

These studies indicate the need to bathe the tumour on a selective basis in order for the activated cells to accumulate and be effective.

The results in clinical trials have substantiated these observations. Patients with metastatic renal cancer who were treated with intravenous injections of IL-2 plus LAK cells followed by repetitive doses of IL-2 have shown temporary regression and stabilisation of pulmonary metastases but no significant improvements in survival have been achieved.

IL-2 and Tumour Infiltrating Lymphocytes (TIL)

There is a group of lymphocytes which are attracted to the site of a developing tumour and begin to infiltrate the mass. They seem to represent NK and LAK cells but are referred to as tumour infiltrating lymphocytes (TIL). Although they are initially cytotoxic, substances produced by the tumour render them ineffective. If these cells are separated from tumour tissue and grown in culture with IL-2, their cytotoxicity is restored. When compared to NK cell activity of PBL, the NK-TIL cells show a marked depression of their activity. The same is true of LAK-TIL cells. Not only can their cytotoxicity be restored in culture, but relatively low doses of IL-2 (15 000 u/kg), given intravenously, can augment TIL NK function and PBL NK activity in vivo.

Anderson et al. (1987, 1988) have shown that there is increased transferrin receptor and HLA-DR expression in the peripheral area of the tumour and increased T-cell infiltration within the tumour in patients receiving intravenous IL-2. In animal models, the adoptive transfer of TIL expanded in IL-2 is 50–100 times more effective in therapeutic potency than are LAK cells.

In humans, these cultured TIL have been shown to have greater cytotoxicity than cultured PBL from the same patient against autologous tumour cells. Kradin et al. (1987) have given expanded TIL to patients with lung cancer and reduced the size of the tumour in 5 of 7 patients. Since expanded TIL are more potent than LAK cells and are sensitised by additional in vitro exposure to IL-2, there is a possibility that fewer cells and lower doses of IL-2 will provide a more efficacious and less toxic therapy for cancer patients.

At present, one of the major problems requiring resolution before the large-scale use of TIL is the difficulty in harvesting and culturing them in sufficient quantities for infusion back into the patient. In approximately 25%–35% of patients, adequate numbers of TIL can be grown. When TIL plus IL-2 can be given, the anti-tumour effect is greatly enhanced by the addition of CTX. Mice with micrometastatic disease can be cured by the use of IL-2 and TIL alone, but when grossly visible tumour is present, this therapy is inadequate. The addition of CTX, given prior to IL-2 plus TIL, results in the complete eradication of large tumour burdens in mice with non-immunogenic tumours.

The usefulness of this approach in the treatment of patients with primary or metastatic disease has yet to be demonstrated. Doses of IL-2 which are relatively low (15 000–30 000 u/kg) can be administered on multiple occasions with minimal toxicity and on an outpatient basis. These doses are adequate to stimulate peripheral NK and LAK activity as well as TIL cytotoxicity.

Interferons

Interferons represent a group of proteins which are elaborated by a large number of cells. They were discovered as a product of virus-infected cells and appear relatively early during these infections. They can be found systemically and in the local environment. There are three major groups: alpha or classical interferon, beta or fibroblast interferon and gamma or immune interferon. Human alpha interferons consist of a family of proteins whose genes are on chromosome 9. Beta interferon is a single protein made by 1–2 genes on chromosome 9. Gamma interferon is made by a single gene on chromosome 6 and there is one expressed protein.

Interferons have a number of biological activities, i.e. they are pleiotropic (Table 3.6). They are also species-specific and receptor-dependent. Their biological activities include anti-viral properties; they are immunomodulatory, inhibit cell proliferation, have an effect on cell differentiation, produce pleiotropic reversions and are involved in oncogene regulation. Their immunoregulatory effects include regulating cytotoxic effector cells, altering cell surface antigen expression and influencing antibody production.

Table 3.6. Biological effects of interferons

Anti-viral activity

Anticellular activity
   Inhibition of cell growth
   Alterations in cell differentiation and phenotype
   Effects on cell cycle
   Interference with oncogene expression

Immunomodulatory activity
   Regulation of cytotoxic effector cells
   Alterations in cell surface antigen expression
   Effects on antibody production

The potential mechanisms for IFN anti-tumour activity include inhibition of cell proliferation, direct killing of neoplastic cells and enhancement of surface antigen expression which may make cancer more immunoreactive. They promote cell differentiation and can cause neoplastic cells to revert to a more normal phenotype. They stimulate the production of various cytokines and promote effector cell cytotoxicity.

The IFN receptor is a high molecular weight glycoprotein (125 000 kd). Cells possess between 350 and 6000 binding sites. These binding sites have a particularly high affinity for IFNa. These receptors can undergo down regulation which is associated with an internalisation of the IFN-receptor complex. Synergistic activity has been demonstrated with combinations of alpha and gamma, alpha and beta, and beta and gamma.

Alpha IFN has been used in the treatment of a large number of human malignancies. There have been positive responses in patients with hairy cell leukemia, chronic myelogenous leukemia, non-Hodgkin's lymphoma, carcinoid, mycosis fungoides, Kaposi's sarcoma, myeloma, melanoma, ovarian carcinoma, renal adenocarcinoma and in Stage T_a, T_1 bladder cancer. There has been no activity demonstrated in breast, colon, or prostate cancer. Non-small cell lung cancer has also failed to show a response.

Colony Stimulating Factors (CSF)

These are substances that stimulate the production of granulocytes, lymphocytes and macrophages. GM-CSF is granulocyte-macrophage CSF which enhances the production of macrophages, neutrophils, eosinophils and, to some extent, red blood cells. M-CSF is macrophage CSF which induces them to proliferate and manufacture GM-CSF. G-CSF is granulocyte CSF which acts primarily on neutrophils. Each growth factor works at specific stages during myeloid cell development. Since the genes producing these agents have been cloned, large enough amounts have been made available for their effects in patients with lymphopenia, immunosuppression, and their interaction with other biological response modifiers to be studied.

Transforming Growth Factor-B (TGF-B)

This is an example of a negative feedback immumodulator which is produced by a number of cells, including those of the immune system. It regulates cellular growth and differentiation and has potent immunosuppressive activity on target cells. TGF-B is 100 000 times more potent than cyclosporin (mole per mole) in suppressing T-cell proliferation.

TGF-B acts as a negative feedback regulator of the interleukins and of lymphokines such as the interferons and tumour necrosis factor. Antigen stimulation initially induces IL-2 production and subsequently TGF-B. IL-2 also induces T-cell proliferation and the development of LAK cells. TGF-B suppresses the proliferative effects of IL-2 leading to homeostatic regulation of T-lymphocyte and LAK cell proliferation.

The regulatory effects of TGF-B on the fibroblast and macrophage function and on angiogenesis involves the formation of the supporting stroma of epithelial tumours. Carcinogenesis is characterised by continuous matrix accumulation due to unregulated secretion of TGF-B. Since tumour growth can result from excessive production of growth promoting factors and from an inadequate supply of growth inhibitory factors, control of TGF-B production represents another method for modulating the host's immune response.

Specific Immunotherapy

Monoclonal Antibodies (MAB)

The advent of hybridoma technology represented a major advance in tumour immunology. The immortalisation of B lymphocytes from immunised hosts fused with myeloma cells allowed the unlimited production of various cell products. Numerous MABs have been generated to most of the human carcinomas. The use of MABs in the management of cancer can be divided into three categories: diagnosis, prognosis and treatment (Fig. 3.3; Tables 3.7, 3.8).

Immunotherapy using MABs can employ a number of different mechanisms. These include effector cell responses, complement, conjugation with chemotherapeutic agents, conjugation with a variety of toxins such as ricin, conjugation with alpha or beta-emitting radionuclides, and immunisation using anti-idiotype immunoglobulins.

Radionuclide conjugates offer some special advantages. The isotopes can kill cells at distances of up to 50 or more cell diameters. Therefore, the MAB-

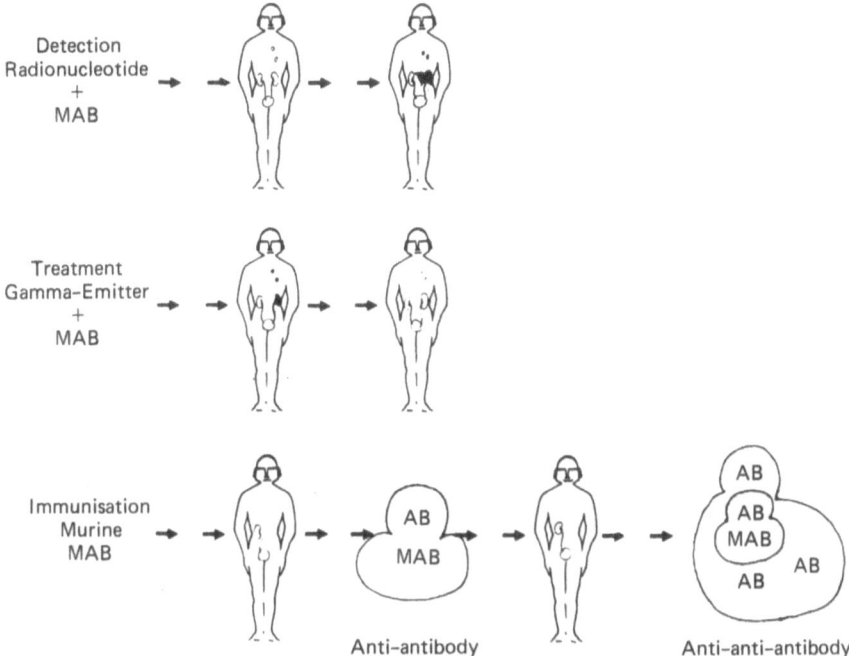

Fig. 3.3. Monoclonal antibodies can be used in a variety of ways in the management of the cancer patient. Immunodiagnosis, immunodetection, therapy and immunisation represent several means of utilising these substances.

Table 3.7. Potential applications of monoclonal antibodies with human carcinomas

---

Diagnosis
1. Screening of body fluids (serum, sputum, effusions, urine, cerebrospinal fluid) and tumour-associated antigens
2. Nuclear scanning with radiolabelled MAB
   a. Detection of primary or metastatic lesions (iv, subepidermal, ip administration of radiolabelled MAB)
   b. Lymphoscintigraphy to detect lymph node involvement
3. Immunopathology
   a. The diagnostic dilemma: malignant against benign
   b. Differential diagnosis of tumour type
   c. Subclassification of tumour based on TAA expression
      Metastatic potential
      Specific favoured sites of metastasis
      Predicted response to specific therapeutic regimen
      Prognosis

Monitoring disease progression
1. Screening of body fluids for TAA
2. Nuclear scanning with radiolabelled MAB
3. Immunopathology for detection of occult metastases
   a. Aspiration cytology
   b. Lymph node or bone marrow biopsy
   c. Cytology of body fluids

Table 3.8. Potential therapeutic applications of monoclonal antibodies in human cancer

---

1. Direct cytotoxicity
     a. complement mediated
     b. cell mediated
2. Combined with chemotherapeutic agents (Adriamycin)
3. Conjugated with toxins (ricin)
4. Conjugated with radionuclides
5. Inhibition of growth factor receptors
6. Immunisation against cancer: administration of anti-idiotype monoclonal antibodies to induce
    specific active immunity to tumour antigens
7. Conjugated with liposomes containing drugs or effector cells

---

radionuclide conjugate does not need to bend to every tumour cell in order to have a therapeutic effect. This may obviate some of the problems associated with tumour cell diversity. Drug conjugates or effector cell mediated mechanisms must be bound to a MAB or group of MABs which can identify specific TAA. Those cells not expressing surface tumour antigens which can be recognised by the MABs would be spared. Many TAAs are stable components of the cell membrane. MAB-TAA complexes on the cell surface do not internalise as do the MAB-lymphocytes antigen cell surface complexes. Since internalisation is necessary to mediate cell killing, these conjugates are likely to have limited effectiveness.

Using MAB-radionuclide conjugates for tumour localisation followed by therapeutic conjugates provides additional benefits. The same MAB conjugate can be used for both purposes by altering the doses or combining different radionuclides. It is also possible that following the radionuclide effects on the cancer cells, a tertiary group of MAB-drug-toxin-effector cell conjugates can be given to destroy those cells which are damaged but are still able to recover. These latter conjugates may have greater efficiency for being internalised while the cells are undergoing recovery.

The ability to develop successful therapy is very difficult. MABs must be selected which have a high affinity for tumour cells with minimal cross reactivity with normal tissues. Appropriate MAB-radionuclide conjugates have to be developed in order to spare normal cells and bone marrow. Two agents which have some promise are ^{90}Y and ^{47}Sc.

Another approach is the use of BRMs or drugs to enhance the expression of tumour antigens of the cell surface. This would augment the antigenicity of the tumour and assist in guiding the MABs to the appropriate targets. This could be a method of managing the antigenic heterogeneity associated with carcinomas. Much of this heterogeneity is associated with the dynamic process of antigenic modulation. This is the turning on and off of the tumour antigenic expression on the cell surface. Factors such as cell cycle, environmental conditions and spatial configuration of the tumour play a role in this type of modulation. BRMs can be used to provide a favourable setting for the action of MABs.

The use of MABs as immunising agents offers some intriguing possibilities. A MAB to a tumour-associated antigen (TAA) or tumour-specific antigen (TSA) is developed and used as an immunogen to prepare a new MAB directed against the antigen binding, idiotypic region of the original MAB. The binding sites of these new anti-idiotype MABs (anti-anti-antibody) provides an "internal image" of the original antigen. A vaccine using such a MAB complex would produce an active and specific response to tumour cells.

Since most MABs are murine derived, there is concern about the use of multiple inoculations of MABs because of the development of human anti-mouse immunoglobulin immune responses (Table 3.9). The vast majority of human anti-murine IgG antibodies are directed against the Fc region of the molecule which would prevent the antibody from binding to cells carrying Fc receptors. One way to obviate this problem is to reduce MABs to very small fragments in order to obtain the minimal binding component. This would eliminate the more immunogenic constant regions on the immunoglobulin molecule. Another method involves cloning the genes coding for individual MABs and reducing them in size with restriction endonucleases and inserting or ligating human immunoglobulin constant regions. Such recombinant chimeric molecules have been formed and have been shown to be effective in some tumour systems. Similar methodology has been developed to ligate metal and drug-binding regions to recombinant immunoglobulin molecules.

Table 3.9.   Problems with monoclonal antibodies as immunoconjugates

1. Human antibodies may destroy murine MAB immunoreactivity
2. Diminution in conjugated drug/toxin site of cytotoxicity
3. Potential decrease in in vivo stability and bioavailability
4. Non-specific uptake
5. Emission of radioenergy beyond the targeted tumour

Conclusion

The immunological basis for human cancer immunotherapy is now well established. Although immunotherapy is not ready to assume a therapeutic role alongside surgery, chemotherapy and radiation therapy, recent advances in the understanding of the immune system and its response to cancer have led to new strategies for cancer management.

Human tumours contain tumour-associated or tumour-specific antigens which elicit a specific anti-tumour immune reponse. Enhancement of the anti-tumour response, diminution of the tumour lymphocyte suppressor response, and specific targeting of drugs, radionuclides, toxins and effector cells present great challenges but also great hope. The immune system is so complex that it is unlikely that a single agent or manipulation will produce a dramatic anti-cancer effect. Instead, the immunotherapist will need to act as an orchestra leader and bring into play the appropriate substances at the correct times and in the proper amounts. The score is represented by the biological interactions between the host and the malignancy with a unique arrangement for each individual.

References

Anderson TM, Ibayashi Y, Holmes EC et al. (1987) Modification of natural killer activity of lymphocytes infiltrating human lung cancers. Cancer Immunol Immunother 25: 65–68

Anderson TM, Iboyashi Y, Tokuda Y et al. (1988) Effects of systemic interleukin-2 on natural killer and lymphokine activated killer activity of human tumor infiltrating lymphocytes. Cancer Res 48: 1180–1187

Balkwell FR, Ward BF, Moodie E, Fiers W (1987) Therapeutic potential of tumor necrosis factor-a and g-interferon in experimental human ovarian cancer. Cancer Res 47: 4755–4758

Bander NH (1987) Monoclonal antibodies in urologic oncology. Cancer [suppl] 60: 658–667

Bugelski PJ, Corwin SP, North SM, Kirsh RL, Nicolson GL, Poste G (1987) Macrophage content of spontaneous metastases at different stages of growth. Cancer Res 47: 4141–4145

Cummings KB, Schmid SM, Bryan GT, Border EC (1986) Antiproliferative activity of recombinant interferons alpha and beta for human renal carcinoma cells: Supra-additive activity with elevated temperature or vinblastine. World J Urol 3:230–233

Droller MJ (1987) Biologic response modifiers in genitourinary neoplasia. Cancer 60 [suppl]: 635–644

Fahey JR, Hines DL (1987) Progressive growth of immunogenic tumors: Relationship between susceptibility of ascites p815 tumor cells to T-cell-mediated lysis and immune destruction in vivo. Cancer Res 47: 4759–4765

Goldstein D, Laszlo J (1986) Interferon therapy in cancer: from imaginon to interferon. Cancer Res 46: 4315–4329

Grups JW, Schmitz-Drager BJ, Ebert T, Ackermann R (1986) Biologic potentials of interferon's relevance in the systemic treatment of superficial bladder carcinoma. World J Urol 3: 224–229

Hersey P, Bindon C, Edwards A, Murray E, Phillips G, McCarthy WH (1981) Induction of cytotoxic activity in human lymphocytes against autologous and allogeneic melanoma cells in vitro by culture with interleukin 2. Int J Cancer 28: 695–703

Kedar E, Ikejiri BL, Timonen T, Bonnard GD, Reid J, Navvarro NJ, Sredni B, Heberman RB (1983) Antitumor reactivity in vitro and in vivo of lymphocytes from normal donors and cancer patients propagated in culture with T-cell growth factor (TCGF). Eur J Cancer Clin Oncol 19: 757–773

Kohler G (1986) Derivation and diversification of monoclonal antibodies. Science 233: 1281–1286

Kradin RL, Boyle LA, Preffer FI et al. (1987) Tumor-derived, interleukin-2-dependent lymphocytes in adoptive immunotherapy of lung cancer. Cancer Immunol Immunother 24: 76–85

Krown SE (1987) Interferon treatment of renal cell carcinoma. Cancer [supplement] 59: 647–651

Lotze MT, Grimm EA, Mazumder A, Strausser JL, Rosenberg SA (1981) Lysis of fresh and cultured autologous tumor by human lymphocytes cultured in T-cell growth factor. Cancer Res 41: 4420–4425

Mazumder A, Rosenberg SA (1984) Successful immunotherapy of natural killer resistant established pulmonary melanoma metastases by the intravenous adoptive transfer of syngeneic lymphocytes activated in vitro by interleukin-2. J Exp Med 159: 495–507

Morales A, Nickel JC (1986) Immunotherapy of superficial bladder cancer with BCG. World J Urol 3: 209–214

Morgan DA, Ruscetti FW, Gallo RC (1976) Growth of thymus derived lymphocytes from human bone marrow. Science 193: 1007–1008

Morita R, Yonese Y, Minato N (1987) In vivo distribution of recombinant interleukin-2-activated autologous lymphocytes administered by intra-arterial infusion in patients with renal cell carcinoma. JNCI 78: 441–447

Nakano E, Yasuharu T, Ichikaw Y et al. (1985) Cytotoxic activity of peripheral blood lymphocytes grown with interleukin-2 against autologous cultured tumour cells in patients with renal cell carcinoma: Preliminary report. J Urol 134: 24–28

Nauts HC (1969) The apparently beneficial effects of bacterial infections on host resistance to cancer: End results in 435 cases. N Y Cancer Res Inst Monogr 8: 1–57

Nossal GJV (1987) The basic components of the immune system. N Engl J Med 316: 320–325

Rabinowich H, Cohen R, Bruderman T et al. (1987) Functional analysis of mononuclear cells infiltrating into tumors: Lysis of autologous human tumor cells by cultured lymphocytes. Cancer Res 47: 173–177

Reif AE (1986) Relationship of success in classical immunotherapy to the relative immunorejective strength of the tumor. JNCI 77: 899–908

Rosenberg SA, Lotze MT, Mool LM et al. (1985) Observations on the systemic administration of autologous lymphokine-activated killer cells and recombinant interleukin-2 to patients with metastatic cancer. New Engl J Med 313: 1485–1492

Rosenberg SA, Spiess P, Lafrenier R (1986) A new approach to the adoptive immunotherapy of cancer with tumor-infiltrating lymphocytes. Science 233: 1318–1321

Sarosdy MF, Pickett SH, Stogdill BJ, Rochester MG, Reynolds RH, Radwin HM, Lamm DL (1986) Immunotherapy and immunodiagnostic studies in carcinoma of the bladder. World J Urol 3: 215–217

Schlom J (1986) Basic principles and applications of monoclonal antibodies in the management of carcinomas. Cancer Res 46: 3225–3238

Schmitz-Drager BJ, Ebert T, Ackermann R (1986): Intravesical treatment of superficial bladder carcinoma with interferons. World J Urol 3: 218–223

Tallberg T, Tykka H (1986) Specific active immunotherapy in advanced renal cell carcinoma: A clinical long-term follow-up study. World J Urol 3: 234–244.

Villasor RB (1965) The clinical use of BCG vaccine in stimulating host resistance to cancer. J Philippine Med Assoc 41: 619–624

Yabro JW (1987) Advance in interferon therapy. Semin Oncol 14 [suppl 2], 1–60

Chapter 4

Carcinoma of the Kidney

T. Ebert and R. Ackermann

Diagnosis and Staging

Introduction

Renal cell carcinoma is the most common malignant tumour of the kidney. It is the third most common urological cancer with an incidence of approximately 5–8 in 100 000 males in most Western countries. The incidence rate is higher in Scandinavian countries (10 in 100 000 males) and smaller in Africa, Asia and South America (1–3 in 100 000 males). The male-to-female ratio is about 2:1 and its peak incidence is in the 5th and 6th decades of life (Paganini-Hill et al. 1983). Electron microscopic and immuno-histochemical studies found the proximal tubular cells to be the most likely origin of renal cell carcinoma (Bander 1985). Tumour spread occurs by direct extension or via the venous or lymphatic system.

The cause of renal cancer is unknown. A number of factors (cadmium, aromatic hydrocarbons, lead, asbestos, hormones, etc.) have been examined in several case-control studies, but a clear correlation could not be established (Paganini-Hill et al. 1983).

Clinical Symptoms

The clinical signs and symptoms of patients with renal cell carcinoma vary considerably. Pain, haematuria, a palpable abdominal mass and hypertension are among the most common. In a survey of 7 different studies Patel and Lavengood (1978) found the classical triad of pain, haematuria and a palpable abdominal mass to be present in 5% to 32%. In about 15% of the patients diagnosis is established incidentally (Oliver et al. 1979; Konnak and Grossman 1985), while 20% present with symptoms related to distant metastases. These lesions occur most commonly in the lungs and bones (Wagle and Scal 1970; McNichols et al. 1981) and may cause shortness of breath or bone pain.

Diagnostic and Staging Procedures

Once diagnosis of renal cell carcinoma has been established the extent of the disease has to be determined. This information, correlated with treatment results, allows for prognostication and may influence the therapeutic approach. Since surgery is pre-eminent in the treatment of renal cell carcinoma (McDonald 1982), the main purpose of preoperative staging in this disease is to separate patients who are likely to benefit from surgical procedures from those who are not. As a consequence of stage-dependent treatment results (see below), diagnostic procedures should be able to distinguish

1. Patients with primary tumours invading adjacent organs from patients with localised disease
2. Patients with multiple metastatic lesions from those with solitary or no metastases
3. Patients with involvement of renal vein and vena cava to allow the planning of an appropriate surgical approach.

Intravenous Urography (IVU)

Intravenous urography is still the primary uroradiological imaging tool satisfying most diagnostic needs. Usually it is the first procedure performed when clinical signs of renal malignancy are evident. Despite adequate imaging of renal masses its specificity in defining the difference between solid and cystic masses remains relatively poor (Lang 1980; Bosniak 1986). Additional tests are necessary to establish the correct diagnosis as well as to determine the extent of an apparently malignant tumour (Sagel et al. 1977; Richie et al. 1983). However, the IVU provides useful preoperative information on morphology and function of the urinary tract. In addition, it contributes to the detection of osseous metastases which are almost always first noted as lytic lesions seen on plain X-ray film (Swanson et al. 1981). Intravenous urography in patients with renal masses is still considered an important part of the preoperative diagnostic work in those patients.

Ultrasonography (US)

In recent years US has become a valuable diagnostic procedure in the evaluation of renal masses. Its accuracy in distinguishing cystic from solid renal masses has approached nearly 100% and usually no further studies need be done, if the sonogram displays all the criteria of a simple cyst (Pollack et al. 1982). However, US is not able to differentiate accurately malignant from solid benign renal masses such as angiomyolipoma, focal fibrolipomatosis, infarction or haemangioma (Baltarowich and Kurtz 1987). In addition, it is of note that US in contrast to other diagnostic modalities such as computed tomography is strongly operator-dependent and reliability is limited to the operator's experience (Mittelstaedt 1987).

Computed Tomography (CT)

CT has been found to be an extremely accurate, operator-independent diagnostic modality. Its accuracy in establishing correct diagnosis in cystic and solid lesions is equal to US (Sagel et al. 1977; Balfe et al. 1982). Its value in determining local extent of the primary tumour is even greater (Levine et al. 1980). In a prospective study, Cronan et al. (1982) correlated preoperative US- and CT-findings to postoperative histological findings. In 21 out of 23 patients (91%) CT provided accurate determination of T- and N-Stage. US and angiography achieved an accuracy of 70% and 61% respectively. Renal vein or vena caval involvement can be detected equally well by CT or angiographic methods (Levine et al. 1979). At the present time CT must be considered as the optimal technique in staging renal cell carcinoma.

Angiography

Angiography was the sine qua non for the evaluation of renal masses prior to the CT/US-era. Now, however, the superiority of CT and US in diagnosis and in staging has been demonstrated in several studies (Weyman et al. 1980; Mauro et al. 1982; Cronan et al. 1982). Although angiography is no longer routinely recommended preoperatively in patients with renal cell carcinoma, it is still necessary in selected cases when accurate definition of vascular anatomy is required, e.g. before intrarenal surgery or vena cava thrombectomy.

Magnetic Resonance Imaging (MRI)

Since only preliminary results are available to date (Leung et al. 1984; Hricak et al. 1985) it is premature to assess the possible role of magnetic resonance imaging in diagnosis and staging of renal cell carcinoma.

Surgical Exploration vs Percutaneous Needle Biopsy

Although computed tomography combined with ultrasound will provide the correct diagnosis in 93%–97% of patients with renal masses, in a small number of patients results of CT and US are inconclusive. Since angiography is not particularly helpful in these patients (Balfe et al. 1982), percutaneous biopsy and cytochemical examination of retrieved material are recommended by several authors (Juul et al. 1985; Parienty et al. 1985). Various reports indicate that diagnosis can be determined in approximately 85% of renal masses by fine needle biopsy (Nosher et al. 1982; Helm et al. 1983). False-positive as well as false-negative results limit the predictive value of the given aspirate. A negative percutaneous biopsy always requires further exploration of suspicious lesions. Though it may occur infrequently, needle tract seeding following aspiration of renal cell carcinoma has been reported (Gibbons et al. 1977; Kiser et al. 1986). Because of the possibility of false-negative or positive findings and of tumour cells spilling into the needle tract, percutaneous biopsy cannot be recommended as a routine procedure.

It is a policy at our institution to perform surgical exploration rather than a biopsy in these patients provided they are fit for a surgical procedure. This approach has been advocated by others as well (Bolton and Vaughan 1977; Stanisic et al. 1977; Murphy and Marshall 1980).

Chest X-ray, Chest-CT

The examination of the lungs by conventional chest X-ray film and/or chest-CT is unanimously considered as a routine part of the preoperative examination of patients with kidney cancer.

Bone Scintigraphy

Since radionucleide bone scanning has demonstrated its superiority to roentgeno-graphic surveys for the early detection of osseous metastases in renal cell carcinoma (Cole et al. 1975; Kim et al. 1983), many institutions have included bone imaging as part of the standard evaluation for all patients with this disease. The largest series of patients with bone metastases was analysed by Swanson et al. (1981). The records of 957 patients with renal cell carcinoma were reviewed identifying 252 (26. 7%) with bone metastases during the clinical course of the disease. Of these, 133 (14%) presented with bone metastases at the time of diagnosis, and 121 out of these 133 patients (91%) had symptoms secondary to the osseous metastases. Rosen and Murphy (1984) concluded from their own data and from analysing the data presented by Swanson et al. that routine bone scanning is unwarranted as a screening method in the absence of skeletal symptoms. This conclusion was supported by the study of Blacher et al. (1985) who evaluated radionucleide bone scans in 85 patients with renal cell carcinoma. Of the patients, 34% were found to have skeletal disease at presentation. Each time the bone scan proved positive for metastatic disease, other routine diagnostic or staging procedures had demonstrated at least one osseous metasta-sis or symptoms had suggested the lesion. Bone scanning was not considered to be an essential screening procedure in asymptomatic patients with renal cell carcinoma.

More recent data suggest that patients with a solitary metastasis may benefit from radical nephrectomy and subsequent surgical removal of the metastatic lesion. In these rare cases the knowledge of an additional asymptomatic bone deposit might alter therapeutic plans and bone scintigraphy should be performed to obtain additional information in order to justify an aggressive surgical approach.

Tumour Classification

Data of staging procedures have been listed in various staging systems (Flocks and Kadesky 1958; Petkovic 1959; Rubin 1968; Robson et al. 1969). The first system was developed by Flocks and Kadesky (1958) and its modification by Robson and associates (1969) is still in widespread use today. The most recent classification is the tumour, nodes, and metastasis (TNM) system defined by the UICC (Hermanek 1986). Since all possible parameters that may affect the treatment history are considered separately, the possible number of subgroups (up to 48) has been considered as a shortcoming of this classification (Bassil et al. 1985).

An apparent shortcoming of Robson's system is the fact that local tumour extent cannot be assessed independently from nodal involvement (Table 4.1).

Table 4.1. Comparison of staging systems for renal cell carcinoma

Extent of tumour	Stage	
	TNM: Hermanek (1986)	Robson et al. (1969)
Tumour confined to the kidney		1
diameter <2.5 cm	T1	
diameter >2.5 cm	T2	
Perinephric fat involvement	T3a	2
Vascular involvement	T3b	2A or 3C
Invasion of adjacent organs	T4	4A
Lymph node involvement		3B or 3C
solitary diameter <2 cm	N1	
solitary/multiple diameter <5 cm	N2	
solitary/multiple diameter >5 cm	N3	
Solitary/multiple distant metastases	M1	4B

Conclusions

In the vast majority of cases computed tomography and ultrasound provide accurate diagnosis in patients presenting with a renal mass. If a definite diagnosis cannot be established, surgical exploration should be given preference over percutaneous biopsy.

CT has demonstrated its superiority as a staging procedure over US and angiography. Preoperative angiography is not routinely recommended in patients with renal cell carcinoma. However, when main renal vein or vena caval involvement are suspected, angiography may provide additional information. In these cases MRI may be of particular help in defining accurately the extent of the thrombus. Arteriography should be part of preoperative diagnosis when intra-renal surgery such as heminephrectomy or tumour excision are proposed.

Chest X-ray films and/or chest-CT are routine radiographic procedures in the evaluation of patients with renal cell carcinoma. At the present time radio-nucleide bone scanning cannot be said to be mandatory for the routine staging of patients without skeletal symptoms.

The use of the TNM-system for accurate staging of renal cell carcinoma as well as for facilitation of information exchange between cancer centres is recommended.

Basic Therapy of Renal Cell Carcinoma

Radical Nephrectomy

Modalities

Radical nephrectomy is the treatment of choice in patients with a normal contralateral kidney and without multiple distant metastases. In contrast to simple nephrectomy this procedure includes complete excision of the kidney including the investing Gerota's fascia and the adrenal gland (Crawford 1982). Radical nephrectomy was first advocated by Chute and associates in 1949. It was found that the direct extension of a tumour into perinephric fat occurs in about 20% of the patients (Beare and McDonald 1949). Others confirmed these findings and reported improved survival rates as compared to simple nephrectomy (Robson et al. 1969; Skinner et al. 1972; Patel and Lavengood 1978). The role of subsequent lymphadenectomy is still controversial and will be discussed separately.

Two main approaches are commonly used for this operation:

1. Anterior transperitoneal
2. Thoraco-abdominal, either intrapleural or extrapleural

Advocates of the thoraco-abdominal modality claim that large upper pole lesions may be removed more easily from this approach, particularly in obese patients. In addition, they stress that the intrapleural procedure allows for palpation of the ipsilateral lung to check for metastases and in the right side for control of the vena cava in the chest in the event of a tumour thrombus in the vena cava (Marshall 1983).

An abdominal incision, however, should be employed in the patient who cannot tolerate the exaggerated flank position required for thoraco-abdominal surgery. An anterior transperitoneal approach (transverse incision, Chevron incision) is ideal, if bilateral renal surgery (bilateral carcinoma) is contemplated or tumour excision is necessary in a solitary kidney. The transperitoneal approach is also preferred when thrombus extraction from the renal vein or vena cava from left renal cell carcinoma is necessary (Das 1982).

Both modalities have been used in large series and operative mortality rates have been reported to range from approximately 2% to 10% for either procedure (Robson et al. 1969; Skinner et al. 1972; Giuliani et al. 1983). Swanson and Borges (1983) analysed data from 193 patients who underwent transperitoneal radical nephrectomy through an upper midline incision. The intraoperative and postoperative complication rates were 20.7% and 19.1%, respectively. It is of note that in 24% of patients with left sided tumours splenectomy was performed because of injury to the spleen. There is no similar report in the literature analysing in detail complications involved with thoraco-abdominal radical nephrectomy.

Results

Survival rates of patients with renal cell carcinoma treated with radical nephrectomy are shown in Fig. 4.1.

Survival has been shown to be dependent on several factors:

1. Local extent of tumour
2. Nodal disease
3. Distant metastases
4. Renal vein/vena caval involvement
5. Histological grading

While there is unanimous agreement in the literature concerning the influence of local extent, nodal and distant metastases, the role of renal vein and vena caval involvement has been controversial. Skinner et al. (1972) studied 309 patients and found no significant difference in survival for patients with renal vein or vena caval involvement compared to those with tumour confined to the kidney, provided perinephric fat and lymph nodes were not involved. Myers et al. (1968) reported that invasion of the renal vein adversely affected prognosis. However, due to the staging system used, the number of patients with concomitant lymph node disease was not recorded. More recent analyses (Cherrie et al. 1982; Sogani et al. 1983; Sosa et al. 1984; Libertino et al. 1987) reported that the level of vena

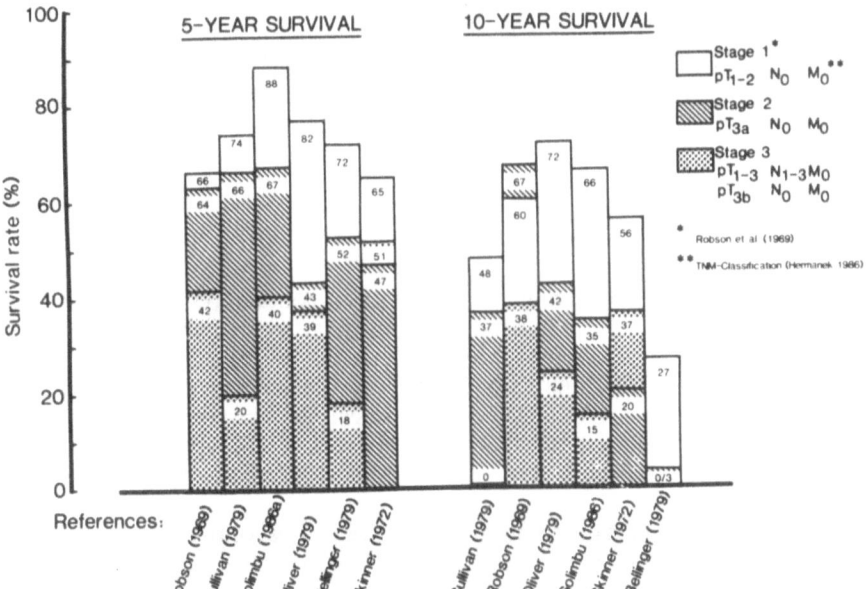

Fig. 4.1. Survival rates following radical nephrectomy for non-metastatic renal cell carcinoma.

caval involvement by tumour thrombus has a prognostic significance. These findings as well as the surgical options for vena cava involvement will be discussed separately.

The importance of tumour grade has been examined only in a limited number of studies (Böttiger 1970; Fuhrman et al. 1982; Nurmi 1984). Though uniform criteria for grading were not employed, results indicated that tumour grade affected survival. Nurmi (1984) showed that the poor prognosis of high grade tumours was even independent of the anatomical extent of the tumour. The cytoplasmic appearance (clear or granular) is not a significant feature relevant to survival of the patient (Boxer et al. 1979). Recent studies investigated nuclear deoxyribonucleic acid (DNA) ploidy of renal cell carcinoma specimens by flow cytometry. A correlation of nuclear DNA content and survival was reported (Ljungberg et al. 1986; Rainwater et al. 1987) and it was concluded that flow cytometry might become a useful modality in the classification and determination of prognosis for patients with kidney cancer (Otto et al. 1984). However, with only a few studies available the importance of the presented data for any individual patient remains to be documented.

Overall survival data indicate that 40%–80% of all patients with renal cell carcinoma will die from disease within 10 years following initial treatment. In the vast majority of cases patients develop distant metastases (McNichols et al. 1981). The interval between initial MO presentation and appearance of metastases may be as short as 1 month (Golimbu et al. 1986b) and as long as 31 years (Kradjian and Bennington 1965). McNichols et al. (1981) reported that of 262 patients with recurrence, 78% developed metastases during the first 5 years postoperatively. In the report of Rafla (1970) the majority of distant metastases occurred in the first two years after nephrectomy, and deKernion et al. (1978) recognised a 21% recurrence rate after 1 year. The most common sites of recurrence are lung and bone (Lokich and Harrison 1975; McNichols et al. 1981; Bassil et al. 1985). Local recurrence is reported to occur in 8%–19% of patients (Waters and Richie 1979; Parienty et al. 1984; Bassil et al. 1985). Generally recurrence indicates a poor prognosis. In the Mayo Clinic series (McNichols et al. 1981) only 50% of the patients who developed a recurrence were alive at 6 months.

Partial Nephrectomy

Renal cell carcinoma occurring bilaterally or in solitary (or sole-functioning) kidneys without evidence of multiple distant metastases represents a challenge for the clinician. The need for preserving renal function limits the surgical options. About 2%–5% of patients will fall into this category (Marberger et al. 1981; Brannen et al. 1983), in which radical nephrectomy would require subsequent renal replacement therapy. The goal of therapy is the complete removal of carcinoma while sparing sufficient renal tissue for a life without dialysis.

Partial nephrectomy is the treatment of choice in most of these patients. Apical or basilar renal tumours may be removed by ligating the appropriate segmental renal arterial branch and excising the involved renal segment at the observed line of demarcation. Frequently, however, the tumour extends across several vascular territories and the only method of removal is a careful excision of the tumour-bearing area with a sufficient margin of normal tissue (Wickham 1975). Though this procedure was initially described by Vermooten in 1950, technical problems and poor control of cancer prevented its widespread use. Technical advances such as local hypothermia following temporary occlusion of the renal artery improved results markedly and over the past 2 decades encouraging data have been reported (Vermillion et al. 1972; Finkbeiner et al. 1976; Malek et al. 1976). In 1981 the European Intrarenal Surgical Society (EIRSS) reported on 72 patients who underwent conservative surgery for renal cell carcinoma (Marberger et al. 1981). The 5-year cancer survival rate for patients with unilateral disease was 78%. Survival for patients with bilateral synchronous and bilateral asynchronous lesions were 48% and 38%, respectively. Topley et al. (1984) described similar results in their study.

In a small subgroup of patients a complex central tumour may prevent a partial nephrectomy. In these cases ex vivo surgery ("bench surgery") for a central wedge excision may be indicated. However, complication rates for bench surgery are considerably increased compared to in situ procedures (Wickham 1975; Marberger et al. 1981) and ex vivo surgery with subsequent renal autotransplantation should be performed only in selected patients when appropriate handling of the situation is not possible in situ (Marshall and Walsh 1984).

Tumour Enucleation

The advantages of this modality compared to partial nephrectomy include reduction of bleeding by not excising the surrounding margin of normal tissue as well as maximal preservation of functional renal parenchyma. However, larger tumours, particularly, frequently infiltrate the surrounding pseudocapsule (Marberger et al. 1981; Rosenthal et al. 1984) and malignant tissue may remain in the renal remnant. Despite an excellent 3-year survival rate of 90% reported by Novick et al. (1986), most urologists believe that every effort should be made to excise a rim of normal cortex around the neoplasm. Though sufficient data are not yet available in this field, the indication for enucleation seems to be rare.

Excision of Metastases

The first successful surgical excision of an apparently solitary lung metastasis in a patient who had undergone nephrectomy for renal cell carcinoma was reported by Barney and Churchill in 1939. This case has prompted other surgeons to treat aggressively apparently solitary metastatic lesions in patients with renal cell carcinoma. Solitary metastases are reported to occur in approximately 1%–3% of patients with this disease (Middleton 1967; Skinner et al. 1971). They are found most commonly in bony tissue and brain (Tolia and Whitmore 1975; O'Dea et al. 1978) and may be present at initial presentation or at any time during the clinical course of the disease.

After reviewing the literature and adding 8 more cases Middleton (1967) reported a 34% 5-year survival rate following nephrectomy and removal of solitary metastases. Tolia and Whitmore (1975) analysed 90 cases treated for solitary metastases and found that 35% of these patients lived 5 years or longer. In more recent reports of deKernion et al. (1978), Swanson et al. (1981) and Golimbu et al. (1986b) similar results have been recorded. The latter studies included even some selected patients with more than 1 metastasis. The spectrum of therapeutic procedures for local treatment of metastases ranges from curettage and intramedullary nailing of isolated skeletal metastases to amputation of limbs, excision of central nervous and pulmonary lesions, cryosurgery, prosthetic replacement and radiotherapy (Marcove et al. 1972; Tolia and Whitmore 1975; deKernion et al. 1978; Swanson et al. 1981; Golimbu et al. 1986b).

Results so far suggest that an aggressive surgical approach may improve survival in patients with solitary metastatic disease.

Adjunctive Nephrectomy

Multiple distant metastases are present in 20%–30% of patients with renal cell carcinoma at time of first presentation. The reported 5-year survival data range from 0%–14.6% (Mims et al. 1966; Rafla 1970; Johnson et al. 1975). Although a prospective randomised study analysing the effect of nephrectomy on survival in these patients has not been performed, some conclusions can be drawn from retrospective analysis of data comparing patients who underwent nephrectomy to those who did not. Results of 4 large studies are shown in Table 4.2.

Table 4.2. Influence of adjunctive nephrectomy on survival in patients with multiple distant metastases

Reference	Median survival (months)	
	Nephrectomy	No nephrectomy
Middleton (1967)	<12	<12
Johnson et al. (1975)	11.3	7.9
Patel and Lavengood (1978)	<12	<12
Swanson et al. (1981)	8	6

A certain benefit of nephrectomy in patients with bony metastases was suggested in 2 studies (Montie et al. 1977a; Bohnenkamp et al. 1980). However, Swanson, analysing data from 252 patients with osseous metastases, stated that the critical factor affecting survival is not whether the metastases are osseous, but whether they are solitary or multiple (Swanson et al. 1981).

Golimbu et al. (1986a) reported 92 patients with disseminated disease who underwent nephrectomy. Two of them survived longer than 5 years, a 5-year survival rate of 2.25%. The therapeutic value of adjunctive nephrectomy seems questionable when this result is compared to a 3.8% 5-year survival of 116 untreated Stage 4 patients in the series of Flocks and Kadesky (1958).

A major argument for nephrectomy in asymptomatic patients is still the possible promotion of spontaneous regression of distant metastases (Giuliani et al. 1983). Spontaneous regression as defined by Everson and Cole (1966) refers to "partial or complete disappearance of a malignant tumour in the absence of all treatment or in the presence of therapy which is considered inadequate". Since Bumpus in 1928 reported the first case of spontaneous regression of pulmonary metastases of renal cell carcinoma, Katz and Schapira (1982) found 68 more well-documented cases in a survey of the literature. In about 30% of these cases actual histological confirmation has been obtained. Those without documented histology could well have had a concomitant benign disease such as sarcoidosis or some collagen or fungal diseases that are known to be capable of producing pulmonary lesions that can appear radiographically indistinguishable from metastases (Middleton 1967; Snow and Schellhammer 1982).

Various factors such as hormonal changes, infection and fever or an altered immune status have been discussed as being possibly involved in spontaneous regression of metastases. However, due to the small numbers, the exact mechanism of regression is still unknown. The incidence has been reported to range from 0.001% to 0.8% in patients with distant metastases following adjunctive nephrectomy (Katz and Schapira 1982). We reviewed 17 large series with regard to the incidence of spontaneous regression and operative mortality (Table 4.3).

Table 4.3. Spontaneous regression of distant metastases and postoperative mortality following nephrectomy

References	No. of patients (M+)	No. of spontaneous regression	Postoperative mortality (%) (all nephrectomies)
Mims et al. (1966)	57	1[a]	5.2
Middleton (1967)	33	0	2.2
Myers et al. (1968)	29	0	4.7
Rafla (1970)	14	0	–
Böttiger (1970)	24	0	9
Skinner et al. (1971)	62	1	10[b]
Johnson et al. (1975)	43	0	2
Lokich and Harrison (1975)	45	0	–
Montie et al. (1977a)	23	0	5.3
Patel and Lavengood (1978)	16	0	2.3
deKernion et al. (1978)	26	0	6[b]
Oliver et al. (1979)	29	0	14[b]
Swanson et al. (1981)	77	0	–
Giuliani et al. (1983)	30	0	10
Nurmi (1984)	54	0	1.9
Bassil et al. (1985)	53	0	–
Golimbu et al. (1986a)	92	1	3.2
Totals	707	3 (0.4%)	$x=5.9\%$

[a] Histologically confirmed
[b] Specified for metastatic disease

Considering the extreme rarity of that event and the mortality from nephrectomy, we conclude that adjunctive nephrectomy is contraindicated for the purpose of promoting spontaneous regression of distant metastases in renal cell carcinoma.

Adjunctive nephrectomy in order to reduce tumour load may be a reasonable procedure in patients who undergo additional systemic treatment for metastatic disease in controlled studies. In our opinion this represents the only indication for nephrectomy in asymptomatic patients with distant metastases.

Palliative Nephrectomy

It is well established that renal cell carcinoma may cause local (haematuria, pain), toxic systemic (fever, anaemia, hypotension, hepatopathy) and endocrine effects (erythrocytosis, hypercalcaemia) (Holland 1973). However, incidence and severity of these symptoms vary considerably (Patel and Lavengood 1978). Problems from the primary tumour that cannot be managed conservatively occur only in a small number of patients with distant metastases (Johnson et al. 1975; Montie et al. 1977a). Since systemic symptoms such as hypercalcaemia, fever, hepatic dysfunction and erythrocytosis may also be produced by the metastases, palliative nephrectomy may be limited to those patients who suffer from intractable haematuria, severe local pain and/or psychological pressure.

Angio-Infarction

Preoperative angio-infarction for metastatic renal cell carcinoma has been advocated by several authors (Swanson et al. 1983; Kaisary et al. 1984) for various reasons:

1. To facilitate subsequent nephrectomy
2. To decrease intraoperative blood loss
3. To "stimulate" an immune response

Since its introduction in the management of metastatic kidney cancer, this procedure has been controversial. No prospective randomised study has yet demonstrated a benefit from angio-infarction. In 1983 Swanson et al. presented the most extensive series with infarction-nephrectomy. Of 100 patients with disseminated renal cell carcinoma who underwent angio-infarction prior to nephrectomy, 7 experienced complete and 8 partial regression of their metastatic lesion(s). In 12 of these 15 patients recurrence or progression occurred within 3 years and the patients subsequently died. More recent reports, also not randomised, could not confirm any beneficial effect of this procedure. In the study of Bakke et al. (1985) survival time was equal whether or not patients underwent angio-infarction. Christensen et al. (1985) did not find significant differences in duration of operation and perioperative blood loss in patients with or without preoperative embolisation of the renal artery. Similar results were reported by Mebust et al. (1984), who did not observe reduction of size in metastatic lesions following renal infarction.

Though arguments for an infarction-nephrectomy in metastatic renal cell carcinoma are weak, embolisation of the renal artery might be worthwhile as a palliative method in patients with intractable bleeding from the primary tumour, when adjunctive nephrectomy is not indicated due to multiple distant metastases.

Management of Vena Caval Involvement

General Considerations

In 4%–9.1% of patients presenting with renal cell carcinoma a tumour thrombus extending into the vena cava inferior will be found (Robson et al. 1969; Waters and Richie 1979; Nurmi 1984; Marshall and Reitz 1985). Vena caval involvement occurs in the majority of cases in right sided tumours (McCullough and Gittes 1974; Kearney et al. 1981) probably because of the shorter right renal vein. Since complete occlusion of the vena cava is rarely found and small collaterals are able to sustain circulation, many patients present without clinical symptoms related to their caval thrombus (Clayman et al. 1980; Cherrie et al. 1982). However, pedal oedema, albuminuria, right or left varicocele, dilated superficial abdominal wall veins or recurrent pulmonary emboli have been described in such patients (McCullough and Gittes 1974; Schefft et al. 1978; Libertino et al. 1987) and always should lead to a meticulous diagnostic investigation.

In days past the prognosis for patients with vena caval involvement was considered to be poor (Riches et al. 1951; Myers et al. 1968). However, in 1972 Skinner et al. presented similar 5- and 10-year survival rates for Stage 1 patients and for patients with vena caval involvement provided they had no nodal or distant metastases. Since then several studies advocating an aggressive surgical approach have shown excellent results in this particular patient group (Schefft et al. 1978; Sogani et al. 1983). Libertino et al. (1987) reported 5-year and 10-year survival rates in patients with caval involvement (N0M0) of 69% and 60% respectively.

Survival in patients with vena caval involvement is significantly associated with capsular invasion, nodal involvement and distant metastases rather than mere presence of a vena caval thrombus (Cherrie et al. 1982; Staehler et al. 1987). These results are supported by the report of Sosa et al. (1984). They found that, in 64% of their patients with thrombus extending to the level of the hepatic veins or beyond, lymph node and/or perinephric fat involvement was present. In contrast, only 2 out of 10 patients (20%) with an infrahepatic vena caval thrombus had extension of tumour into the perinephric fat and none had involvement of the regional lymph nodes. The 2-year survival rates were 21% and 80% for suprahepatic and infrahepatic thrombus extension respectively.

The level of caval involvement determines the surgical approach. In order to assess the cranial extent of the tumour thrombus in the vena cava, inferior venacavography is indicated when caval involvement is suspected on any imaging modality (CT, US, IVU). In patients who demonstrate complete occlusion of the vena cava, superior venacavography or even a right atriography might be necessary.

Surgical Procedures

Venacavotomy

This is the most common technique to remove a free floating tumour thrombus from the vena cava. The vena caval incision is extended from the orifice of the renal vein cephalad and the thrombus is extracted in continuity with the tumour. When the tumour thrombus extends beyond the main hepatic veins (supradiaphragmatically), the cephalad control of the cava is usually best done after opening the pericardium. In these cases Abdelsayed et al. (1978) recommended isolating the liver from its blood supply by the Pringle manoeuvre. A thoracoabdominal or midline abdominal incision with or without a median sternotomy is usually performed for best exposure.

Atriotomy

The presence of tumour within the right atrium requires the use of atriotomy and cardiopulmonary bypass. A Chevron incision combined with median sternotomy is recommended as providing the best exposure by Libertino et al. (1987). After removal of the intraatrial part of the thrombus, the infradiaphragmatic portion is extracted by venacavatomy.

Partial Mural Venacavectomy/Segmental Venacavectomy

When renal cell carcinoma invades the wall of the vena cava a simple thrombectomy cannot be performed. If a small part of the caval wall is invaded, this portion can be resected with thrombus and kidney en bloc. Subsequently the vena cava is reconstructed.

A complete cylindrical resection of the vena cava is performed when the major part of the caval circumference has been invaded by tumour thrombus. This procedure is less complicated in right sided tumours, since the extensive collateral drainage of the left renal vein often allows its ligation during venacavectomy without significant compromise of left renal function. When caval resection is performed for tumour invasion from left sided tumours the venous drainage of the right kidney must be reconstructed, because of the absence of sufficient collaterals. The reconstruction may be achieved by interposition of a saphenous vein graft to join the right renal vein to the remaining vena cava or by a renal vein-to-portal vein interposition graft (Kearney et al. 1981; McDonald 1982).

Marshall and Reitz (1985) reported on a successful vena caval reconstruction with a patch of pericardium following a partial caval resection. They also described a possible method of total reconstruction of a caval segment with the use of pericardium forming a tubular graft.

If sufficient venous drainage of the remaining kidney cannot be achieved with one of these modalities, renal autotransplantation might be another option.

It must be underlined that none of these procedures should be performed without the ready availability of a cardiovascular surgeon and a cardiopulmonary bypass team. The operative mortality rate is reported to range from 0% to 16% (Abdelsayed et al. 1978; Schefft et al. 1978; Clayman et al. 1980; Heney and Nocks 1982; Sogani et al. 1983; Sosa et al. 1984; Pritchett et al. 1986; Libertino et al. 1987). Postoperative complications include temporary renal dysfunction, cardiac or respiratory arrhythmias, pulmonary embolism, hyperbilirubinaemia, prolonged ileus, adrenal insufficiency and deep vein thrombosis.

Conclusions

Vena caval involvement in patients with renal cell carcinoma, but without evidence of nodal or distant metastases does justify an aggressive surgical approach. Reported survival rates are similar to N0M0 patients who do not present with caval involvement. An accurate evaluation of the extent of the tumour thrombus is absolutely mandatory for planning the appropriate surgical procedure. Experience in vascular surgery is a prerequisite in managing vena caval thrombus. In selected cases cooperation with a cardiovascular surgeon is necessary.

Lymphadenectomy in Patients with Renal Cell Carcinoma

In patients with malignant tumours there may be two reasons for recommending a lymphadenectomy:

1. For the purpose of staging the extent of the malignancy
2. For the possible therapeutic benefit of removal of metastatic lesions

As documented in many studies lymph node metastases will be found in approximately 20%–30% of the patients with renal cell carcinoma when a formal lymphadenectomy is performed (Hultén et al. 1969; Robson et al. 1969; Giuliani et al. 1983). To assess the role of lymphadenectomy in patients with this disease, one has first to define the area of interest.

Anatomical and Pathological Considerations

In 1935 Parker investigated the lymphatics of the genitourinary system. Injecting a colouring fluid into the parenchyma of the kidneys she was able to study its distribution in the draining lymph vessels and nodes. The regional lymph nodes of the right kidney were found to be the interaortocaval, the paracaval, the pre- and postcaval and other occasional nodes. For the left kidney the left lateral lumbar nodes and the pre- and postaortic nodes were defined as regional nodes. However, it was also noted, that through various connecting vessels even hypogastric and external iliac nodes as well as nodes of the sacral promontory were stained.

It was not until 1969 that Hultén et al. documented an accurate anatomical description of the location of lymph node metastases from renal cell carcinoma. In a more recent report, Giuliani et al. (1983) described the pattern of lymph node metastases in 15 patients. So far, an exact mapping of positive nodes has been reported in 22 patients (Fig. 4.2). According to these observations it seems not uncommon that regional nodes may be skipped and nodal metastases develop in different areas.

Staging Lymphadenectomy

To determine the role of this procedure the impact of nodal status on prognosis and treatment has to be examined. All reports in the literature clearly demonstrate a poor prognosis for patients with positive lymph nodes. In most studies 5-year survival rates range from approximately 10%–20% in this patient group (Rafla 1970; Skinner et al. 1972; Nurmi 1984; Bassil et al. 1985).

To address the question of how radical a lymphadenectomy should be for staging purposes one has again to study the distribution of positive nodes. In 8 out

Patient*	Iliacal	Lumbal Ipsilat.	Lumbal Contral.	Post-caval	Post-aortal	Inter-aorto-caval	Mediast.	Supra-clavic.
1	+							
2	+							
3								+
4		+						
5		+						
6		+	+				+	+
7		+						
8		+						
9		+						
10		+		+				
11		+		+				
12		+		+				
13		+		+				
14		+						
15		+						
16		+						
17		+				+		
18						+		
19						+		
20						+		
21						+		
22					+			

* 1–7: Hultén *et al.* (1969)
8 –22: Giuliani *et al.* (1983)

Fig. 4.2. Localisation of lymph node metastases in 22 patients with renal cell carcinoma.

of 22 mapped patients nodal disease would not have been revealed if only a regional node dissection as proposed by deKernion (1980) had been performed. In 5 of these 8 cases an extended procedure as described by Marshall and Powell (1982) would have detected lymph node disease (Fig. 4.3). As a consequence a strong argument could be made for the extended staging lymphadenectomy, if information on "lymph node metastasis" would definitely alter treatment programmes. At present, with no effective adjuvant therapy available, the diagnosis of microscopic lymph node metastases has only prognostic value and a bilateral retroperitoneal lymphadenectomy cannot be recommended as a routine staging procedure in renal cell carcinoma.

Therapeutic Lymphadenectomy

The first report of markedly improved survival rates in patients with lymphatic disease was that of Robson et al. (1969). In their patients a radical bilateral retroperitoneal lymph node dissection ranging from the diaphragm to the aortal bifurcation had been performed. For patients with positive lymph nodes, both the 5-year and 10-year survival rates were approximately 35%. This improvement over previous results may be accounted for by several factors: All patients underwent a mediastinoscopy and biopsy prior to lymphadenectomy. Patients with mediastinal metastases were excluded. This patient selection decreased the probability of including patients with distant tumour dissemination. In addition, a remarkably high percentage of patients (61%) had grade I lesions. Furthermore, only Stage 3 patients *without* renal vein involvement were included.

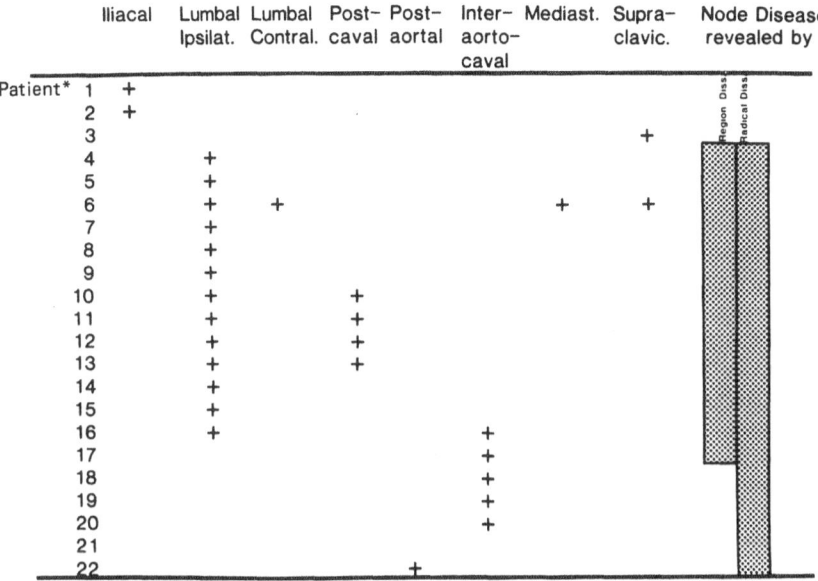

* 1-7: Hultén et al. (1969)
8-22: Giuliani et al. (1983)

Fig. 4.3. Correlation of extent of lymphadenectomy and revealing node disease in 22 patients with renal cell carcinoma.

Peters and Brown (1980) did not find a difference when they compared survival of patients with lymphadenectomy to survival of those without, in Stage 1 and Stage 2 disease. In Stage 3 patients the 5-year survival rate was approximately 45% for those with lymphadenectomy and 25% for those without. However, the authors pointed out that apart from their small numbers, bias might be introduced since the operator decided what group patients should be assigned to intraoperatively rather than preoperative randomisation. In 1983 Giuliani et al. examined a series of 104 consecutive patients with renal cell carcinoma. The 5-year survival for patients with lymph node metastases only (N+M0) was 34.6%, similar to that reported by Robson et al. The authors concluded that the improved survival rate compared to 14% 5-year survival in the report of Skinner et al. (1972) was probably due to the far more extended lymphadenectomy in their series. However, if one looks at the identical group of patients (N+M0) in the study of Skinner, one finds that 3 out of 9 (33%) survived 5 years or longer although an extended lymphadenectomy was not performed in these patients. Herrlinger et al. (1984) presented retrospective data on 381 patients without distant metastases who underwent either a "partial" or complete retroperitoneal lymph node dissection. The 5-year survival rate in patients with Stage 2 were reported to be 92% ± 10% for complete and 45% ± 25% for "partial" node dissection. It was concluded that the radical procedure should be applied in patients with non-metastatic renal cell carcinoma. However, the statistically significant observed survival difference in Stage 2 patients (without node disease by definition) only indicates that patients with unrecognised nodal disease must have been included in the group with partial dissection. It certainly does not prove that the extended procedure (removing more negative lymph nodes) is responsible for longer survival. Evaluating Stage 3 patients (including patients with node metastases) the authors were not able to find a difference in survival between both groups. A beneficial therapeutic effect of systemic lymph node dissection could not be demonstrated in this study.

In a recent study Golimbu et al. (1986a) found evidence to support radical lymphadenectomy. Of patients with Stage 1 tumours who underwent lymph node dissection, 90% survived free of disease for 5 years compared with 88% without node dissection. In Stage 2 patients survival rates were 80% against 65% and in Stage 3 patients (vein involvement only) the numbers were 60% against 57%. The authors concluded that the improved survivals were probably due to removal of micrometastases during lymphadenectomy. Unfortunately they included only patients with histologically proved *negative* nodes in the lymphadenectomy group, while 26 patients with positive nodes were excluded. From the report of Waters and Richie (1979), it seems very likely that several patients with grossly negative lymph nodes in the no-dissection group had microscopic lymph node disease. Waters and Richie found that 5 out of 16 patients (30%), who had no clinical evidence of metastases at exploration had histologically positive nodes. Consequently it is very conceivable that patients with histologically negative nodes have a better prognosis than patients with a 30% chance of positive nodes. The improved survival rates reported by Golimbu et al. (1986a) might be due to patient selection rather than dissection of negative nodes.

Opposite results were reported by Bassil et al. (1985). They found similar 5-year survival rates for T2-patients with or without lymph node dissection. Almost 50% of their T3 patients were alive 5 years following radical nephrectomy regardless of whether a node dissection had been performed or not. The authors concluded that lymphadenectomy has no therapeutic effect in patients with renal cell carcinoma. Again, this was a retrospective study and these results might be influenced by disease unrelated factors.

Conclusions

From the data available a definite statement regarding the prognostic and therapeutic value of lymphadenectomy for renal cell carcinoma cannot be made. However, data suggest that regional rather than radical lymph node dissection provides sufficient prognostic information. No therapeutic impact of lymphadenectomy has been clearly documented in any study. The reported improved survival rates of patients who underwent radical lymphadenectomy might be due to factors in patient selection rather than to the surgical procedure. As in other malignancies, lymph node metastases may reflect systemic disease that demands systemic treatment rather than a local surgical approach.

Adjuvant Therapy in Renal Carcinoma

Radiotherapy

The role of adjuvant radiotherapy has long been controversial. In 1951 Riches et al. showed in a retrospective series that postoperative irradiation increased the survival rates at the 5-year and 10-year periods. Similar results were reported by Flocks and Kadesky (1958). However, Arner et al. (1966) did not observe any improvement in the prognosis of renal carcinoma, when patients underwent postoperative radiation therapy. Postoperative irradiation even worsened the prognosis of these patients in the study presented by Peeling et al. (1969). Since none of these studies were randomised trials, the place of postoperative radiotherapy could not be evaluated on an accurate basis.

A prospective randomised trial was undertaken, and Finney reported on its results in 1973. The 5-year survival rate for patients who had been treated with nephrectomy alone was 44%, while only a 36% survival rate was noted for patients who received postoperative irradiation. It was found that radiotherapy did not influence the incidence of local recurrence or distant metastases. However, several irradiated patients died from coincidental causes including radiation liver damage. In various, more recent reports (Patel and Lavengood 1978; McNichols et al. 1981; Bassil et al. 1985) the absence of any therapeutic benefit of postoperative irradiation has been stated.

Preoperative irradiation was first reported by Waters in 1935. This form of adjuvant therapy was recommended later by others as well (Riches et al. 1951; Cox et al. 1970; Rost and Brosig 1977). It was claimed that due to preoperative radiation the tumour would become smaller and the operation might become easier. Cox et al. (1970) demonstrated arteriographically a reduction in tumour size in 8 of 14 patients who underwent preoperative irradiation. Rafla (1970), however, found that the change in the size of the tumour following irradiation was often not remarkable.

It was not until van der Werf-Messing in 1973 and Juusela et al. in 1977 that prospective randomised trials assessed the role of preoperative irradiation in patients with renal carcinoma. The results of both studies documented clearly that preoperative irradiation did not improve the 5-year survival rates of patients with renal carcinoma.

The most important aim of an adjuvant therapy is to improve the prognosis of the disease. Both preoperative and postoperative radiotherapy failed to show improved survival compared to patients treated with nephrectomy alone. For that reason neither procedure can be recommended routinely in the treatment of patients with renal carcinoma.

Chemotherapy

The urgent need for adjuvant therapy has prompted clinicians to test a broad variety of chemotherapeutic drugs in patients with advanced renal cell carcinoma. More than 30 different drugs have been administered as single agents but results were generally disappointing. In a survey of the literature, Hrushesky and Murphy (1977) found that treatment with vinblastine had resulted in the highest response rate of all tested drugs. A 25% response rate was documented in 135 patients treated with this substance. Alkylating drugs such as Cytoxan, Nitrosureas or Thiotepa demonstrated poor response rates ranging from 0%–10%. Similar results were achieved with antimetabolites (5-Fluorouracil, Mercaptopurin). Only small numbers of patients had received methotrexate, adriamycin, actinomycin-D, mitomycin-C, bleomycin or cis-platinum. No responses were reported for any of these drugs.

More recently agents such as methotrexate-citrovorum factor (MTC-CF), methyl-glyoxal bis-guanylhydrozone (M-GAG), estramustine phosphate (EMCYT) and neocarzinostatin have been evaluated (Baumgartner et al. 1980; Todd et al. 1981; Swanson and Johnson 1981; Zeffren et al. 1981; Satake et al. 1985). Response rates ranged from 0% (EMCYT) to 16% (M-GAG).

Due to the lack of effective and well-evaluated agents few studies investigating the effect of a multiple agent chemotherapy have been performed. In most of these studies vinblastine was included in the combined treatment regimen. Response rates were similar to those achieved with vinblastine as a single agent (Olver and Leavitt 1984).

To date, no single or multiple agent chemotherapy can be considered as clearly effective in patients with renal cell carcinoma. Though – mostly temporary – regression of metastatic lesions has been reported, no study is yet available documenting an improvement in prognosis for patients treated with chemotherapy. Further development of potent cytotoxic drugs hopefully will provide agents that can evade the apparent resistance of renal cell carcinoma to this form of therapy. To substantiate beneficial effects of chemotherapy these highly toxic drugs should be administered only within clearly defined protocols.

Hormone Therapy

In 1959 Kirkman described the induction of kidney tumours in Syrian hamsters by oestrogen. Since non-gonadectomised female animals and all animals receiving progesterone together with oestrogen did not develop kidney tumours, it was suspected that progesterone prevented tumour induction. Since then, various studies have been performed examining the effect of hormonal therapy in renal cell carcinoma.

In their review of the literature Hrushesky and Murphy (1977) noted that the early enthusiasm for androgenic and progestational therapies was generated by studies that seldom clearly separated subjective from objective response data. Since objective response criteria were ill-defined in most early series, Hrushesky and Murphy (1977) compared studies prior to 1972 with subsequent reports. They found an average response rate of 17% (ranging from 7%–33%) in early studies, but only 2% of the patients in 6 series between 1972 and 1977 presented an objective response following hormonal treatment (0% to 7%).

In 1978 Concolino et al. tried to correlate the efficiency of progestational therapy with the presence of renal cancer steroid receptors. Oestradiol and progesterone receptors were determined in 18 patients who received adjuvant medroxyprogesterone acetate (MPA) treatment following nephrectomy. All but 1 patient were free of lymph node and distant metastases. No significant difference in survival for patients who expressed oestrogen and/or progesterone receptors and those negative for receptors could be observed. Mukamel et al. (1984) found a low content of progesterone and oestrogen receptors in renal cell carcinoma compared to normal kidney. In only 25% of Stage 1/2 tumours were progesterone receptors observed, while in all normal autologous renal specimens this receptor was present. The survival of 19 patients treated with adjuvant hormonal therapy did not compare favourably with historic controls treated by radical nephrectomy alone. No correlation was found between survival and content of oestrogen or progesterone receptors. The authors concluded that hormonal therapy for the individual patient with renal cell carcinoma remains largely empirical.

In 1984 Nakano et al. presented a study analysing hormone receptors in cytosols from 41 renal cell carcinoma specimens. Oestrogen, progesterone and androgen receptors were detected in 11%, 11% and 13% of the specimens respectively. Though no complete or partial regression in tumour size was observed, the survival rate of patients with 1 or more receptors was significantly higher than that of patients negative for receptors. However, the authors pointed out that this observation might be due to a higher biochemical differentiation of cells positive for hormone receptors rather than the mere presence of hormone receptors.

At present, no hormonal treatment regimen has proved to prolong survival in patients with renal cell carcinoma. The tumour generally expresses lower levels of hormone receptors than normal kidney tissue. However, hormonal therapy which usually has no severe side effects might offer a degree of palliative relief to some patients with metastatic disease.

Immunotherapy

For generations an altered homeostasis in which the host's response to an oncogenic challenge is insufficient has been regarded as a possible explanation for the origin of neoplastic diseases. Since the late 1800s efforts have been made to treat cancer by stimulating the host's immune system (Coley 1891). However, it was not until recent advances in molecular biology that manipulation of biological responses has become a more realistic goal for therapy.

Various immunotherapeutic approaches to renal cell carcinoma have been employed and are listed in Table 4.4.

Table 4.4. Immunotherapeutic modalities in renal cell carcinoma

	"Specific"	"Non-specific"
Active	Antigen vaccination	Bacillus Calmette-Guerin
		Coumarin/Cimetidine
		Interferon
		Interferon-Inducer
Adoptive	Immune-RNA	Transfer-Factor
	Lymphokine-activated	
	killer cells	
Passive	Serotherapy[a]	

[a] Only anecdotal cases reported.

Bacillus Calmette-Guerin (BCG)

Active non-specific immunostimulants have been the most commonly used agents in immunotherapy, especially BCG. In animal models a marked stimulation of cell-mediated cytotoxicity following BCG administration and a subsequent rejection of implanted syngeneic tumours were observed (Old et al. 1959;

Alexander 1973). These results were the basis for numerous trials with BCG in tumour patients (Bluming et al. 1972; Powles et al. 1973; Ziegler and Magrath 1973; Morales et al. 1976). In 1976 Morales and Eidinger reported on 10 patients with disseminated renal cell carcinoma treated with BCG. Objective responses were recorded in 4 patients. Others observed response rates ranging from 0% to 32%. In a more recent study Morales et al. (1982) found 4 partial responses in 20 patients. There was no statistically significant difference in survival for patients treated with BCG and a concurrent control group.

Active "Specific" Immunisation

As a consequence of the findings by Tallberg (1974) that insoluble antigenic polymer particles caused an immune response in experimental animals, Tykkä et al. (1978) performed a controlled, non-randomised clinical trial in patients with advanced renal cell carcinoma. They reported a 26% 5-year survival rate in patients who had been injected with autologous tumour material and an adjuvant (tuberculin and/or Candida antigen). In contrast, only a 3% 5-year survival rate was observed in their contemporary control group. In 11 of 21 (52%) patients with lung metastases who underwent immunotherapy, an objective regression was reported. Neidhart et al. (1980) found 4 out of 30 (13%) patients responding to active immunisation. Similar results were noted by McCune et al. (1981). In 1986 Fowler observed only 2 minimal responses in 23 actively immunised patients with metastatic renal cell carcinoma.

Transfer Factor (TF)

The phenomenon of transfer of cell-mediated responses from immune donors to non-immune recipients with lymphoid cells was first recognised in guinea pigs by Landsteiner and Chase in 1942. Lawrence (1969) used the term "transfer factor" to designate the specific factor/factors in leukocytes responsible for the transfer of delayed hypersensitivity. Transfer factor has been used in the treatment of several immune-deficiency diseases and certain chronic infectious diseases (Kirkpatrick and Gallin 1974). Montie et al. (1977b) treated 10 patients with metastatic renal cell carcinoma with TF. TF was obtained from donor leukocytes that had shown inhibitory effects on renal carcinoma cell lines in vitro. No objective clinical regression was noted in any patient. In 1979 Bukowsky et al. reported 1 complete response in 9 treated patients.

Xenogeneic Immune Ribonucleic Acid (I-RNA)

The transfer of antitumour activity by ribonucleic acid extracted from the lymphoid tissues of immunised syngeneic or xenogeneic animals has been demonstrated in a variety of animal systems (Fishman and Adler 1967; Deckers and Pilch 1970). In 1976 Skinner et al. described the first results of I-RNA treatment in patients with renal cell carcinoma. I-RNA was obtained from sheep immunised with human renal cell carcinoma. None of the patients with measurable metastatic disease showed a complete (CR) or partial response (PR) according to the WHO Response Criteria (WHO Handbook for Reporting Results of Cancer Treatment 1979). In subsequent reports (deKernion and Ramming 1980) a total of 25 patients were analysed and a CR or PR could not be observed in any patient. Richie et al. (1981) observed 1 CR and 2 PR in their first 6 patients treated with I-RNA (50% response rate). However, in a subsequent report (Richie et al. 1984) on 21 more patients (Stage 3 and 4) only 3 partial responses in 16 (18.7%) patients with measurable metastases could be documented. The side effects of the above mentioned procedures usually were minor and included fatigue, low-grade fever, occasional nausea and skin-induration at the side of injection.

Interferon (IFN)

Interferons are glycoproteins produced by leukocytes (IFN-alpha), fibroblasts (IFN-beta) and lymphocytes and monocytes (IFN-gamma). They have been demonstrated to have antiviral and antineoplastic activity which seems to be mediated by direct tumour cytotoxicity and/or indirect cytotoxicity through alteration of immune responses (Oldham and Smalley 1983). IFN-alpha was the first interferon that successfully could be produced by recombinant genetic techniques. For that reason IFN-alpha has been used in most clinical trials to date. Response rates range from 7% to 31% (Trump et al. 1984; Quesada et al. 1985; Muss et al. 1987; Sarna et al. 1987). Sarna et al. (1987) reviewing 84 patients with renal cell carcinoma treated with IFN-alpha at UCLA found that response to therapy was linked to prolonged survival, but it was not clear whether response to therapy merely selected out patients with better initial prognosis or actually led to improved survival.

Rinehart et al. (1986) reported on the results of a phase I/II trial of human recombinant IFN-beta in patients with renal cell carcinoma. Of the 15 patients evaluable, 2 (13%) demonstrated partial responses. In a recent study 1 (2.4%) complete and 3 (7.3%) partial responses were observed in 41 evaluable patients treated with interferon gamma. Median duration of response was 6 and 9 months respectively (Garnick et al. 1988).

Recently, Droller (1987) used polyinosinic-polycytidylic acid, a potent inducer of IFN production, to treat 11 patients with disseminated renal cell carcinoma. Complete or partial response was not observed in any patient, though 2 patients demonstrated regression of isolated metastases, but in both metastases at other sites progressed. Side effects of IFN therapy include malaise, weakness, fever, chills, leukopenia and peripheral nervous system toxicity. All patients with brain metastases treated with the IFN inducer experienced lethargy and coma during treatment.

Lymphokine Activated Killer (LAK)-Cells plus Interleukin-2

A very recent immunotherapeutic approach to neoplastic diseases has been developed by Rosenberg et al. (1985). They observed that human peripheral blood lymphocytes incubated with interleukin (IL-2) were able to lyse fresh, natural-killer-cell-resistant tumour cells, but not normal cells. These activated lymphoid cells were termed LAK cells. The adoptive transfer of these LAK cells plus recombinant Il-2 has been shown to mediate the regression of metastases in animal models (Mazumder and Rosenberg 1984). Subsequently the efficiency of this approach was tested for immunotherapy of human cancers. Twenty five patients with various solid cancers were treated with autologous LAK cells and recombinant IL-2. In all of the 3 patients with renal cell carcinoma partial regression of pulmonary metastases was observed (Rosenberg et al. 1985). In a more recent report on 36 patients with renal cell carcinoma treated with LAK cells and IL-2, 4 complete responses and 8 partial responses (response rate 33%) were documented (Rosenberg et al. 1987).

Severe fluid retention, dyspnoea, fever, malaise, and nausea were the most common side effects of the therapy (Rosenberg et al. 1987). A reduction of some of the toxicity was achieved by the administration of dexamethasone. However, none of the dexamethasone-treated patients demonstrated an objective response. It was suspected that this substance may play an inhibitory role in the mechanism of this form of immunotherapy (Vetto et al. 1987). Though the first results are encouraging larger subsequent trials with extended follow-up are required to determine the role of this modality in the therapy of neoplastic diseases.

Coumarin/Cimetidine

Coumarin either as a single agent or in combination with cimetidine has demonstrated antitumour activity against human melanoma (Thornes et al. 1982; Borgström et al. 1982). At present, the exact mechanism of antineoplastic action of both substances is not completely understood. Coumarin may act as a macrophage stimulant (Piller 1976) and cimetidine seems to inhibit a variety of functions mediated by T-suppressor cells in vitro (Damle and Gupta 1981). Marshall et al. (1987) recently reported on 45 patients with metastatic renal cell carcinoma who were treated with coumarin (1,2-benzopyrone) and cimetidine. A response rate of 33% (3 complete and 11 partial responses) was observed in 42 evaluable patients. No severe toxicity was noted. To define the therapeutic value of this regimen the authors have instituted a randomised, blinded, placebo-controlled study in patients with Stage 2/3 disease.

Conclusions

Despite a number of encouraging early reports no form of immunotherapy ever initiated for renal cell carcinoma has stood the test of time. Due to the relatively limited knowledge of the basic mechanisms of the immune system, immunotherapy trials have been empirical in approach. Though tumour-specific cytotoxicity has been claimed for several modalities the presumptive target antigens are yet to be defined precisely in human cancer. Hybridoma monoclonal antibody technology will certainly improve our understanding of cell differentiation and of cancer biology by better identifying differences between the neoplastic cell and its normal counterpart.

Bander (1987) reported in detail on the contribution of monoclonal antibodies to recent advances in immunology. Several antigenic systems in renal cell carcinoma could successfully be defined by monoclonal antibodies; however, most of the antigens were also present in normal tissue. Old (1981) presumed that, in order to use the body's potential for selective elimination of cancer cells it will be necessary to direct the "full force of specific immunity against tumour cells". To achieve this goal, tumour specific antigens, if present, have still to be defined.

So far, no form of adjuvant therapy has improved survival rates in patients with renal cell carcinoma compared to surgery alone. Surgical procedures are still pre-eminent in the treatment of this malignancy and most effective in low stage disease. Early detection of the tumour and development of effective adjuvant therapy are mandatory goals in the management of renal cell carcinoma.

References

Abdelsayed MA, Bissada NK, Finkbeiner AE, Redman JF (1978) Renal tumors involving the inferior vena cava: plan for management. J Urol 120: 153–155

Alexander P (1973) Activated macrophages and the antitumor action of BCG. Natl Cancer Inst Monogr 39: 127–133

Arner O, Edsmyr F, von Schreeb T, Sundbom L (1966) Renal adenocarcinoma. Postoperative radiation therapy. Acta Chir Scand 132: 377–383

Bakke A, Goethlin J, Hoisaeter PA (1985) Renal malignancies: Outcome of patients in Stage 4 with or without embolization procedure. Urology 26: 541–543

Balfe DM, McClennan BL, Stanley RJ, Weyman PJ, Sagel SS (1982) Evaluation of renal masses considered indeterminate on computed tomography. Radiology 142: 421–428

Baltarowich OH, Kurtz AB (1987) Songraphic evaluation of renal masses. Urol Radiol 9: 79–87

Bander NH (1985) Study of the normal human kidney and kidney cancer with monoclonal antibodies. Uremia Invest 8: 263–273

Bander NH (1987) Monoclonal antibodies: State of the art. J Urol 137: 603–612

Barney JD, Churchill EJ (1939) Adenocarcinoma of the kidney with metastasis to the lung. J Urol 42: 269–276

Bassil B, Dosoretz DE, Prout GR jr (1985) Validation of the tumor, nodes and metastasis classification of renal cell carcinoma. J Urol 134: 450–454

Baumgartner G, Heinz R, Arbes H, Lenzhofer R, Pridun N, Schüller J (1980) Methotrexate-citrovorum factor used alone and in combination chemotherapy for advanced hypernephromas. Cancer Treat Rep 64: 41–46

Beare JB, McDonald JR (1949) Involvement of the renal capsule in surgically removed hypernephroma: A gross and histopathologic study. J Urol 61: 857–861

Bellinger MF, Koontz WW, Smith MJV (1979) Renal cell carcinoma: twenty years of experience. Va Med 106: 819–824

Blacher E, Johnson DE, Haynie TP (1985) Value of routine radionuclide bone scans in renal cell carcinoma. Urology 26: 432–434

Bluming AZ, Vogel CL, Ziegler JL, Mody N, Kamya G (1972) Immunological effects of BCG in malignant melanoma: two modes of administration compared. Ann Intern Med 76: 405–411

Bohnenkamp B, Rhomberg W, Sonnentag W, Feldmann U (1980) Metastasierungstyp und Prognose beim hypernephröiden Carcinom der Niere. Cancer Res Clin Oncol 96: 105–114

Bolton WK, Vaughan ED jr (1977) A comparative study of open surgical and percutaneous renal biopsies. J Urol 117: 696–698

Borgström S, Eyben von FE, Flodgren P, Axelsson B, Sjögren HO (1982) Human leukocyte interferon and cimetidine for metastastic melanoma. N Engl J Med 307: 1080–1081

Bosniak M (1986) The current radiological approach to renal cysts. Radiology 158: 1–10

Böttiger LE (1970) Prognosis in renal carcinoma. Cancer 26: 780–787

Boxer RJ, Waisman J, Lieber MM, Mampaso FM, Skinner DG (1979) Renal carcinoma: Computer analysis of 96 patients treated by nephrectomy. J Urol 122: 598–601

Brannen GE, Correa RJ, Gibbons RP (1983) Renal cell carcinoma in solitary kidneys. J Urol 129: 130–131

Bukowski RM, Groppe C, Reimer R, Weick J, Hewlett JS (1979) Immunotherapy (IT) of metastatic renal cell carcinoma. Proc Am Soc Clin Oncol 20: 402

Bumpus HC jr (1928) The apparent disappearance of pulmonary metastasis in a case of hypernephroma following nephrectomy. J Urol 20: 185–191

Cherrie RJ, Goldman DG, Lindner A, DeKernion JB (1982) Prognostic implications of vena caval extension of renal cell carcinoma. J Urol 128: 910–912

Christensen K, Dyreborg U, Andersen JF, Nissen HM (1985) The value of transvascular embolization in the treatment of renal carcinoma. J Urol 133: 191–193

Chute R, Soutter L, Kerr WS (1949) The value of the thoracoabdominal incision in the removal of kidney tumors. New Engl J Med 241: 951–960

Clayman RV, Gonzalez R, Fraley EE (1980) Renal cell cancer invading the inferior vena cava: Clinical review and anatomical approach. J Urol 123: 157–163

Cole AT, Mandell J, Fried FA, Stabb EV (1975) The place of bone scan in the diagnosis of renal cell carcinoma. J Urol 114: 364–365

Coley WB (1891) Contribution to the knowledge of sarcoma. Ann Surg 14: 199–220

Concolino G, Marocchi A, Conti C, Tenaglia R, Di Silverio F, Bracci U (1978) Human renal cell carcinoma as a hormone-dependent tumor. Cancer Res 38: 4340–4344

Cox CE, Lacy SS, Montgomery WG, Boyce WH (1970) Renal adenocarcinoma: 28-year review with emphasis on rationale and feasibility of preoperative radiotherapy. J Urol 104: 53–61

Crawford ED (1982) Radical nephrectomy: Thoracoabdominal intrapleural approach. In: Crawford ED, Borden TA (eds) Genitourinary cancer surgery. Lea and Febiger, Philadelphia, pp 41–46

Cronan JJ, Zeman RK, Rosenfield AT (1982) Comparison of computerized tomography, ultrasound and angiography in staging renal cell carcinoma. J Urol 127: 712–714

Damle NK, Gupta S (1981) Autologous mixed lymphocyte reaction in man. II. Histamine-induced suppression of the autologous mixed lymphocyte reaction by T-cell subsets defined with monoclonal antibodies. J Clin Immunol 1: 241–249

Das S (1982) Radical nephrectomy: Thoracoabdominal extrapleural approach. In: Crawford ED, Borden TA (eds) Genitourinary cancer surgery. Lea and Febiger, Philadelphia, pp 30–40

Deckers PJ, Pilch YH (1970) Transfer of tumor immunity with ribonucleic acid. Surg Forum 21: 124–126

deKernion JB (1980) Lymphadenectomy for renal cell carcinoma. Urol Clin North Am 7: 697–703

deKernion JB, Ramming KP (1980) The therapy of renal adenocarcinoma with immune RNA. Invest Urol 17: 378–381

deKernion JB, Ramming KP, Smith RB (1978) The natural history of metastatic renal cell carcinoma: A computer analysis. J Urol 120: 148–152

Droller MJ (1987) Immunotherapy of metastatic renal cell carcinoma with polyinosinic-polycytidylic acid. J Urol 137: 202–206

Everson TC, Cole WH (1966) Spontaneous regression of cancer. WB Saunders, Philadelphia, p. 4

Finkbeiner A, Moyad R, Herwig K (1976) Bilateral simultaneously-occurring adenocarcinoma of the kidney. J Urol 116: 26–28

Finney R (1973) The value of radiotherapy in the treatment of hypernephroma – A clinical trial. Br J Urol 45: 258–269

Fishman M, Adler FL (1967) The role of macrophage-RNA in the immune response. Cold Spring Harbor Symp Quant Biol 32: 343–347

Flocks RH, Kadesky MC (1958) Malignant neoplasms of the kidney: An analysis of 353 patients followed five years or more. J Urol 79: 196–201

Fowler JE jr (1986) Failure of immunotherapy for metastatic renal cell carcinoma. J Urol 135: 22–25

Fuhrman SA, Lasky LC, Limas C (1982) Prognostic significance of morphologic parameters in renal cell carcinoma. Am J Surg Pathol 6: 655–663

Garnick MB, Reich SD, Maxwell B, Coval-Goldsmith S, Richie JP, Rudnick SA (1988) Phase I/II study of recombinant interferon gamma in advanced renal cell carcinoma. J Urol 139: 251–255

Gibbons RP, Bush WH jr, Burnett LL (1977) Needle tract seeding following aspiration of renal cell carcinoma. J Urol 118: 865–867

Giuliani L, Martorana G, Giberti C, Pescatore D, Magnani G (1983) Results of radical nephrectomy with extensive lymphadenectomy for renal cell carcinoma. J Urol 130: 664–668

Golimbu M, Joshi P, Sperber A, Tessler A, Al-Askari S, Morales P (1986a) Renal cell carcinoma: Survival and prognostic factors. Urology 27: 291–301

Golimbu M, Al-Askari S, Tessler A, Morales P (1986b) Aggressive treatment of metastatic renal cancer. J Urol 136: 805–807

Helm CW, Burwood RJ, Harrison NW, Melcher DH (1983) Aspiration cytology of solid renal tumours. Br J Urol 55: 249–253

Heney NM, Nocks BN (1982) The influence of perinephric fat involvement on survival in patients with renal cell carcinoma extending into the inferior vena cava. J Urol 128: 18–20

Hermanek P (1986) Neue TNM/pTNM-Klassifikation und Stadieneinteilung urologischer Tumoren ab 1987. UrologeB 26: 193–197

Herrlinger A, Sigel A, Giedl J (1984) Methodik der radikalen transabdominalen Tumornephrektomie mit fakultativer oder systematischer Lymphdissektion und deren Ergebnisse an 381 Patienten. UrologeA 23: 267–274

Holland JM (1973) Cancer of the kidney – natural history and staging. Cancer 32: 1030–1042

Hricak H, Demas BE, Williams RD, McNamara MT, Hedgcock MW, Amparo EG, Tanagho EA (1985) Magnetic resonance imaging in the diagnosis and staging of renal and perirenal neoplasms. Radiology 154: 709–715

Hrushesky WJ, Murphy GP (1977) Current status of the therapy of advanced renal carcinoma. J Surg Oncol 9: 277–288

Hultén L, Rosencrantz M, Seeman T, Wahlqvist L, Åhrén C (1969) Occurrence and localization of lymph node metastases in renal carcinoma. Scand J Urol Nephrol 3: 129–133

Johnson DE, Kaesler KE, Samuels ML (1975) Is nephrectomy justified in patients with metastatic renal carcinoma? J Urol 114: 27–29

Juul N, Torp-Pedersen S, Gronvall S, Holm HH, Koch F, Larsen S (1985) Ultrasonically guided fine needle aspiration biopsy of renal masses. J Urol 133: 579–581

Juusela H, Malmio K, Alfthan O, Oravisto KJ (1977) Preoperative irradiation in the treatment of renal adenocarcinoma. Scand J Urol Nephrol 11: 277–281

Kaisary AV, Williams G, Riddle PR (1984) The role of preoperative embolization in renal cell carcinoma. J Urol 131: 641–646

Katz SE, Schapira HE (1982) Spontaneous regression of genitourinary cancer – An update. J Urol 128: 1–4

Kearney GP, Waters WB, Klein LA, Richie JP, Gittes RF (1981) Results of inferior vena cava resection for renal cell carcinoma. J Urol 125: 769–773

Kim EE, Bledin AG, Gutierrez C, Haynie TP (1983) Comparison of radionuclide images and radiographs for skeletal metastases from renal cell carcinoma. Oncology 40: 284–286

Kirkman H (1959) Estrogen-induced tumors of the kidney. IV. Incidence in female Syrian hamsters. Natl Cancer Inst Mongr 1: 59–91

Kirkpatrick CH, Gallin JI (1974) Treatment of infectious and neoplastic diseases with transfer factor. Oncology 29: 46–73

Kiser GC, Totonchy M, Barry JM (1986) Needle tract seeding after percutaneous renal adenocarcinoma aspiration. J Urol 136: 1292–1293

Konnak JW, Grossman HB (1985) Renal cell carcinoma as an incidental finding. J Urol 134: 1094–1096

Kradjian RM, Bennington JL (1965) Renal carcinoma recurrent 31 years after nephrectomy. Arch Surg 90: 192–195

Landsteiner K, Chase MW (1942) Experiments on transfer of cutaneous sensitivity to simple compounds. Proc Soc Exp Biol Med 49: 688–690

Lang EK (1980) Roentgenologic approach to the diagnosis and management of cystic lesions of the kidney: Is cyst exploration mandatory? Urol Clin North Am 7: 677–688

Lawrence HS (1969) Transfer factor. Advances Immunol 11: 195–266

Leung AWL, Bydder GM, Steiner RE, Bryant DJ, Young IR (1984) Magnetic resonance imaging of the kidneys. AJR 143: 1215–1227

Levine E, Lee KR, Weigel J (1979) Preoperative determination of abdominal extent of renal cell carcinoma by computed tomography. Radiology 132: 395–398

Levine E, Maklad NF, Rosenthal SJ, Lee KR, Weigel J (1980) Comparison of computed tomography and ultrasound in abdominal staging of renal cancer. Urology 16: 317–322

Libertino JA, Zinman L, Watkins E jr (1987) Long-term results of resection of renal cell cancer with extension into inferior vena cava. J Urol 137: 21–24

Ljungberg B, Stenling R, Roos G (1986) Prognostic value of deoxyribonucleic acid content in metastastic renal cell carcinoma. J Urol 136: 801–804

Lokich JJ, Harrison JH (1975) Renal cell carcinoma: Natural history and chemotherapeutic experience. J Urol 114: 371–374

Malek RS, Utz DC, Culp OS (1976) Hypernephroma in the solitary kidney: Experience with 20 cases and review of the literature. J Urol 116: 553–556

Marberger M, Pugh RCB, Auvert J, Bertermann H, Costantini A, Gammelgaard PA, Petterson S, Wickham JEA (1981) Conservative surgery of renal carcinoma: The EIRSS experience. Br J Urol 53: 528–532

Marcove RC, Sadrieh J, Huvos AG, Grabstald H (1972) Cryosurgery in the treatment of solitary or multiple bone metastases from renal cell carcinoma. J Urol 108: 540–547

Marshall FF (1983) Editorial comment. J Urol 129: 707

Marshall FF, Powell KC (1982) Lymphadenectomy for renal cell carcinoma: Anatomical and therapeutic considerations. J Urol 128: 677–681

Marshall FF, Reitz BA (1985) Supradiaphragmatic renal cell carcinoma tumor thrombus: Indications for vena caval reconstruction with pericardium. J Urol 133: 266–268

Marshall FF, Walsh PC (1984) In situ management of renal tumors: Renal cell carcinoma and transitional cell carcinoma. J Urol 131: 1045–1049

Marshall ME, Mendelsohn L, Butler K, Riley L, Cantrell J, Wiseman C, Taylor R, MacDonald JS (1987) Treatment of metastatic renal cell carcinoma with Coumarin (1,2-Benzopyrone) and cimetidine: A pilot study. J Clin Oncol 5: 862–866

Mauro MA, Wadsworth DE, Stanley RJ, McClennan BL (1982) Renal cell carcinoma: Angiography in the CT era. AJR 139: 1135–1138

Mazumder A, Rosenberg SA (1984) Successful immunotherapy of natural killer-resistant established pulmonary melanoma metastases by the intravenous adoptive transfer of syngeneic lymphocytes activated in vitro by interleukin 2. J Exp Med 159: 495–507

McCullough DL, Gittes RF (1974) Vena cava resection for renal cell carcinoma. J Urol 112: 162–167

McCune CS, Schapira DV, Henshaw EC (1981) Specific immunotherapy of advanced renal carcinoma: evidence for the polyclonality of metastases. Cancer 47: 1984–1987

McDonald MW (1982) Current therapy for renal cell carcinoma. J Urol 127: 211–217

McNichols DW, Segura JW, DeWeerd JH (1981) Renal cell carcinoma: Long-term survival and late recurrence. J Urol 126: 17–23

Mebust WK, Weigel JW, Lee KR, Cox GG, Jewell WR, Krishnan EC (1984) Renal cell carcinoma – angioinfarction. J Urol 131: 231–235

Middleton RG (1967) Surgery for metastatic renal cell carcinoma. J Urol 97: 973–977

Mims MM, Christenson B, Schlumberger FC, Goodwin WE (1966) A 10-year evaluation of nephrectomy for extensive renal cell carcinoma. J Urol 95: 10–15

Mittelstaedt, CA (1987) Abdominal ultrasound. Churchill Livingstone, New York, p 356

Montie JE, Stewart BH, Straffon RA, Banowsky LHW, Hewitt CB, Montague DK (1977a) The role of adjunctive nephrectomy in patients with metastatic renal cell carcinoma. J Urol 117: 272–275

Montie JE, Bukowksi RM, Deodhar SD, Hewlett JS, Stewart BH, Straffon RA (1977b) Immunotherapy of disseminated renal cell carcinoma with transfer factor. J Urol 117: 553–556

Morales A, Eidinger D (1976) Bacillus Calmette-Guerin in the treatment of adenocarcinoma of the kidney. J Urol 115: 377–380

Morales A, Eidinger D, Bruce AW (1976) Intracavitary Bacillus Calmette-Guerin in the treatment of superficial bladder tumors. J Urol 116: 180–183

Morales A, Wilson JL, Pater JL, Loeb M (1982) Cytoreductive surgery and systemic Bacillus Calmette-Guerin therapy in metastatic renal cancer: A phase II trial. J Urol 127:230–235

Mukamel E, Bruhis S, Nissenkorn I, Servadio C (1984) Steroid receptors in renal cell carcinoma: Relevance to hormonal therapy. J Urol 131: 227–230

Murphy JB, Marshall FF (1980) Renal cyst versus tumor: A continuing dilemma. J Urol 123: 566–570

Muss HB, Costanzi JJ, Leavitt R, Williams RD, Kempf RA, Pollard R, Ozer H, Zekan PJ, Grunberg SM, Mitchel MS, Caponera M, Gavigan M, Ernest ML, Venturi C, Greiner J, Spiegel RJ (1987) Recombinant alfa-interferon in renal cell carcinoma: A randomized trial of two routes of administration. J Clin Oncol 5: 286–291

Myers GH jr, Fehrenbaker LG, Kelalis PP (1968) Prognostic significance of renal vein invasion by hypernephroma. J Urol 100: 420–423

Nakano E, Tada Y, Fujioka H, Matsua M, Osafune M, Kotake T, Sato B, Takaha M, Sonoda T (1984) Hormone receptor in renal cell carcinoma and correlation with clinical response to endocrine therapy. J Urol 132: 240–245

Neidhart JA, Murphy SG, Hennick LA, Wise HA (1980) Active specific immunotherapy of stage IV renal carcinoma with aggregated tumor antigen adjuvant. Cancer 46: 1128–1134

Nosher JL, Amorosa JK, Leiman S, Plafker J (1982) Fine needle aspiration of the kidney and adrenal gland. J Urol 128: 895–899

Novick AC, Zincke H, Neves RJ, Topley HM (1986) Surgical enucleation for renal cell carcinoma. J Urol 135: 235–238

Nurmi MJ (1984) Prognostic factors in renal carcinoma. An evaluation of operative findings. Br J Urol 56: 270–275

O'Dea MJ, Zincke H, Utz DC, Bernatz PE (1978) The treatment of renal cell carcinoma with solitary metastasis. J Urol 120: 540–542

Old LJ, Clarke DA, Benacerraf B (1959) Effect of Bacillus Calmette-Guerin infection on transplanted tumours in the mouse. Nature 184: 291–292

Old LJ (1981) Cancer immunology: The search for specificity – G. H. A. Clowes memorial lecture. Cancer Res 41: 362–375

Oldham RK, Smalley RV (1983) Immunotherapy: The old and the new. J Biol Resp Modif 2: 1–37

Oliver JA, Laplante MP, Reid EC, Schual RS (1979) Results of radical nephrectomy in 178 cases of renal cell adenocarcinoma. Can J Surg 22: 409–412

Olver IN, Leavitt RD (1984) Chemotherapy and immunotherapy of disseminated renal cancer. In: Javadpour N (ed) Cancer of the kidney. Thieme-Stratton, New York, pp 109–120

Otto U, Baisch H, Huland H, Klöppel G (1984) Tumor cell deoxyribonucleic acid content and prognosis in human renal cell carcinoma. J Urol 132: 237–239

Paganini-Hill A, Ross RK, Henderson BE (1983) Epidemiology of kidney cancer. In: Skinner DG (ed) Urological cancer. Grune and Stratton, New York, pp 383–407

Parienty RA, Pradel J, Parienty I (1985) Cystic renal cancers: CT characteristics. Radiology 157: 741–744

Parienty RA, Richard F, Pradel J, Vallancien G (1984) Local recurrence after nephrectomy for primary renal cancer: Computerized tomography recognition. J Urol 132: 246–249

Parker AE (1935) Studies on the main posterior lymph channels of the abdomen and their connections with the lymphatics of the genito-urinary system. Am J Anat 56: 409–443

Patel NP, Lavengood RW (1978) Renal cell carcinoma: Natural history and results of treatment. J Urol 119: 722–726

Peeling WB, Mantell BS, Shepheard BGF (1969) Post-operative irradiation in the treatment of renal cell carcinoma. Br J Urol 41: 23–31

Peters PC, Brown GL (1980) The role of lymphadenectomy in the management of renal cell carcinoma. Urol Clin North Am 7: 705–708

Petkovic SD (1959) An anatomical classification of renal tumors in the adult as a basis for prognosis. J Urol 81: 618–623

Piller NB (1976) The ineffectiveness of Coumarin treatment on thermal oedema of macrophage-free rats. Br J Exp Path 57: 170–178

Pollack HM, Banner MP, Arger PH, Peters J, Mulhern CB, Coleman BG (1982) The accuracy of gray-scale renal ultrasonography in differentiating cystic neoplasms from benign cysts. Radiology 143: 741–745

Powles RL, Crowther D, Bateman CJT, Beard MEJ, McElwain TJ, Russel J, Lister TA, Whitehouse JMA, Wrigley PFM, Pike M, Alexander P, Fairley GH (1973) Immunotherapy for acute myelogenous leukaemia. Br J Cancer 28: 365–376

Pritchett TR, Lieskovsky G, Skinner DG (1986) Extension of renal cell carcinoma into the vena cava: Clinical review and surgical approach. J Urol 135: 460–464

Quesada JR, Rios A, Swanson D, Trown P, Gutterman JU (1985) Antitumor activity of recombinant-derived interferon alpha in metastatic renal cell carcinoma. J Clin Oncol 3: 1522–1528

Rafla S (1970) Renal cell carcinoma. Natural history and results of treatment. Cancer 25: 26–40

Rainwater LM, Hosaka Y, Farrow GM, Lieber MM (1987) Well differentiated clear cell renal carcinoma: Significance of nuclear deoxyribonucleic acid patterns studied by flow cytometry. J Urol 137: 15–20

Riches EW, Griffiths IH, Thackray AC (1951) New growths of the kidney and ureter. Br J Urol 23: 297–356

Richie JP, Wang BS, Steele GD, Wilson RE, Mannick JA (1981) In vivo and in vitro effects of xenogeneic immune ribonucleic acid in patients with advanced renal cell carcinoma. A phase I study. J Urol 126: 24–28

Richie JP, Garnick MB, Seltzer S, Bettmann MA (1983) Computerized tomography scan for diagnosis and staging of renal cell carcinoma. J Urol 129: 1114–1116

Richie JP, Steele GD Jr, Wilson RE, Ervin T, Wang BS, Mannick JA (1984) Current treatment of metastatic renal cell carcinoma with xenogeneic immune ribonucleic acid. J Urol 131: 236–238

Rinehart J, Malspeis L, Young D, Neidhardt J (1986) Phase I/II trial of human recombinant β-interferon serine in patients with renal cell carcinoma. Cancer Res 46: 5364–5367

Robson CJ, Churchill BM, Anderson W (1969) The results of radical nephrectomy for renal cell carcinoma. J Urol 101: 297–301

Rosen PR, Murphy KG (1984) Bone scintigraphy in the initial staging of patients with renal cell carcinoma: Concise communication. J Nucl Med 25: 289–291

Rosenberg SA, Lotze MT, Muul LM, Leitman S, Chang AE, Ettinghausen SE, Matory YL, Skibber JM, Shiloni E, Vetto JT, Seipp CA, Simpson C, Reichert CM (1985) Observations on the systemic administration of autologous lymphokine-activated killer cells and recombinant interleukin-2 to patients with metastatic cancer. N Engl J Med 313: 1485–1492

Rosenberg SA, Lotze MT, Muul LM, Chang AE, Avis FB, Leitman S, Linehan WM, Robertson CN,

Lee RE, Rubin JT, Seipp CA, Simpson CG, White DE (1987) A progress report on the treatment of 157 patients with advanced cancer using lymphokine-activated killer cells and interleukin-2 or high-dose interleukin-2 alone. N Engl J Med 316: 889–897

Rosenthal CL, Kraft R, Zingg EJ (1984) Organ-preserving surgery in renal cell carcinoma: Tumor enucleation versus partial kidney resection. Eur Urol 10: 222–228

Rost A, Brosig W (1977) Preoperative irradiation of renal cell carcinoma. Urology 10: 414–417

Rubin P (1968) Cancer of the urogenital tract: Kidney. JAMA 204: 127–128 [Apr 15]

Sagel SS, Stanley RJ, Levitt RG, Geisse G (1977) Computed tomography of the kidney. Radiology 124: 359–370

Sarna G, Figlin R, DeKernion J (1987) Interferon in renal cell carcinoma. The UCLA experience. Cancer 59: 610–612

Satake I, Tari K, Yamamoto M, Nishimura H (1985) Neocarzinostatin-induced complete regression of metastatic renal cell carcinoma. J Urol 133: 87–89

Schefft P, Novick AC, Straffon RA, Stewart BH (1978) Surgery for renal cell carcinoma extending into the inferior vena cava. J Urol 120: 28–31

Skinner DG, Colvin RB, Vermillion CD, Pfister RC, Leadbetter WF (1971) Diagnosis and management of renal cell carcinoma. Cancer 28: 1165–1177

Skinner DG, Vermillion CD, Colvin RB (1972) The surgical management of renal cell carcinoma. J Urol 107: 705–710

Skinner DG, deKernion JB, Brower PA, Ramming KP, Pilch YH (1976) Advanced renal cell carcinoma: treatment with xenogeneic immune ribonucleic acid and appropriate surgical resection. J Urol 115: 246–250

Snow RM, Schellhammer PF (1982) Spontaneous regression of metastatic renal cell carcinoma. Urology 20: 177–181

Sogani PC, Herr HW, Bains MS, Whitmore WF jr (1983) Renal cell carcinoma extending into inferior vena cava. J Urol 130: 660–663

Sosa RE, Muecke EC, Vaughan ED jr, McCarron JP jr (1984) Renal cell carcinoma extending into the inferior vena cava: The prognostic significance of the level of vena caval involvement. J Urol 132: 1097–1100

Staehler G, Liedl B, Kreuzer E, Sturm W, Schmiedt E (1987) Nierenkarzinom mit Cavazapfen: Einteilung, Operationsstrategie und Behandlungsergebnisse. UrologeA: 26: 46–50

Stanisic TH, Babcock JR, Grayhack JT (1977) Morbidity and mortality of renal exploration for cyst. Surg Gynecol Obstet 145: 733–736

Sullivan LD, Westmore DD, McLoughlin MG (1979) Surgical management of renal cell carcinoma at the Vancouver General Hospital: 20-year review. Can J Surg 22: 427–431

Swanson DA, Borges PM (1983) Complications of transabdominal radical nephrectomy for renal cell carcinoma. J Urol 129: 704–707

Swanson DA, Johnson DE (1981) Estramustine phosphate (EMCYT) as treatment for metastatic renal carcinoma. Urology 17: 344–346

Swanson DA, Orovan WL, Johnson DE, Giacco G (1981) Osseous metastases secondary to renal cell carcinoma. Urology 18: 556–561

Swanson DA, Johnson DE, von Eschenbach AC, Chuang VP, Wallace S (1983) Angioinfarction plus nephrectomy for metastatic renal cell carcinoma – An update. J Urol 130: 449–452

Tallberg T (1974) Cancer immunotherapy by means of polymerized autologous tumor tissue with special reference to some patients with pulmonary tumor. Scand J Resp Dis [Suppl] 89: 107–122

Thornes RD, Lynch G, Sheehan MV (1982) Cimetidine and Coumarin therapy of melanoma. Lancet II: 322

Todd RF III, Garnick MB, Canellos GP, Richie JP, Gittes RF, Mayer RJ, Skarin AT (1981) Phase I-II trial of methyl-GAG in the treatment of patients with metastatic renal adenocarcinoma. Cancer Treat Rep 65: 17–20

Tolia BM, Whitmore WF jr (1975) Solitary metastasis from renal cell carcinoma. J Urol 114: 836–838

Topley M, Novick AC, Montie JE (1984) Long-term results following partial nephrectomy for localized renal adenocarcinoma. J Urol 131: 1050–1052

Trump D, Harris J, Tuttle R, Oken M, Bennett J, Magers C, Davis T (1984) Phase II trial of high dose human lymphoblastoid interferon (Wellferon) in advanced cell carcinoma (aRCC): An ECOG pilot. Proc Am Soc Clin Oncol 3: 153

Tykkä H, Oravisto KJ, Lehtonen T, Sarna S, Tallberg T (1978) Active specific immunotherapy of advanced renal cell carcinoma. Eur Urol 4: 250–258

Vermillion CD, Skinner DG, Pfister RC (1972) Bilateral renal cell carcinoma. J Urol 108: 219–222

Vermooten V (1950) Indications for conservative surgery in certain renal tumors: A study based on the growth pattern of the clear cell carcinoma. J Urol 64: 200–208

Vetto JT, Papa MZ, Lotze MT, Chang AE, Rosenberg SA (1987) Reduction of toxicity of interleukin-2 and lymphokine-activated killer cells in humans by the administration of corticosteroids. J Clin Oncol 5: 496–503

Wagle DG, Scal DR (1970) Renal cell carcinoma – A review of 256 cases. J Surg Oncol 2: 23–32

Waters CA (1935) Preoperative irradiation of cortical renal tumors. AJR 33: 149–164

Waters WB, Richie JP (1979) Aggressive surgical approach to renal cell carcinoma: Review of 130 cases. J Urol 122: 306–309

van der Werf-Messing B (1973) Carcinoma of the kidney. Cancer 32: 1056–1061

Weyman PJ, McClennan BL, Stanley RJ, Levitt RG, Sagel SS (1980) Comparison of computed tomography and angiography in the evaluation of renal cell carcinoma. Radiology 137: 417–424

Wickham JEA (1975) Conservative renal surgery for adenocarcinoma. The place of bench surgery. Br J Urol 47: 25–36

World Health Organization (1979) WHO Handbook for Reporting Results of Cancer Treatment. World Health Organization, Geneva, Offset Publication No. 48

Zeffren J, Yagoda A, Watson RC, Natale RB, Blumenreich MS, Chapman R, Howard J (1981) Phase II trial of methyl GAG in advanced renal cancer. Cancer Treat Rep 65: 525–527

Ziegler JL, Magrath IT (1973) BCG immunotherapy in Burkitt's lymphoma: Preliminary results of a randomized clinical trial. Natl Cancer Inst Monogr 39: 199–202

Chapter 5

Intravesical Treatment of Superficial Bladder Cancer

W.W. Bonney

Introduction

Transitional cell carcinoma most commonly presents as superficial bladder cancer, a disease of heightened importance because of the invasive cancer that can follow.

Despite years of careful study, the relationship between superficial and invasive cancers remains uncertain. In some ways they seem to be separate diseases, yet invasive cancer does show up later in a significant percentage of cases. This suggests at least a concurrence of factors leading to both and perhaps still the possibility of a true progression from one to the other. Among superficial bladder cancers, certain characteristics predict the subsequent appearance of invasive tumour.

Superficial bladder cancer treatment must therefore be evaluated in terms of ability to prevent "progression", to alter the natural history of this disease. It is not enough to consider just the reduction or delay of recurrence. The present article will attempt to review intravesical therapy in regard to these issues, an approach implied by previous authors (Fosså 1985).

Literature Review Methods

In the choice of papers for review, an attempt was made to select for substantial patient numbers, mucosal biopsy and cytology reports, uniformity and complete description of tumour status at entry, prospective randomised study design, and accession of consecutive eligible cases with exclusions documented. This well-intentioned effort falls far short of a comprehensive review.

Included were stage Ta–T1 tumours with the presence of carcinoma in situ clarified whenever possible. Histological grades 1–3 were usually present in roughly similar proportions. Tables 5.1 to 5.5 were simplified as follows: prior transitional carcinoma, prior chemotherapy, and presence of carcinoma in situ were each "positive" if applicable to more than half of cases, otherwise marked "negative", with clarification in the text.

In randomised control and prophylactic treatment groups each patient was assumed to have no evident disease (NED) at completion of the initial TUR, unless otherwise noted. (In fact, the matter was not always specifically mentioned. Furthermore, some studies omitted mucosal biopsies and cytology while others included both among the requirements for NED status.)

For present purposes, percentage recurrence was defined as the proportion of patients with at least one tumour on follow up cytoscopy, percentage progression those with subsequent metastases or recurrent tumour of stage T2–4. Tumours unresponsive to induction treatment (TUR or chemotherapy) were included – mainly because early recurrence was not always distinguishable from non-response.

Recurrence rate and progression rate were used or calculated whenever feasible, representing either number of positive cytoscopies or number of tumours per 100 follow-up months, ideally in patients observed well beyond the first recurrence (methodological details were not always available).

Among the reviewed papers there was a wide variety of innovative ways to present data, which partially blocked the attempt to extract comparative information. Previous authors (Sylvester 1985) have offered suggestions for standardisation.

Transurethral Resection Alone

In addition to its diagnostic value, transurethral resection (TUR) is the initial treatment in the large majority of superficial tumours. After TUR alone, with tumour status known at that point, data about recurrence and progression provide the background for evaluation of additional treatment (Table 5.1).

Greene et al. (1973) reported 100 consecutive cases of newly diagnosed superficial tumour. Pagano et al. (1987) described 200 cases, "unselected" and therefore presumably a mixture of newly diagnosed and recurrent tumours. Althausen et al. (1976) reported 129 cases (182 with exclusion of 53 lost to follow-up or dead of other disease earlier than the specified minimal observation period).

Torti et al. (1987) reported percentage progression in 252 consecutive patients after exclusion of patients with CIS and those followed less than 3 months. Further, setting aside the 11 patients with T2 initial tumour, progression to T3 tumour was still seen in 16%.

Lutzeyer et al. (1982) followed 315 patients after TUR or open resection (data

Table 5.1. TUR alone

Ref	Grade	Stage	n	FU[a]	Recurrence			Progression		
					%[b]	Rate[c]	DFI[d]	%	Rate	DFI
Greene et al. (1973)	1	Ta–T1	100	15+[e]	73	3.3	–	10	0.06	8.0
Pagano et al. (1987)	1–3	Ta–T1	200	3.3	83	2.1	–	20	0.5	–
Althausen et al. (1976)	1–2	Ta–T1	129	5+	80	–	–	30	–	36
Torti et al. (1987)	1–4	Ta–T2	252	5.2	–	–	–	17	–	–
Cutler et al. (1982)	1–3	Ta–T1	154	3+	54	–	31	–	–	–
Heney et al. (1983)	1–3	Ta–T1	243	3.3	53	–	–	–	–	–
Heney et al. (1983)	1–3	Ta–T1	201	3.3	–	–	–	12	–	–
Jakse et al. (1987)	1–3	Ta–T1	172	8.8	–	–	–	8	–	39

[a] Follow-up in years, mean value unless otherwise indicated.
[b] Percentage of patients with at least one recurrence.
[c] Number of recurrences/100 months follow-up.
[d] Disease-free interval in months, mean value.
[e] Minimal follow-up in years.

not included in Table 5.1). In relation to initial stage, percentage recurrence was Ta 52%, T1 69%, T2 77%; newly diagnosed 45%, prior tumour 84%. Percentage progression to T3 or higher was Ta 19%, T1 34%, T2 46%; newly diagnosed 24%, prior tumour 56%.

Cutler et al. (1982) gave 3-year follow-up data on National Bladder Cancer patients rendered NED by TUR plus other treatment in some cases. Progression occurred in 4 (3%) of 120 stage Ta and 19 (24%) of 78 stage T1. In Table 5.1, data represent 154 patients NED by TUR alone. From the same patient group subsequent data were presented (Heney et al. 1983) for those NED by TUR alone.

Jakse et al. (1987) presented comparative recurrence rates and DFI for specific stages and grades without summary data.

The above references convey some idea about the natural history or long-term outlook for superficial bladder cancer after TUR alone. Many of these patients were newly diagnosed and (for this and other reasons) at low risk for recurrence and progression. However, intravesical chemotherapy patients are frequently a higher risk group. It is therefore difficult to judge whether chemotherapy produces better long-term results – except by prospective, randomised trials with late observations.

Intravesical Chemotherapy, Therapeutic

By definition, this section concerns the treatment of patients with documented superficial cancer present in the bladder, after TUR or otherwise (Table 5.2). As a general rule they are at higher risk than the TUR-alone group by virtue of multiple prior recurrences, bulky disease, or associated carcinoma in situ.

Jakse et al. (1984) gave late follow-up on 15 patients, 10 of whom responded completely to intravesical treatment.

Soloway (1985, 1987) treated 70 patients, 18 with recurrent but previously untreated tumour and 57 previously treated with thiotepa (including 39 treatment failures). CIS was present in 12 cases, grade 3 tumour in 25. Complete response

Table 5.2. Intravesical chemotherapy, therapeutic

Ref	Rx	Prior		CIS[a]	n	Fu[b] yr	CR[c] %	Recurrence			Progression		
		TCC	Rx					%[d]	Rate[e]	DFI[f]	%	Rate	DFI
Jakse et al. (1984)	ADR[g]	–	0	+	15	4.2	67	53	–	(1.0)	–	–	–
Soloway (1985, 1987)	MMC[h]	+	+	0	70	2.3	36	70	–	19	32	–	–
Fitzpatrick et al. (1979)	EPO[i]	+	0	+	64	(5)	63	69	–	(34)	53	–	–
Koontz (1981)	TTP[j]	+	0	0	95	(1.0)	47	(72)	–	(3)	–	–	–
Somerville et al. (1985)	MMC[k]	+	+	0	22	2.0	77	41	–	–	27	–	–
Stricker et al. (1987)	MMC[l]	+	0	+	19	1.8	78	42	2.6	6.4	5	0.2	24

[a] Carcinoma in situ present in majority of patients.
[b] Follow-up in years after entry, mean value.
[c] Complete response to treatment, percentage of patients.
[d] Failures to respond *plus* responders with recurrence, per cent of patients.
[e] No. of recurrences or positive cystoscopies/100 months follow-up, mean value.
[f] Disease-free interval in months, from entry until recurrence.
[g] Doxorubicin 40 mg biweekly or 80 mg monthly for 2 years.
[h] Mitomycin C 30–40 mg weekly (× 8), then 40 mg monthly for responders.
[i] Epodyl 1 g weekly (× 12), then monthly (× 12), then every 3 months.
[j] Thiotepa 30–60 mg (× 4), one or two courses.
[k] Mitomycin C 20 mg (× 21) over 7 weeks.
[l] Mitomycin C 30 mg weekly (× 8).

was defined as NED with negative cytology and seen in 20% of patients with prior TTP, 61% with no prior treatment.

Fitzpatrick et al. (1979) reported patients given longterm treatment, which produced complete responses as late as 2 years on continuing therapy. Entries in parentheses were estimated here from tabular or other data.

Koontz et al. (1981) reported thiotepa treatment in 95 patients and prophylaxis in 93. CIS was the only disease present in 11 and coexisted with papillary tumour in another 8. Forty-five patients were judged complete responders, 27 after one course and another 18 after the second course, with cytology negative in half and positive in another third of those patients. In Table 5.2 the treatment-response data represent the original 95 patients. The recurrence data (in parentheses) represent the original non-responders plus 30 responders who moved on into the prophylaxis study.

Somerville et al. (1985) gave late follow-up on 22 of the 23 patients reported earlier (Harrison et al. 1983). CIS initially present in 6, prior chemo- or radiotherapy in 16. Cytology was not used to define complete response. Progression ultimately seen in 5 of 17 complete responders and 1 of 6 induction failures.

Stricker et al. (1987) reported 19 patients, 4 with CIS alone and 15 CIS plus papillary tumour, none with prior chemotherapy. Complete response included negative cytology.

Intravesical Chemotherapy, Prophylactic

By definition, this was adjuvant therapy given immediately or soon after the patient was rendered free of all known disease (NED) by TUR (Table 5.3). These patients have not necessarily been at higher risk than those traditionally managed by TUR alone.

Schulman et al. (1982) reported a large, well balanced prophylactic trial of 2 agents against control. Carcinoma in situ was not mentioned and therefore presumably not present in most subjects. Bladder cancer was newly diagnosed in 62%, recurrent in 38%. Cytology was not reported. Of 308 evaluable patients, 23 (7.5%) progressed locally and none had metastases. None were followed beyond first recurrence.

Table 5.3. Intravesical chemotherapy, prophylactic

Ref	Rx	Prior TCC	Rx	CIS[a]	n	Fu[b] yr	Recurrence %[c]	Rate[d]	DFI[e]	Progression %	Rate	DFI
Schulman et al. 1982	Con	0	0	0	104	1.3	69	8.9	8.8	–	–	–
Schulman et al. 1982	TTP[f]	0	0	0	105	1.5	59	5.4	13.0	–	–	–
Schulman et al. 1982	VM26[g]	0	0	0	99	1.4	69	6.7	8.0	–	–	–
Kurth et al. 1984	Con	0	0	0	69	1.0	47	7.6	–	–	–	–
Kurth et al. 1984	Epo[h]	0	0	0	85	1.0	22	3.0	–	–	–	–
Kurth et al. 1984	ADR[i]	0	0	0	86	0.9	22	4.1	–	–	–	–
MRC 1985	Con	0	0	0	123	1.0	37	3.8	7.9	2	–	–
MRC 1985	TTP[j]	0	0	0	124	1.0	42	4.6	8.9	2	–	–
MRC 1985	TTP[k]	0	0	0	120	1.0	38	4.6	10.0	3	–	–
Prout et al. 1983	Con	+	0	0	45	(2.0)	76	–	–	13	–	–
Prout et al. 1983	TTP[l]	+	0	0	45	(2.0)	87	–	–	18	–	–
Huland and Otto 1985	Con	0	0	0	31	2.9	54	–	–	26	–	–
Huland and Otto 1985	MMC[m]	0	0	0	54	2.8	11	–	–	4	–	–
Byar et al. 1977	Con	–	0	–	48	2.6	60	5.6	–	–	–	–
Byar et al. 1977	Pyr[n]	–	0	–	32	2.6	47	5.8	–	–	–	–
Byar et al. 1977	TTP[o]	–	0	–	38	2.6	47	3.8	–	–	–	–
Rubben et al. 1988	Con	0	0	0	82	(2)	61	2.7	18.6	12	–	–
Rubben et al. 1988	ADR[p]	0	0	0	79	(2)	55	2.5	18.9	16	–	–
Rubben et al. 1988	ADR[q]	0	0	0	59	(2)	57	2.3	21.9	11	–	–

[a] Carcinoma in situ present in majority of patients.
[b] Follow-up in months after entry, mean value.
[c] First recurrence, per cent of patients.
[d] No. of recurrences or positive cystoscopies/100 months follow-up, mean value.
[e] Disease-free interval, in months, from entry until recurrence.
[f] Thiotepa 30 mg weekly ($\times$ 4), then monthly ($\times$ 11).
[g] VM26 (epipodophyllin derivative) 50 mg weekly ($\times$ 4), then monthly ($\times$ 11).
[h] Ethoglucid 1.13 g weekly ($\times$ 4), then monthly ($\times$ 11).
[i] Doxorubicin 50 mg weekly ($\times$ 4), then monthly ($\times$ 11).
[j] Thiotepa 30 mg immediately after TUR.
[k] Thiotepa 30 mg immediately after TUR and every 3 months ($\times$ 4).
[l] Thiotepa 30 or 60 mg monthly ($\times$ 24) or until recurrence.
[m] Mitomycin C 20 mg biweekly for 1 year, then monthly for 1 year.
[n] Pyridoxine 25 mg tablet daily for study duration.
[o] Thiotepa 60 mg weekly ($\times$ 4), then monthly for study duration.
[p] Doxorubin 50 mg twice weekly ($\times$ 12).
[q] Doxorubicin 50 mg twice weekly ($\times$ 12), then semi-monthly/monthly for 1 year.

Kurth et al. (1982) reported a randomised trial of 2 agents against control. Entered were 149 newly diagnosed cancer patients and 91 with recurrent disease, apparently none with prior chemotherapy. Carcinoma in situ was present alone in 9 cases and not mentioned in the others. Follow-up extended through the treatment year and beyond until the first recurrence (the earliest recurrence came during treatment). Disease-free intervals were presented in Kaplan–Meier probability curves with statistically significant differences documented between ethoglucid and control, mainly in newly diagnosed disease. Recurrence rates were significantly different between treated patients and controls but not between the 2 treatments. There were no data on progression.

The MRC Working Party (1985) reported a randomised trial of 2 thiotepa dose schedules against control, with patient assignment well analysed in regard to prognostic factors. All patients were newly diagnosed. Cytology and random mucosal biopsy data were not mentioned, nor was the presence of carcinoma in situ. As presented in Table 5.3, the disease-free intervals were roughly calculated from available data.

Prout et al. (1983) studied patients randomised between treatment and control. All of the original 93 patients were NED at entry, 63 after TUR and 30 after prior thiotepa treatment (90 were reported in this paper). There was no difference between the 2 dose levels, so the patients were reported as one group. Twenty-two had positive cytology at entry, equally divided between treatment and control arms. Patients were removed from study at first recurrence, otherwise removed from treatment at 2 years, and followed to 4 years. Mean follow-up time was not provided but estimated by the present author to be something less than 2 years. Available data included patients free from recurrence at 4 years: prior thiotepa continued on treatment 52%, prior thiotepa control 29%, post TUR on treatment 23%, post TUR control 13%. Mean disease-free interval and interval to progression could not be calculated from available data.

Huland and Otto (1985) reported a randomised study of mitomycin C against control. Just under half of the patients had one or more prior bladder tumours. Carcinoma in situ was initially present in 2 cases. None had prior chemotherapy. NED status was confirmed at entry in all cases; the T1 patients had repeat TUR with biopsies and cytology before randomisation.

Byar and Blackard (1977) reported a randomised study of oral placebo, oral pyridoxine, and intravesical thiotepa. Patients were all NED by cystoscopy and biopsy at entry with no prior treatment. There is no information about prior tumour or carcinoma in situ at entry and no data on progression.

Rubben et al. (1988) studied patients who all received intravesical doxorubicin at TUR and were then randomised to control against short term or longterm doxorubicin. At entry 72% had newly diagnosed bladder cancer. All were visually NED at conclusion of TUR, but 11% had dysplasia and 17% positive cytologies. Mean follow-up was not mentioned, but median follow-up was roughly 2 years in all treatment arms.

Bacillus Calmette-Guerin (BCG)

Since its early use in bladder cancer (Morales et al. 1976), BCG has provided alternative treatment for superficial tumours resistant to other intravesical agents, in part due to a substantially different mechanism of action (Lamm 1987).

That mechanism, however, still eludes precise definition. Non-specific stimulation of host immunity remains a controversial point. Positive BCG skin test conversion accompanies tumour response in many cases (Lamm 1987), but not all data support the significance of that association (Orihuela et al. 1987). Altered circulating leukocyte levels and similar assays simply miss the mark. Another possibility is tumour-specific sensitisation from a local Freund's adjuvant effect. This concept came from classical animal models, all of which involve chemicals and tissues of proven antigenic strength in the host of interest. Autochthonous human tumours, however, lack proven antigenicity. About one point, at least, all authors agree: a severe local granulomatous inflammatory reaction invariably appears with complete local tumour response, as if both neoplastic and normal epithelium were destroyed in a sort of bystander effect and replaced by regenerating new urothelium.

Intravesical BCG, Therapeutic

Herr et al. (1986) emphasised carcinoma in situ, giving late follow-up data on 47 patients given BCG for residual CIS after TUR. Of those 47, 23 were studied in a randomised trial of BCG against TUR alone with residual CIS. All had multiple prior TCC, and over half had prior intravesical chemotherapy. Progression was defined as metastatic disease (2 control patients, 2 BCG) or cystectomy (17 control, 5 BCG). Cystectomy was done for prostatic CIS (3 patients, all BCG group), small capacity with inability to retain BCG (3), widespread uncontrolled T1 tumour (4), and stage T2+ recurrence.

Kavoussi et al. (1988) described several simultaneous or overlapping therapy trials, reported as phase II studies. All patients had prior TCC with prior chemotherapy not specified. The first listed treatment group (Table 5.4) had residual papillary tumour alone, the second group carcinoma in situ with or without papillary tumour. In the third group, all patients had recurrent tumour after BCG, failures from the other 2 listed treatment groups and other sources. Evaluation included cystoscopy, biopsies and cytology.

Brosman (1985) resected all visible tumour and treated weekly until NED status was achieved by cystoscopy, biopsy and cytology. The patients then began monthly maintenance treatment to 2 years. All patients had prior TCC and all had carcinoma in situ, with prostatic urethral involvement in 7 and associated papillary tumour in 18. Of the 33 patients, 27 had failed thiotepa, mitomycin C and/or doxorubicin, and 3 had failed external radiation 4500–6500 rads. Six patients tolerated weekly treatment poorly and withdrew after 6–10 instillations; 4 of these achieved durable complete responses and 2 failed with 1 progression. The other 27 continued until achieving NED: 18 for 12 weeks, 6 for 18 weeks, and 3 for 24 weeks. Of these 27, 4 had late recurrent tumour with at least 1 progression. This is debatably the most intensive treatment schedule ever reported, also a group of patients at notably high risk for recurrence and progression. Systemic side effects were minimised by isoniazide and antihistamines, bladder irritation by indomethacin and anticholinergics. Serial bladder capacities were not reported.

Table 5.4. Intravesical BCG, therapeutic

Ref	Rx	Prior TCC	Rx	CIS[a]	n	Fu[b] yr	CR[c] %	Recurrence %[d]	Rate[e]	DFI[f]	Progression %	Rate	DFI
Herr et al. 1986	Con	+	+	+	26	4.3	–	(100)–	–	–	73	–	–
Herr et al. 1986	BCG[g]	+	+	+	47	4.1	68	55 –	–	–	17	–	–
Kavoussi et al. 1988	BCG[h]	+	0	0	17	2.5	41	59 –	–	–	–	–	–
Kavoussi et al 1988	BCG[h]	+	0	+	32	2.0	37	63 –	–	–	–	–	–
Kavoussi et al. 1988	BCG[i]	+	+	0	57	1.5	60	40 –	–	–	–	–	–
Brosman 1985	BCG[j]	+	+	+	33	4.2	94	18 –	10.5	–	6	–	–
Badalament et al. 1987	Con[k]	+	0	+	46	1.8	63	53 0.15	–	–	13	–	–
Badalament et al. 1987	BCG[l]	+	0	+	47	1.8	64	50 0.07	–	–	13	–	–
Soloway 1987	BCG[m]	+	+	0	30	1.3	70	30 –	–	–	17	–	–

[a] Carcinoma in situ present in majority of patients.
[b] Follow-up in years after entry, mean value.
[c] Complete response to treatment, percentage of patients.
[d] Failures to respond *plus* responders with recurrence, percentage of patients.
[e] No. of recurrences or positive cystoscopies/100 months follow-up, mean value.
[f] Disease-free interval in months, from entry until recurrence.
[g] BCG Pasteur 120 mg weekly (× 6) (half also received intradermal Tice).
[h] BCG Pasteur 120 mg weekly (× 6).
[i] BCG Pasteur 120 mg weekly (× 6), then cross over to repeat weekly (× 6).
[j] BCG Tice (1 ampoule) weekly (× 6–24), then monthly to 2 years.
[k] BCG Pasteur 120 mg weekly (× 6) (control arm).
[l] BCG Pasteur 120 mg weekly (× 6), then monthly to 2 years (maintenance arm).
[m] BCG Tice (1 ampoule) weekly (× 6), then monthly to 1 year.

Badalament et al. (1987) reported treatment of existing tumour (6 week induction) followed by restaging TUR and randomisation to control against 2 year maintenance. At entry all patients had recurrent TCC (visible 60%, carcinoma in situ 78%) after prior intravesical chemotherapy in 36%. At the post-induction, pre-randomisation TUR 36% still had positive biopsies and/or cytology.

Soloway (1987) reported induction and maintenance treatment of patients who had all failed prior treatment, both thiotepa and mitomycin C in most cases. Of the 30, 9 had carcinoma in situ and all had existing tumour. NED criteria included cystoscopy, biopsies and cytology. NED status was achieved by 50% after induction and by 70% after maintenance.

Hillyard (1988) reported 8 patients treated for bladder carcinoma in situ involving the prostatic urethra. After 6 weekly instillations by ordinary technique, 7 patients achieved NED status including negative prostatic urethral biopsies. The remaining patient, and one other with subsequent progression in the bladder, went on to surgical treatment.

Intravesical BCG, Prophylactic

Pinsky et al. (1985) reported patients rendered visually NED by initial TUR, then randomised to BCG against control (Table 5.5). Of the evaluable 86 patients, 19 had prior intravesical chemotherapy and 49 had CIS on initial biopsy (distributed equally between BCG and control). Subsequent NED status was defined by cystoscopy, biopsy, and cytology. Disease-free intervals were presented in Kaplan–Meier curves with differences between BCG and control $P=0.001$ for recurrence, $P=0.01$ for progression (to cystectomy for invasive disease). Pre- and post-protocol recurrence rates changed with a significant overall difference between BCG and control.

Table 5.5. Intravesical BCG, prophylactic

Ref	Rx	Prior		CIS[a]	n	Fu[b] yr	Recurrence			Progression		
		TCC	Rx				%[c]	Rate[d]	DFI[e]	%	Rate	DFI
Pinsky et al. 1985	Con	+	0	+	43	2.5	95	1.7	–	63	–	–
Pinsky et al. 1985	BCG[f]	+	0	+	43	2.5	70	1.0	–	33	–	–
Lamm 1985	Con	+	0	0	27	2.5	52	–	24	–	–	–
Lamm 1985	BCG[g]	+	0	0	30	2.5	20	–	48	–	–	–
Kavoussi et al. 1988	BCG[h]	+	0	0	55	1.8	64	–	–	5	–	–
Hudson et al. 1987	BCG[h]	+	0	0	21	1.4	29	–	12	–	–	–
Hudson et al. 1987	BCG[i]	+	0	0	21	1.4	33	–	15	–	–	–

[a] Carcinoma in situ present in majority of patients.
[b] Follow-up in months after entry, mean value.
[c] First recurrence, percentage of patients.
[d] No. of recurrences or positive cystoscopies/100 month follow-up, mean value.
[e] Disease-free interval, in months, from entry until recurrence.
[f] BCG Pasteur 120 mg weekly ($\times$ 6).
[g] BCG Pasteur 120 mg weekly ($\times$ 6), also Pasteur intradermal weekly ($\times$ 6).
[h] BCG Pasteur 120 mg weekly ($\times$ 6).
[i] BCG Pasteur 120 mg weekly ($\times$ 6), then every 3 months maintenance.

Lamm (1985) reported patients visually NED after TUR, then randomised to BCG against control. All had prior TCC ("stage B" in 5 cases) without other notable high risk factors. Prior chemotherapy and CIS were not detailed. Regular follow-up cystoscopy was supplemented by mucosal biopsies and cytology "as indicated".

Kavoussi et al. (1988) reported this prophylactic trial as a phase II study. All had prior TCC and were NED with negative biopsies and cytology at entry. No mention was made of prior chemotherapy.

Hudson et al. (1987) reported a randomised trial of longterm maintenance therapy against control. Eighty patients were randomised and then evaluated by cystoscopy, biopsy, and cytology after all had received a preliminary 6-week course of BCG. Twenty-one were judged evaluable in each treatment arm, 42 total, of which 26 were NED at entry, 11 had CIS, and 5 had visible papillary tumour (all stratified between treatment arms).

Discussion

In the short term perspective, intravesical therapy offers the only conservative way to treat carcinoma in situ. It also postpones recurrence of superficial papillary tumours, although not necessarily in a better way than TUR for those tumours that return in low number and frequency. However, the longterm issue of interest remains progression to invasive and metastatic disease.

In the data presented here there is little convincing evidence that intravesical therapy has altered the natural history and outcome of superficial bladder cancer. As pointed out by Fosså (1985), more longterm follow-up is needed to support a conclusion. These same patients might be followed-up and reported further by the same centres with recurrences treated under appropriate protocols to provide outcome data.

Prophylactic treatment seems to delay or prevent recurrence best when continued on a longterm maintenance basis. This effect apparently extends to invasive recurrences, so that progression patterns might be favourably altered with considerable cost and patient involvement in each case so managed. A suitable strategy might therefore employ longterm intravesical treatment on a selective basis. Previous authors (Rubben et al. 1988; Jakse et al. 1987) have suggested that standard prognostic factors be used after TUR to identify those patients at greatest risk for metastatic progression and therefore appropriate candidates for intensive treatment. This might provide a cost-effective solution to the apparent dilemma.

References

Althausen AF, Prout GR Jr, Daly JJ (1976) Non-invasive papillary carcinoma of the bladder associated with carcinoma in situ. J Urol 116: 575–579

Badalament RA, Herr HW, Wong GY, Gnecco C, Pinsky CM, Whitmore WF Jr, Fair WR, Oettgen HF (1987) A prospective randomized trial of maintenance versus non-maintenance intravesical Bacillus Calmette-Guerin therapy of superficial bladder cancer. J Clin Oncol 5: 441–449

Brosman SA (1985) The use of Bacillus Calmette-Guerin in the therapy of bladder carcinoma in situ. J Urol 134: 36–39

Byar D, Blackard C, The Veterans Administration Cooperative Urological Research Group (1977) Comparisons of placebo, pyridoxine, and topical thiotepa in preventing recurrence of stage I bladder cancer. Urol 10: 556–561

Cutler SJ, Heney NM, Friedell GH (1982) Longitudinal study of patients with bladder cancer: factors associated with disease recurrence and progression. In: Bonney WW, Prout GR Jr (eds) Bladder cancer. Williams and Wilkins, Baltimore, pp 35–46

Fitzpatrick JM, Khan O, Oliver RTD, Riddle PR (1979) Long-term follow-up in patients with superficial bladder tumours treated with intravesical epodyl. Br J Urol 51: 545–548

Fosså S (1985) The need for long-term follow-up studies after treatment of superficial bladder cancer. In: Schroeder FH, Richards B (eds) Superficial bladder tumors. Alan R. Liss, New York, pp 31–38 (Progress in Clinical and Biological Research vol. 185B)

Greene LF, Hanash KA, Farrow GM (1973) Benign papilloma or papillary carcinoma of the bladder? J Urol 110: 205–207

Harrison GSM, Green DF, Newling DWW, Richards B, Robinson MRG, Smith PH (1983) A phase II study of intravesical mitomycin C in the treatment of superficial bladder cancer. Br J Urol 55: 676–679

Heney NM, Ahmed S, Flanagan MJ, Frable W, Corder MP, Hafermann MD, Hawkins IR for National Bladder Cancer Collaborative Group A (1983) Superficial bladder cancer: progression and recurrence. J Urol 130: 1083–1086

Herr HW, Pinsky CM, Whitmore WF Jr, Sogani PC, Oettgen HF, Melamed MR (1986) Long-term effect of intravesical Bacillus Calmette-Guerin on flat carcinoma in situ of the bladder. J Urol 135: 265–267

Hillyard RW Jr, Ladaga L, Schellhammer PF (1988) Superficial transitional cell carcinoma of the bladder associated with mucosal involvement of the urethra: results of treatment with intravesical Bacillus Calmette-Guerin. J Urol 139: 290–293

Hudson MA, Ratliff TL, Gillen DP, Haaff EO, Dresner SM, Catalona WJ (1987) Single course versus maintenance Bacillus Calmette-Guerin therapy for superficial bladder tumors: a prospective, randomized trial. J Urol 138: 295–299

Huland H, Otto U (1985) Use of mitomycin as prophylaxis following endoscopic resection of superficial bladder cancer. Urol 26 [Supplement to Number 4]: 32–35

Jakse G, Hofstadter F, Marberger H (1984) Topical doxorubicin hydrochloride therapy for carcinoma in situ of the bladder: a followup. J Urol 131: 41–42

Jakse G, Loidl W, Seeber G, Hofstadter F (1987) Stage T1, Grade 3 transitional cell carcinoma of the bladder: an unfavorable tumour? J Urol 137: 39–43

Kavoussi LR, Torrence RJ, Gillen DP, Hudson MA, Haaff EO, Dresner SM, Ratliff TL, Catalona WJ (1988) Results of 6 weekly intravesical Bacillus Calmette-Guerin instillations on the treatment of superficial bladder tumors. J Urol 139: 935–940

Koontz WW Jr, Prout GR Jr, Smith W, Frable WJ, Minnis JE (1981) The use of intravesical thio-tepa in the management of non-invasive carcinoma of the bladder. J Urol 125: 307–312

Kurth KH, Schroder FH, Tunn U, Ay R, Pavone-Macaluso M, Debruyne F, de Pauw M, Dalesio O, ten Kate F, Members of the EORTC Genitourinary Tract Cancer Cooperative Group (1982) Adjuvant chemotherapy of superficial transitional cell bladder carcinoma: preliminary results of an EORTC randomized trial comparing doxorubicin hydrochloride, ethoglucid and transurethral resection alone. J Urol 132: 258–262

Lamm DL (1985) Bacillus Calmette-Guerin immunotherapy for bladder cancer. J Urol 134: 40–46

Lamm DL (1987) BCG immunotherapy in bladder cancer. In: Rous SN (ed) Urology annual. Appleton & Lange, Norwalk, Connecticut, pp 67–86

Lutzeyer W, Rubben H, Dahm H (1982) Prognostic parameters in superficial bladder cancer: an analysis of 315 cases. J Urol 127: 250–252

Morales A, Eidinger D, Bruce AW (1976) Intracavitary Bacillus Calmette-Guerin in the treatment of superficial bladder tumors. J Urol 116: 180–184

MRC Working Party on Urological Cancer, London (1985) The effect of intravesical thiotepa on the recurrence rate of newly diagnosed superficial bladder cancer. Br J Urol 57: 680–685

Orihuela E, Herr HW, Pinsky CM, Whitmore WF Jr (1987) Toxicity of intravesical BCG and its management in patients with superficial bladder tumors. Cancer 60: 326–333

Pagano F, Garbeglio A, Milani C, Bassi P, Pegoraro V (1987) Prognosis of bladder cancer. Eur Urol 13: 145–149

Pinsky CM, Camacho FJ, Kerr D, Geller NL, Klein FA, Herr HA, Whitmore WF Jr, Oettgen HF (1985) Intravesical administration of Bacillus Calmette-Guerin in patients with recurrent superficial carcinoma of the urinary bladder: report of a prospective, randomized trial. Cancer Treat Rep 69: 47–53

Prout GR Jr, Koontz WW Jr, Coombs LJ, Hawkins IR, Friedell GH for National Bladder Cancer Collaborative Group A (1983) Long-term fate of 90 patients with superficial bladder cancer randomly assigned to receive or not to receive thiotepa. J Urol 130: 677–680

Rubben H, Lutzeyer W, Fischer N, Deutz F, Lagrange W, Giani G, Members of the Registry for Urinary Tract Tumors (1988) Natural history and treatment of low and high risk superficial bladder tumors. J Urol 139: 283–285

Schulman CC, Robinson M, Denis L, Smith P, Viggiano G, de Pauw M, Dalesio O, Sylvester R, Members of the EORTC Genito-Urinary Tract Cancer Cooperative Group (1982) Prophylactic chemotherapy of superficial transitional cell bladder carcinoma: an EORTC randomized trial comparing thiotepa, an epipodophyllotoxin (VM26) and TUR alone. Eur Urol 8: 207–212

Soloway MS (1985) Treatment of superficial bladder cancer with intravesical mitomycin C: analysis of immediate and long-term response in 70 patients. J Urol 134: 1107–1109

Soloway MS (1987) Selecting initial therapy for bladder cancer. Cancer 60: 502–513

Somerville JJF, Newling DWW, Richards B, Robinson MRG, Smith PH (1985) Mitomycin C in superficial bladder cancer: 24–month follow-up. Br J Urol 57: 686–689

Stricker PD, Grant ABF, Hosken BM, Taylor JS (1987) Topical mitomycin C therapy for carcinoma of the bladder. J Urol 138: 1164–1166

Sylvester R (1985) The analysis of results in prophylactic superficial bladder cancer studies. In: Schroeder FH, Richards B (eds) Superficial bladder tumors. Alan R. Liss, New York, pp 3–11 (Progress in Clinical and Biological Research vol. 185B)

Torti FM, Lum BL, Aston D, MacKenzie N, Faysel M, Shortliffe LD, Freiha F (1987) Superficial bladder cancer: the primacy of grade in the development of invasive disease. J Clin Oncol 5: 125–130

Chapter 6

Management of Invasive Bladder Neoplasms

Cora N. Sternberg and H.I. Scher*

Infiltrating bladder tumours encompass a broad clinical spectrum exhibiting varied biological potential. While the term can be applied biologically to any tumour that extends beyond the in situ category, urologically it implies muscle infiltration and uniform recommendations concerning management are lacking. Once infiltration is documented, the ability to control the disease by transurethral resection diminishes, thus, radical surgery, with or without radiation therapy is commonly recommended. Clinical trials reporting the results of these approaches vary with respect to case selection criteria for the given treatment, the extent of pretreatment staging and restaging, and time to and specific site(s) of relapse. More important is that few studies are randomised, the number of patients actually receiving the planned therapy is small and follow-up time too short to assess the impact of a particular strategy on either local control or survival. Frequently neglected is the fact that these diseases occur in an older population with a variety of intercurrent medical problems which preclude an aggressive combined modality approach. Death rates from non-cancer-related causes can be significant and are rarely factored in to the reported results.

The impact of infiltration on prognosis, despite the inherent inaccuracies of the clinical staging system (Table 6.1 and Fig. 6.1) is well recognised (Jewett and Strong 1946; Marshall 1952). The physician treating a patient with an invasive tumour has a variety of treatment options with differing morbidity and impact on quality of life (Table 6.2). These range from transurethral methods (including

*Dr. Sternberg and Dr. Scher are recipients of The American Cancer Society Clinical Oncology Career Development Awards.

Table 6.1. TNM classification of bladder tumours*

The classification applies to epithelial tumours and papillomas are excluded. All biopsies should be submitted to the reference pathologist who should note whether the material contains lamina propria and muscle so that invasion can be assessed. The assignment of a TNM category is based on the following minimum requirements. If an accurate assessment cannot be made then the following designation is used $T_xN_xM_x$.

T stage: Physical examination, excretory urography, examination under anaesthesia with biopsy or transurethral resection of tumour if feasible.

N stage: Physical examination and imaging studies as indicated (excretory urography, lymphography, ultrasound and computed tomography).

M stage: Physical examination, biochemical profiles and imaging studies. These usually include chest radiographs, hepatic ultrasound, bone scan and CT scan of the abdomen and pelvis.

Primary tumour
- T_x Minimum requirements to assess the primary tumour cannot be met.
- T_0 No evidence of primary tumour.
- T_{is} Carcinoma in situ.
  - u   ureter
  - pu   prostatic urethra
  - pd   prostatic ducts
  - fem u   female urethra
- T_a Papillary non-invasive carcinoma.
- T_1 Carcinoma without histological evidence of invasion beyond the lamina propria. On bimanual examination a freely mobile mass may be felt; this should not be felt after complete transurethral resection of the lesion.
- T_2 Histological evidence of invasion of superficial muscle of the bladder. On bimanual examination there may be induration of the bladder wall, which is mobile. There is no residual induration after complete transurethral resection of the lesion.
- T_3 On bimanual examination there may be induration or a nodular mass palpable in the bladder wall that persists after transurethral resection. There is microscopic evidence of deep muscle invasion (T_{3a}) or extension into perivesical fat (T_{3b}).
- T_4 Histological evidence of muscle invasion with tumour fixed or invading adjacent structures.
  - T_{4a} Extension into prostate, uterus or vagina.
  - T_{4b} Tumour fixed to the pelvic and/or abdominal wall.

Nodal sites
Includes lymph nodes in the true pelvis. All others are considered distant nodes.
- N_x Minimum requirements to assess the regional nodes cannot be met.
- N_0 No involvement of regional nodes.
- N_1 Involvement of a single homolateral regional lymph node.
- N_2 Involvement of contralateral, bilateral, or multiple regional lymph nodes.
- N_3 A fixed mass on the pelvic wall with a free space between it and the primary tumour.
Juxtaregional lymph nodes are considered in the distant metastases (M_1) category.

Distant metastases
- M_x Minimum requirements to assess the presence of distant metastases cannot be met.
- M_0 No (known) distant metastasis.
- M_1 Distant metastases present.

*The 1978 classification is quoted, as the 1988 version is not yet uniformly accepted for use in clinical trials.

laser therapy) which have the least morbidity but a higher risk of inadequate control, to more radical procedures with or without radiation therapy. More recently, chemotherapeutic regimens have been developed and some patients previously thought to be incurable, are enjoying long-term survival (Sternberg

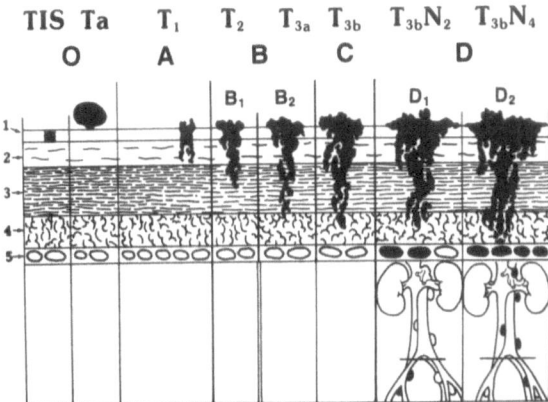

Fig. 6.1. Classification of bladder tumours. TNM classification compared to the Jewett/Strong/ Marshall system for bladder cancer. 1. Mucosa: 2. Lamina propria. Note presence of isolated muscle fibres, muscularis mucosae, that may be involved in superficially invasive cancer: 3. Muscularis propria: 4. Perivesical fat: 5. Lymph nodes.

Table 6.2. Treatment options for invasive bladder tumours

Local control	Problems
Transurethral resection	Inadequate local control
Laser	
Segmental resection	Selection of treatment
Radiation therapy	
Cystectomy ± node dissection	
Irradiation + salvage cystectomy	Metastasis
Integrated radiation + surgery	
Chemotherapy: M-VAC, CMV, DDP, 5-FU, CAP	
Intra-arterial chemotherapy	
Chemotherapy + radiation	
Chemotherapy + surgery	
Chemotherapy + radiation + surgery	

Modified after Whitmore (1986)

et al. 1985; Harker et al. 1985; Logothetis et al. 1985a; Stoter et al. 1987). These observations, coupled with the dissatisfaction with aggressive local therapies such as radical surgery and/or radiation therapy have led to the widespread and perhaps ill-advised use of these combinations in patients with localised disease.

Is improvement in survival with muscle-infiltrating bladder cancer possible? Is bladder preservation a realistic therapeutic goal? Can treatment morbidity be reduced and quality of life factored into the therapeutic equation? This chapter will outline the dynamic role of the combined modality treatment team in the management of invasive bladder cancer. The impact of newly designed integrated chemotherapy and radiotherapeutic approaches will be discussed along with current clinical trials designed to assess the place for these approaches in individual patient management. Ultimately, a better understanding of biological prognostic factors based on immunohistochemistry, flow cytometry and molecular probes may allow more rational individualisation of treatment.

Role of the Urologist

Of the 45 000 new cases of bladder cancer in the United States, 75% present with superficial lesions, 20% with invasive tumours and 5% present with de novo metastatic disease. The management of superficial tumours has been discussed. Of those with invasive tumours, 65% present with no antecedent history while the other 35% will have progressed following treatment for less invasive tumours (Prout et al. 1976; Whitmore 1979). The latter represents an extremely heterogeneous group.

Most patients with urinary symptoms, and in particular haematuria, first present to the urologist. Thus his evaluation is central to future management decisions. Although details of the endoscopic procedure are beyond the scope of this discussion, the evaluation should include a careful bimanual examination under anaethesia, urine sampling or barbotage bladder wash for cytological examination, and a careful bladder map labelling the location, appearance, size and number of visible tumours. At a minimum, the report should detail the number and location of lesions, their endoscopic appearance, and the presence or absence of an in situ component (as determined from histological study).

Selected-site biopsies should be performed particularly when large and/or high grade and/or multiple tumours are visible (Friedell 1987). The examination should also include an inspection and possible biopsy of the prostatic urethra, particularly in patients who have been treated intravesically for in situ disease and have a high risk for extravesical recurrence. A transperineal or transrectal biopsy of the prostate may be performed to allow the distinction between tumour in the urethra versus ducts versus stroma versus the glands of the prostate.

The pathological review allows assignment of a final clinical T category. This is illustrated in Table 6.1. Histological subtype(s) along with the presence or absence of carcinoma in situ are recorded. Controversies do exist with respect to assignment of grade and the significance of papilloma (Mostofi 1979, 1985). However, the report must include a statement as to whether or not muscle is present in the specimen so that invasion can be assessed. Inadequate specimens justify resampling. It is important to recognise the presence of the muscularis mucosa, which is a small muscle layer present in the lamina propria and is distinct from the deeper muscle layers. Tumours in this category fall in the T_1 stage, and can frequently be managed by endoscopic means (Ro et al. 1987).

While the majority of bladder neoplasms are pure transitional cell tumours, other subtypes include squamous, adenocarcinoma and small cell tumours. Frequently, a mixed histology of transitional plus squamous or transitional plus adenocarcinoma is observed. This has prognostic importance when potentially bladder-sparing strategies with pre-operative chemotherapy are being considered (Logothetis et al. 1985b; Scher et al. 1988a). Incidental carcinoma of the prostate is not infrequent in this population and may be found on prostatic biopsies (Winfield et al. 1987; Neumann and Limas 1986). This must be distinguished from primary and metastatic bladder tumours which are managed differently.

The final T category has been shown to correlate with prognosis. However, it must be recognised that cystoscopic evaluations frequently understage the disease. In one series reported by Whitmore et al. 38% were understaged (Whitmore 1979), while Skinner et al. (1984) reported only a 52% correlation between clinical T stage and pathological P stage. Staging is least accurate in distinguishing T2 from T3 lesions, where treatment choices range from local TUR alone with preservation of bladder function, to more debilitating radical procedures. However, as noted by Skinner, the accuracy of clinical staging is probably not as important to the patient as the ability to differentiate those tumours that require aggressive therapy from those that can be satisfactorily managed by more conservative methods (Skinner and Lieskovsky 1988).

Other non-invasive procedures that may help with appropriate treatment selection include transabdominal ultrasonography (Dershaw and Scher 1987), CT scans and MRI (magnetic resonance imaging) (Hryniuk 1987). Ultrasonography is relatively inexpensive and can allow an assessment of the depth of invasion, particularly transmural tumours that extend into perivesical fat. The transrectal approach may permit assessment of extension into the prostatic urethra. CT scanning, when performed with proper distension of the bladder with air and contrast media, can allow visualisation of tumours as small as 5–10 mm, as well as an assessment of transmural disease. Both of these modalities, however, are relatively non-specific in distinguishing tumours confined to the submucosa from those with superficial and/or deep muscle invasion. This distinction can be particularly difficult in patients who have undergone repeated transurethral resections of the bladder, where cystitis and bladder wall oedema are present. MRI permits images in the sagittal, transverse and coronal planes. Extension into the bladder, perivesical fat and adjacent structures can be well visualised. It has limited capability in distinguishing tumour from oedema and remains expensive considering the lack of specificity and sensitivity. It should be emphasised that these procedures are not routinely utilised in the TNM classification, but are becoming increasingly important and should be reported when included in a clinical trial. As will be discussed, the routine use of these modalities can significantly alter the reported outcome independent of the therapy.

Some of the treatment options for patients with invasive tumours are highlighted in Table 6.2. Categorical statements regarding the "optimal" treatment are not possible, but are based primarily on the results of the clinical evaluation outlined above. Selection is based on a consideration of the ability to control the disease within the bladder with the least morbid approach coupled with an assessment of the risk of development of metastases. Performing a radical procedure in a patient destined to die of metastases in a few months, is clearly not optimal therapy. While the depth of invasion correlates with an increasing incidence of nodal positivity, it is unknown what percentage of patients with invasive disease develop metastatic disease without first involving the regional lymph nodes. Identified vascular or lymphatic invasion may correlate with this occurrence (Wolf et al. 1986). This group is difficult to identify in reported surgical series because complete restaging including scans is not routinely performed at the time of relapse in one site, be it local or distant. For example, when a patient develops pulmonary nodules on routine chest X-ray films following radical surgery, a CT scan of the pelvis to assess for a concurrent pelvic recurrence is generally not performed. Location of tumour is also an important factor in selecting therapy. For example, a patient with carcinoma in situ documented in the prostatic urethra, with a significant chance of extension into the prostate, may require a radical cystoprostatectomy despite the lack of an invasive component. A tumour located near the bladder neck may not be suitable for segmental resection, where an adequate margin of normal bladder is essential, whereas a lesion on the dome might be. Using strict criteria of case selection, only 5%–12% of patients with muscle infiltrating tumours had tumours that were considered amenable to segmental resection (Utz et al. 1973; Novick and Stewart 1976; Skinner and Lieskovsky 1988).

Surgery

In the United States, the standard therapy for muscle infiltrating bladder tumours not amenable to endoscopic resection remains radical surgery. Other experiences with results reporting the use of TUR alone, partial cystectomy or radiation therapy alone or as part of a combined modality approach, must be compared against this standard. These comparisons can be difficult for several reasons. First, the criteria for cystectomy are not universal. At Memorial Hospital, indications for cystectomy include:

1. Muscle-invading tumours not deemed suitable for segmental resection regardless of grade
2. Low stage tumours that are unsuitable for conservative management because of multicentricity, frequent recurrences, high grade, or prostatic urethral involvement
3. High grade tumours associated with carcinoma in situ
4. Rapidly recurring multifocal high grade tumours or carcinoma in situ
5. Severe irritative bladder symptoms, e.g. frequency or haemorrhage, unresponsive to intravesical chemotherapy

Retrospective analyses of older cystectomy series in comparison with contemporary reports are not valid due to improvements in surgical technique, the availability of modern era antibiotics and anaesthesia, and improved preoperative staging. Surgical mortality has decreased from 10%–20% in older series, to <5% in more recent reports. Further, the percentage of patients dying from causes other than bladder cancer is usually not reported. In sequential series at Memorial Hospital, 13%–28% of patients treated by radical surgery died of causes other than their primary bladder tumours (Whitmore and Batata 1984). These factors are rarely considered in the choice of treatment. More important is that most studies report projected actuarial survival distributions, usually to 5 years. The number of patients actually followed for this time period is frequently small, resulting in large confidence limits toward the latter portion of the survival curves.

The choice of a radical procedure must be weighed against the impact on quality of life and associated morbidity of the treatment. These include possible incontinence, loss of sexual potency, and impairment of self-image. Intense interest has recently been generated by reports of continent urinary diversions

(Camey and Le Duc 1979; Camey 1985; Kock et al. 1978; Montie et al. 1987; Skinner and Lieskovsky 1988). Potency can also be preserved in selected cases. Controversies exist concerning the details of the procedure and the anatomical source of the "bladder" reservoir or diverting loop. Some have questioned the adequacy of these approaches as a "cancer" operation and complication rates remain high, particularly in inexperienced hands. Long-term follow-up for these various modifications will be required before they can be recommended routinely.

Interpretation of reported results is also hindered by differences in case selection and the surgical technique employed. Some patients may require cystectomy for control of local disease, such as diffuse T1 or Tis disease refractory to intravesical therapy, even though there is little risk of metastatic disease. Inclusion of these patients in overall reporting will "improve" 5-year survival results independent of treatment. The actual surgical procedure is variable. In some series, lymph node sampling is performed while in others a formal node dissection is the standard practice. Careful pathological review, with serial step sections of each lymph node, may identify microscopic disease that can be missed on more routine examination. This can alter survival distributions independent of case selection, disease natural history, and treatment.

While reports based on the actual pathological stage of the cystectomy specimen are more accurate than those based on clinical T stage, the latter impact more directly on individual patient management. Results of therapy are difficult to compare due to the recognised inaccuracies of the clinical staging system, especially in the assessment of T3 lesions. Routine use of CT and MRI scans may allow exclusion of un-resectable T4 lesions and identify a subset of patients with node-positive disease who might not be considered for radical surgery.

Careful case selection can identify a subgroup of patients whose disease can be controlled by local transurethral resection alone. At Memorial Hospital, patients routinely have a repeat endoscopic procedure performed as part of the initial evaluation. This permits more consistent restaging. Those found to have no tumour on repeat transurethral biopsy, even if muscle infiltration was identified in submitted material, may simply be re-evaluated in 6–12 weeks and not entered on clinical protocols. This allows identification of subgroups that may be susceptible to more conservative management. Herr recently reported a series of consecutively treated patients with muscle infiltrating tumours, documented by pathological review of submitted biopsy material, seen at Memorial Hospital (Herr 1987). Of 217 patients, 172 (79%) were judged to have invasive tumours not amenable to local resection and underwent radical surgery. Of these, 89 (52%) are alive and free of disease. The other 45 (22%) were selected for conservative management because restaging showed no tumour (T0) in 20, carcinoma in situ only in 17, T1 in 4, and T2 in 4 patients. With follow-up of 5.1 years (range 3–7 years) 30/45 (67%) are free of disease. Of these, 9 have required no further therapy while 21 have required repeat TUR with or without intravesical therapy for recurrent superficial but non-muscle infiltrating bladder tumours. Of the 15 failures, 11 required cystectomy from 9–30 months after initial restaging for subsequent development of a muscle-infiltrating tumour (8 patients) or rapidly recurrent superficial bladder tumours refractory to conservative measures (3 patients). The overall disease-free survival at 5.1 years is 37/45 (82%), 67% (30/45) of whom have a functional bladder with continued close surveillance and often intense local endoscopic and topical intravesical therapy.

Reports of selected series evaluating 5-year survival by pathological stage are listed in Table 6.3. Most reflect actuarial survival. The number of patients entered, reported follow-up period, percentage of patients with no disease in the bladder and percentage who died of other causes are listed. Five-year survivals range from 25%–88% for those with muscle infiltration (P2, P3a) and 11%–50% for those with disease infiltrating perivesical fat (P3b). In most series, about 10% of patients are unresectable (Montie et al. 1981).

Table 6.3. Reported 5-year survival with surgery alone

Author	Year	P2	P3a	P3b	P4N[+]
Poole-Wilson and Barnard	1971	25%	12%	–	–
Richie et al.	1975	40%	40%	20%	–
Prout	1976	31%	31%	21%	–
Whitmore et al.	1977	60%	26%	11%	–
Pearse et al.	1978	–	–	50%	11%
Bredael et al.	1980	53%	36%	11%	–
Mathur et al.	1981	88%	57%	11%	–
Montie et al.	1982	50%	63%	29%	–
Skinner and Lieskovsky	1988	83%	69%	29%	26%

Fifteen to 25% will have metastases to the regional lymph nodes. The role of lymph node dissection remains controversial. In a series at Memorial Hospital, 20% of 662 patients who underwent radical cystectomy with or without preoperative radiation therapy had positive nodes. Only 7% (9/134) of patients with microscopic nodal disease after radical cystectomy survived 5 years; 82% died from cancer. The actuarial survival ranged from 7 months for patients with N_4 (disease above the common iliac bifurcation) to 22 months for patients with N_1 disease (single nodal metastasis below the common iliac bifurcation) (Smith and Whitmore 1981). More recently, Skinner and co-workers reported a projected 5-year survival of 31% for patients with node-positive disease who underwent en bloc lymph node dissection and radical cystectomy. Further follow-up will be required (Skinner and Lieskovsky 1988).

At Memorial Hospital, when grossly positive nodal disease is documented at the time of exploration, a radical cystectomy is not performed and the patient is referred for systemic chemotherapy. At M. D. Anderson Hospital, the radical procedure is completed and the patient referred for postoperative "adjuvant" chemotherapy. While some reports suggest a benefit for patients treated with postoperative chemotherapy, the approach must still be considered investigational (Logothetis et al. 1987b; Skinner and Lieskovsky 1988).

Radiation Therapy

In the United States, radiation therapy alone is not considered adequate therapy for muscle-infiltrating bladder tumours. Although the approach has been in use for over 25 years, its role in the preoperative (2000 or 40 Gy), postoperative or as full dose (definitive – 50–75 Gy) treatment with or without a salvage cystectomy, remains controversial. Often neglected is that the selection criteria for treatment using radiation therapy are predominantly negative: patients are often "medically unfit" for cystectomy or have large bulky tumours deemed to be unresectable (Shipley and Rose 1985; Shipley et al. 1987). With these caveats, the results of selected radiation therapy plus cystectomy series are included in Table 6.4 and for radiation therapy alone in Table 6.5. For T2–3 lesions 33%–65% and for T4 lesions, 0%–25% survive five years.

Table 6.4. Reported 5-year survival for surgery with radiation therapy

Author	Year	Dose and Time	T2	T3a	T3b	T4
Miller et al.	1973	50 Gy 5 wk			53%	0%
van der Werf Messing	1975	40 Gy 4 wk			50%	
Prout et al.	1976	45 Gy 4.5 wk	65%		38%	6%
Reid et al.	1976	20 Gy 4 days			34%	
Wallace et al.	1976	40 Gy 4 wk			33%	
Whitmore et al.	1977	40 Gy 4 wk	50%	34%	33%	0%
Boileau et al.	1980	50 Gy 5 wk	38%	51%	57%	
Whitmore + Batata	1984	20 Gy 5 days	41%	49%		
Skinner et al.	1982	15 Gy	52%	37%		25%
Whitmore et al.	1984	20 Gy 1 wk	45%	42%	33%	0%

Table 6.5. Reported 5-year survival for radiation therapy alone

Author	Year	Dose/Time	Pts	T2	T3a	T3b	T4
Miller and Johnson	1973	70 Gy/7 wk	109		20%		
Goffinet et al.	1975	70 Gy/7 wk	218		28%		
Morrison	1975	50 Gy/4 wk	40		33%		
Greiner et al.	1977	70 Gy/7 wk	195	28%			
Blandy et al.	1980	55 Gy/4 wk	352	34%			
Goodman et al.	1981	50 Gy/3 wk	450	38%			
Bloom et al.	1982	60 Gy/6 wk	91		25%		
Shipley et al.	1985	68.4 Gy/7 wk	37	39%			
Timmer et al.	1985	60–65 Gy/7 wk	76	42%	32%		
Miller and Johnson	1973	70 Gy/7 wk	128				13%
Goffinet et al.	1975	70 Gy/7 wk	65				8%
Greiner et al.	1977	70 Gy/7 wk	30				1%
Blandy et al.	1980	55 Gy/4 wk	258				9%
Goodman et al.	1981	50 Gy/3 wk	110				7%
Shipley et al.	1985	68.4 Gy/7 wk	18				6%

Modified after Shipley (1986) with additions.

Two randomised trials have compared preoperative radiation therapy (50 Gy) and cystectomy against definitive radiation therapy alone. At M. D. Anderson Hospital 51% of patients with clinical T3 disease treated with the combined modality approach survived 5 years compared to 13% for the radiation therapy alone (Miller and Johnson 1973). At the Institute of Urology in London, 40-Gy preoperative radiation therapy and cystectomy against 60-Gy alone were compared. A 5-year survival benefit, 44% against 24%, was demonstrated for the combined therapy (Bloom et al. 1981).

The difficulties in performing clinical trials in this group of patients are highlighted by the experience of the National Surgical Adjuvant Bladder Project (Prout 1976) which compared 40-Gy preoperative radiation therapy plus cystectomy to cystectomy alone. Of 246 patients randomised to receive preoperative radiation therapy and cystectomy, only 123 (50%) actually completed the protocol. Similarly, of 229 patients randomised to receive cystectomy alone, only 133 (58%) completed the treatment. Overall, 244 patients with clinical T2-3 disease were evaluable. The 5-year survival was 37% for the combined and 31% for the surgery alone group.

A strategy of irradiation followed by cystectomy at time of failure, "salvage cystectomy" has been recommended by some authors (Blandy et al. 1980). From prognostic analyses of radiation therapy trials, complete disappearance of disease (clinical T0 following treatment) is associated with improved longterm survival. In the London Hospital series, 43% of 220 stage T3 patients who were T0 after treatment had an actuarial survival of 72% compared to only 17% for partial or non-responders. In a report from the Massachusetts General Hospital of patients with stage T2–3 tumours receiving full-dose radiation therapy, the probability of survival in the 19 patients who did not develop local recurrence was 79% vs. 11% for the 18 patients who did (Shipley et al. 1987). Other prognostic factors included tumour size, whether the lesion was papillary or sessile, the presence or absence of ureteral obstruction and the extent of resection of the primary tumour. It can be argued that radiation therapy alone may allow the identification of patients with a good response (clinical T0 following treatment) and perhaps a good prognosis, reserving salvage cystectomy for treatment failures. This approach must be weighed against the observation that few patients, in actuality <10% (Blandy et al. 1980) actually underwent definitive surgical therapy.

Preoperative radiation therapy is no longer considered routine practice in the United States. The rationale was based on the theoretical possibility of reducing the metastatic potential of localised cells and the eradication of microextensions of cancer not excised with the surgical specimen. The initial reports seemed to indicate a decrease in the number of local recurrences and a beneficial effect on survival, particularly in those patients whose tumours were observed to undergo downstaging following radiation therapy (Batata et al. 1981; Whitmore and Batata 1984). A decrease in the number of pelvic recurrences from 37% without to 24% with preoperative radiation therapy and a subsequent increase in 5-year survival from 20% to 38% with preoperative radiation was reported (Whitmore and Batata 1984). Similarly, van der Werf Messing showed a significant decrease in the number of pelvic recurrences using interstitial irradiation (van der Werf Messing 1984).

More recent analyses, albeit retrospective, coupled with reports of contemporary cystectomy results, suggest that only a small subset of patients could actually benefit from this approach. The Cleveland Clinic reported a 20-year experience of radical cystectomy in 99 cases who did not receive preoperative radiation therapy. Five-year survival in patients with T3 and T4a lesions was 40%, and the pelvic recurrence rate only 9% (Montie and Whitmore 1984). At UCLA, 297 patients treated by surgery alone (197 patients) or surgery plus radiation therapy (100 patients) were evaluated. Surgery involved a single stage radical cystectomy with pelvic lymph node dissection and urinary diversion as definitive therapy (Skinner and Lieskovsky 1984) and radiation a minimum of 16 Gy preoperatively

(Skinner et al. 1984; Skinner and Lieskovsky 1988). No benefit was demonstrated for the use of preoperative radiation therapy. An analysis of the pattern of failure in patients treated with surgery, suggests that the majority of patients succumb to metastatic disease. Thus any local therapy, in particular radiation therapy, would be expected to have little impact on survival when used as an adjunct to cystectomy.

Whitmore pointed out that for those with nodal disease, more effective systemic therapy is required before any impact on survival will be realised. As noted previously, at Memorial Hospital patients who are found to have grossly positive nodes at the time of surgery, do not have a cystectomy performed, but are referred for systemic chemotherapy. Following completion of chemotherapy, a re-exploration is performed to resect residual disease if present, followed by 2 additional cycles of chemotherapy (vide infra).

While the use of radiation therapy in combination with cystectomy is no longer routine, it does play a role in the patient who cannot tolerate radical surgery or for control of local symptoms such as haemorrhage. Some of the newer uses of radiation therapy, in particular in conjunction with chemotherapy, will be discussed below.

Criteria for Response and Evaluation

Before discussing some of the newer integrated treatment strategies for invasive bladder cancer, it is important to recognise a change in response criteria, as suggested by the First International Consensus Development Conference on Bladder Cancer held in Antwerp, Belgium in June, 1985 (Yagoda 1985; Van Oosterom et al. 1986). Thus response assessments based on cystoscopic evaluations only are considered as clinical restaging and not pathological restaging. Further, with the more widespread use of non-invasive staging procedures such as CT scanning, sonography – both transabdominal and transurethral – and magnetic resonance imaging, some standardisation of reporting is essential to permit comparisons between clinical trials. Using the UICC TNM staging classification, complete remission has been expanded to incorporate non-invasive procedures. A prefix $_c$, is utilised to denote clinical restaging, including cystoscopy and biopsy, with no other surgical procedures. Using these designations, a $_cCR$ includes a normal physical examination, normalisation of previously abnormal CT, radionuclide scans and sonograms with a *normal cystoscopy and biopsy* with no carcinoma in situ (T_{is}), and normal urinary cytology. Thus, a patient who presents with muscle infiltrating (T_{2-4}) disease on cystoscopic biopsy with a thickened bladder wall on CT scan, who is found after treatment to have a negative cystoscopy and biopsy (T_0) with persistent bladder wall thickening on CT scan would not be a $_cCR$, but rather a $_cPR$. The importance of these clarifications will become apparent when comparing results of neo-adjuvant treatment strategies.

A prefix $_p$ in a response classification, signifies surgical or pathological staging was undertaken. A $_pCR$ indicates that restaging by exploratory laparotomy with biopsies of sites of known previous disease, such as a pulmonary nodule, pelvic node or bladder mass revealed no tumour. In the example cited above, persistent bladder wall thickening on CT scan in a patient with a negative cystoscopic examination (T0) is classified as a $_c$PR. At surgery, if no disease is found, the final classification would be $_p$CR, whereas if residual disease documented, the patient would remain a $_p$PR. At Memorial Hospital, the postscript $_s$ is used when residual disease, present after induction chemotherapy, is completely removed following a surgical procedure. In the previous example, if residual disease were removed, the patient would be classified first as a $_p$PR and then subsequently as a CR$_s$. These designations are important when one considers the inaccuracies of clinical staging. Prior to surgical restaging such CR$_s$ and $_p$PR cases may have been clinically characterised as $_c$CR, $_c$MR, $_c$STAB or $_c$PROG. Since response rates for combination regimens have now reached the 40%–70% range, attainment of CR has gained increasing importance, and becomes critical in the interpretation of neo-adjuvant trials.

Neo-Adjuvant Therapy

The identification of a number of active single and combination chemotherapy programmes (Table 6.6), in particular the demonstration of complete responses with chemotherapy alone or chemotherapy plus surgery in patients with advanced nodal and metastatic disease (Harker et al. 1985; Sternberg et al. 1985, Logothetis et al. 1985; Carmichael et al. 1985; Hillcoat and Raghavan 1986; Stoter et al. 1987), has led to the use of chemotherapy as initial therapy (neo-adjuvant chemotherapy) in patients with muscle-infiltrating tumours. Before using this approach, it was important to identify active chemotherapeutic regimens. In a series of phase II disease-site specific trials for advanced urothelial tract cancer at Memorial Hospital in patients selected for bidimensionally measurable indicator lesions, cisplatin (DDP), methotrexate (MTX), adriamycin (ADM) and vinblastine sulphate (VLB) induced complete and partial clinical remission in 30%, 29%, 17% and 18% of cases respectively (Yagoda 1987; Sternberg and Scher 1987). Following 2 additional trials using MTX + VLB and ADM + DDP the 4 agents were combined to produce the M-VAC regimen in 1983. Using this combination, 37% of 83 patients with metastatic (M+) and/or non-resected nodal (N$_{2-4}$) disease achieved complete remission either with chemotherapy alone or in combination with surgery (Sternberg et al. 1988). With a median follow-up of 43 months (range 11–49+ months), 17 of 31 complete responders are alive, free of disease. The estimated probabilities of survival were 71% at 2 years and 55% at 3 years for this group. The overall complete and partial remission rate was 69% (95% confidence intervals 59%–79%).

The strategy of chemotherapy as initial therapy has the immediate advantage of providing an in vivo marker of chemosensitivity, where full doses of chemotherapy can be used. Occult micrometastases, which theoretically may be more responsive than clinically established lesions, can also be treated. Tolerance to chemotherapy may also be better in the preoperative than in the postoperative setting. Ideally, non-responders can be considered for alternative treatment and be spared ineffective therapy, while responders can receive maximal doses. In the

Table 6.6. Complete response rates to combination chemotherapy in metastatic bladder tumours

	No. Pts		No. CR+PR	%CR+PR	95% confidence
Single agents					
Cisplatin	320		90	30	(25–35)
Methotrexate	236		68	29	(23–25)
Adriamycin	274		47	17	(13–22)
Vinblastine	38		6	16	(4–28)

	No. Pts	CR(%)	PR(%)	%CR+PR	95% confidence
Cisplatin and methotrexate combinations					
Stoter (1987)	43	10 (23%)	10 (23%)	47%	(32–61)
Stoter (1987)	40	4 (10%)	6 (15%)	25%	(12–38)
Carmichael (1985)	19	4 (21%)	9 (47%)	68%	(48–89)
Oliver (1986)	21	3 (14%)	7 (33%)	48%	(26–69)
Hillcoat (1986)	49	3 (6%)	19 (38%)	44%	(31–59)
	172	24 (14%)	51 (30%)	44%	(36–51)
Harker (1985) CMV	50	14 (28%)	14 (28%)	56%	(42–70)
Sternberg (1988) M-VAC	83	31 (37%)	26 (26%)	69%	(59–79)
Cisplatin/adriamycin/cyclophosphamide (CAP = CISCA)					
Mulder EORTC (1982)	42	5 (12%)	11 (27%)	39%	(29–49)
Khandekar ECOG (1985)	45	10 (22%)	5 (11%)	33%	(0–47)
Troner SEG (1987)	46	5 (12%)	3 (8%)	21%	(20–47)
Al Sarraf SWOG (1984)	23	2 (9%)	8 (34%)	43%	(23–64)
Schwartz MSKCC (1985)	28	2 (7%)	11 (39%)	46%	(28–64)

CMV, Cisplatin, methotrexate, vinblastine
M-VAC, Methotrexate, vinblastine, adriamycin, cisplatin.
CISCA, Cyclophosphamide, adriamycin, cisplatin.
MDAH, M. D. Anderson Hospital
EORTC, European Organization for the Research and Treatment of Cancer
ECOG, Eastern Cooperative Oncology Group
SEG, Southeast Group
SWOG, Southwest Oncology Group
MSKCC, Memorial Sloan-Kettering Cancer Center

long term, if complete local control is achieved, patients may be spared a more radical procedure. Possible criteria for bladder preservation can also be identified.

The approach, however, is not without hazard. The results of surgical series demonstrate 5-year survivals in 20%–40% of cases with muscle infiltrating tumours. For this subgroup, chemotherapy is unnecessary. Further, the choice of chemotherapy is not based on in vivo sensitivity, as the prediction of response is beyond the scope of present clinical capabilities. Thus many patients may be exposed to ineffective and potentially toxic treatment. Case selection is based on a clinical staging system, where it is hard to predict which patients are at greatest risk for developing metastatic disease and would most benefit from this approach. Finally, the false interpretation of response may result in a delay or refusal of potentially curative therapy and possibly jeopardise survival. At present, "neoadjuvant" chemotherapy must be considered investigational and if it is employed, it should be used cautiously, ideally in the context of controlled clinical trials.

Attempting to assess the role of neo-adjuvant therapy, based on present reports, is difficult. Clinical trial design is variable. Few investigations have clearly defined endpoints for analysis, most report a short median follow-up time and few trials are randomised. Known prognostic factors such as the histology of the primary lesion, the presence or absence of urethral obstruction and the extent of surgical resection of the primary lesion prior to entry are not uniformly reported. Patients who are resected and clinically "free of disease" before treatment, cannot be evaluated for "response", only for time to recurrence. For example, in a study by Hall et al. complete endoscopic tumour resection, prior to high-dose methotrexate administration, was accomplished in 59/63 patients, of whom 59% became clinically tumour-free and 36 (62%) showed no evidence of residual invasive cancer at 6 months (Hall 1986). With a median follow-up of 42 months, 47/58 (81%), 33/55 (60%) and 16/31 (52%) were alive at 1, 2 and 3 years respectively. Three-year survivals were similar to historical series using radical cystectomy or curative radiotherapy (Hall 1987). Of importance, bladder preservation was achieved.

The response rates reported for various chemotherapy regimens are variable. Complete remissions ranged from 13% (2/15) for MTX/DDP (Hall 1986) to 60% (9/15) using a 3-drug combination given by the IA and IV route (Logothetis et al. 1985b) (Table 6.8). The time to reassessment of response varies from 1 week to as long as several months and the extent and degree of clinical restaging is also variable. Few routinely incorporate non-invasive testing, such as CT scanning, transabdominal ultrasound and MRI. Some investigators emphasise the "CR rate" within the bladder, yet few include true pathological restaging with laparotomy. Meyers et al. (1985) described 6 CR in 17 evaluable patients treated with CMV; 4 of 17 were restaged with cystoscopy and only 2 had a laparotomy with biopsy. Five additional patients attained $_c$CR, confirmed cystoscopically, after receiving local radiation therapy to the bladder.

At Memorial Hospital, 71 patients with $T_{2-4}N_0M_0$ bladder tumours were treated in a pilot phase I–II trial with 1–6 (median 3) cycles of M-VAC (Scher et al. 1989). Pretreatment evaluation included TURB, CT scan and/or sonogram and urinary cytology. The criteria for response are outlined in Table 6.7. Responses were observed by TURB (T0) in 48%, cytology in 54%, and by all non-invasive procedures in 21%.

Twenty-three (32%) patients did not undergo surgical staging within three months of completion of M-VAC. Of these, 11 were clinical T_0 (7 have no evidence of disease, 3 developed new invasive lesions at 8, 18 and 28 months, and 1 had M+ disease). In 7 patients with residual Tis, one is disease-free after treatment with intravesical BCG, 3 developed M+ disease and 3 are alive with in-situ disease on cystoscopic biopsy. One with disease, resected at the start, was not evaluable.

In 48 surgically staged patients, 13 had a partial cystectomy (10 alive with a functional bladder), 19 radical cystectomy, 5 were unresectable and 1 died of unrelated causes and was Po at autopsy. Pathologically, 11 (22%; 5 with partial and 6 radical cystectomy) were Po, 4 Pis and 1 Pl. Two cases, felt to be completely resected endoscopically prior to M-VAC, were not considered in the evaluation of response. Of 30 patients with residual invasive (25 cases) or unresectable (5 cases) disease at surgery, 14 (tumour at surgery) (47%) have relapsed at distant sites at a median follow-up of 16 months (range 2 to 34+ months). In all 71 cases, 40 are alive and disease-free including 19 (27%) with functional bladder. In this study, non-invasive radiological testing was too non-specific to distinguish fibrosis

Table 6.7.   Response criteria at Memorial Sloan-Kettering Cancer Center

---

Complete Remission (CR)
   Complete disappearance of all clinical evidence of tumour on physical examination, X-ray films and biochemical evaluation for one month

   Clinical ($_c$CR)
      Clinically proved disappearance of all tumour by physical examination, radiography, cytology, and cystoscopy both visually and by biopsy (including T_{is}, as defined by the UICC TNM staging system)

   Pathological ($_p$CR)
      Complete remission, pathologically proved at laparotomy or biopsy of areas of known prior disease as defined by the UICC TNM System. (For disease confined to the bladder ($T_{2-4}N_0M_0$, surgical staging may include either a radical or partial cystectomy and/or pelvic lymph sampling with biopsy of the serosal surface of the bladder.)

   Surgical (CR$_s$)
      Similar to $_p$CR except all remaining disease surgically removed (no evidence of disease after surgery)

Partial Remission (PR)
   Greater than 50% decrease upon physical examination or radiography of the summed products of the perpendicular diameters of all measured lesions. No simultaneous increase in size of any lesion or the appearance of any new lesions may occur

Minor Response (MR)
   25%–49% decrease in the summed products of diameters of measured lesions.

Stabilisation (STAB)
   Less than 25% decrease or increase in tumour size of biochemical abnormalities for a minimum of 3 months

Progression (PROG)
   Less than 25% decrease in tumour size for less than 3 months or greater than 25% increase in the sum of all measured lesions, appearance of new lesions or mixed response

---

or oedema from residual disease, crucial to the accurate evaluation of response. While M-VAC chemotherapy alone produced downstaging with maintenance of bladder function, follow-up is required to monitor for the development of new tumours. Further non-responding patients appear to have a distinctly poor prognosis (Splinter et al. 1989; Scher et al. 1989).

At present all patients with invasive bladder tumours are entered on a clinical protocol comparing M-VAC alone with M-VAC plus radiation therapy. Two cycles of chemotherapy are administered followed by a complete re-evaluation including cystoscopy and biopsy, urinary cytology and non-invasive procedures. Non-progressing patients are continued on treatment for a total of 4 cycles followed by restaging as outlined. At this point, patients are randomised to receive no additional therapy or radiation to the primary site. All patients ultimately undergo surgical exploration including selected lymph node sampling and transmural bladder biopsy. Those patients judged to be pathologically free of tumour at the time of exploration do not undergo radical surgery. If residual disease is documented, a radical cystectomy is performed and two additional cycles of therapy administered. This approach must still be considered investigational. While the goal of bladder preservation is a desirable endpoint, compromising potentially curative surgery by reliance on inaccurate staging could have a deleterious effect on survival.

The routine adaptation of more non-invasive staging techniques, including ultrasound of the bladder and CT scan of the abdomen and pelvis, introduces another variable that can affect the reported outcome of a trial – "lead time bias"

Table 6.8. Neo-adjuvant strategies for invasive bladder tumours

Reference[a]	Therapy	T Stage[b]	Time to re-evaluation[c]	Operation[d]	No. Pts	CR (%)[f]	95%
Raghavan (1985)	DDP+RT	B2–D1	10–12 w	y	49	31 (63)	(50–77)
Torti (1985)	DDP+RT	N.S.	22 d	y	22	6 (27)	(9–46)
Coppin (1985)	DDP+RT	T3b–T4a	4–6 w	21/29	29	22 (76)	(60–91)
Herr (1985)	DDP+RT	T3–T4	8 d	18/24	24	5 (21)	(5–37)
Shipley (1985)	DDP+RT	T3	16 w	y	10	8 (80)	(55–99)
	DDP+RT	T4		y	5	2 (29)	(38–99)
Jakse (1985)	DDP+ADM+RT	T3–T4	12 w	y	25	20 (80)	(64–96)
Fosså (1987)	MTX+DDP+RT	T2	9 w	y	9	2 (22)	
Raghavan (1985)	DDP	B2–D1	6–8 w	y	49	8 (16)	(6–27)
Logothetis (1985)	DDP/ADR/CTX	T4b	5.7[g]	n	12	5 (42)	(14–70)
		T4N3	cycles	n	15	9 (60)	(35–85)
Hall (1986)	MTX/DDP	T3	12 w	y	15	2 (13)	(0–30)
Scher (1989)	M-VAC	T2–T4	4–8 w	y	22[h]	11 (50)	(29–71)
					48[i]	11 (24)	(12–36)
Simon (1986)	M-VAC	T3	12 w	y	12	4 (33)	(7–60)
Zincke (1988)	M-VAC	T2–T4b	Q cycle	y	16	8 (50)	(21–79)
Hall (1986)	MTX	T2–T3b	24 w	res[e]	57	33 (67)	(45–71)
Hall (1986)	MTX/DDP	T3	12 w	res	14	11 (79)	(57–99)
Splinter (1988)	MTX/DDP	T3–T4	2 cycles	y	32	9 (28)	(13–44)
			4 cycles	y	23	9 (39)	(19–59)

[a] Individual references should be consulted for treatment doses and schedules.
[b] T Stage, clinical staging for inclusion into study.
[c] Time to re-evaluation, time from start of treatment to time of first restaging (w, weeks, d, days, [g], median number of cycles, [h], considers only clinically staged patients found to be To, [i], considers only pathologically staged patients).
[d] Operation, patients entered were resectable by radical cystectomy (y, yes; n, no).
[e] res, all visible disease resected at the start of treatement).
[f] CR, complete remission, 95% = 95% confidence interval for the observed complete remission rate.

(Feinstein et al. 1985). This can "extend" the statistical life of a patient without improving survival. By more careful pre-operative staging, fewer patients with metastatic disease are included in the "early stage" categories, resulting in an apparent increase in survival and making it appear that a given therapy is impacting favourably on survival. Similarly, the inclusion of more patients with clinically silent metastatic disease in the advanced category will "improve" the survival of this group as well. The survival of the entire group would be unchanged, but the statistical artefact would become apparent in the subgroup analysis. This has been termed stage migration or the "Will Roger's Phenomenon," and is particularly important in the comparison of "neo-adjuvant" protocols.

In an attempt to increase the CR rate within the bladder and to preserve bladder function, several groups are evaluating the synergy of cisplatin and radiation therapy. A summary of several studies using chemotherapy alone and chemotherapy plus radiation is listed in Table 6.8. The endpoint evaluated was the CR rate, which is listed along with calculated confidence intervals. In most cases a CR classification was based on cystoscopic examination as the sole criteria. Also included is the initial stage, the operability – i.e., were patients resectable at the start of therapy, the degree of initial resection of the primary lesion – complete or incomplete – and the time from the start of therapy to evaluation of response or disease recurrence. Two studies using cisplatin and radiation prior to cystectomy produced $_p$CR in 21% and 27% of cases respectively when evaluated 8–22 days after treatment (Herr 1983; Torti et al. 1986). This rate is similar to that reported for TUR alone prior to cystectomy (Neumann and Limas 1986). In the former study, 75% of patients were alive at 28 months (median follow-up 22 months, range 13–34 months) (Herr 1985). As noted in the table, the $_c$CR rate increases to 63%–80% when the re-evaluation is performed at 6–16 weeks (Coppin et al. 1986; Jakse et al. 1987; Raghavan et al. 1985; Shipley et al. 1984). In the Canadian series, the CR rate was 76% and 3-year survival 82%, a significant improvement over a historical control group treated with radiation therapy alone where the CR rate and 3-year survival were 24% and 49% respectively (Coppin et al. 1985). The 3-year survival, reported with a minimum follow-up of 4 years, for the Australian series was 50% (Raghavan 1987) for the first 50 patients. Most relapses occurred in the bladder or pelvis (Raghavan et al. 1985) which may reflect the clinical staging used. To date, a total of 100 patients have been studied. Also noteworthy is the observation that 6 (15%) of 38 longterm survivors have developed myocardial infarctions. This highlights the importance of randomised trial designs and the potential for unusual late toxicities in this population. At Memorial Hospital, a prospective randomised trial of chemotherapy alone against chemotherapy plus radiation therapy is in progress (*vide supra*).

The National Bladder Cancer Cooperative Group A evaluated cisplatin and radiation therapy in a multi-institution study. A complete response rate of 77% was reported in 62 patients who completed the planned radiation therapy. Among the complete responders, 73% are currently maintained and a higher 4-year survival rate was noted than in those not having CR or with recurrence (57% against 11%). Evaluated by stage, 88% of cT2, 84%, 84% of cT3 and 50% of cT4 responded (Shipley et al. 1987). Without prospective randomised trials, these data are difficult to interpret.

Intra-arterial chemotherapy has also been employed in highly selected series (Jacobs et al. 1984, Schulman et al. 1985; Maatman et al. 1986). The approach has the advantage of increasing the local concentration of the administered agent. For example, Montie et al. noted a 1.5–2 fold increase in DDP concentration when given by the IA route. The reported series vary with respect to: dose, schedule, stop flow vs. pulsatile administration, concurrent adjunctive therapy, angiotensin to constrict "normal" vs. tumour vasculature thereby minimising local toxicity, chemoembolisation, use of hyperthermia or radiation therapy, site and position of catheter, regional vs. local blood flow and vascularity of tumour. Further, it is unclear whether steady state vs. peak drug levels are important for maximal antitumor effect (Montie 1987). Toxicities can be significant and include skin sloughing, tissue necrosis and severe neuropathy (Logothetis et al. 1985b; Montie 1987). It is therefore difficult to recommend this approach outside the clinical trial setting.

At present, based on published data, some conclusions on the role of neo-adjuvant therapy can be made:

1. Chemotherapy alone or in combination with radiation therapy can produce significant tumour regression of intravesical and locoregional transitional cell carcinoma

2. Bladder function can be maintained and may be used as an endpoint in future trials

3. The presence of an extensive in situ component, or a mixed histology lesion, may preclude attempts at possible bladder sparing as complete responses are rare in such settings

4. The similarity in response rates for locoregional and metastatic disease suggests no intrinsic biological differences with respect to drug sensitivity between primary and metastatic tumour.

However, the ultimate question is whether large prospective randomised neo-adjuvant studies will negate the heterogeneity inherent in these trials.

Table 6.9. Study questions to assess role for integrated therapy in invasive bladder cancer

---

A. Bladder preservation: Endpoint of clinical CR ($_cCR$) in the bladder
1. Chemotherapy alone vs. chemotherapy plus radiation therapy.
2. Chemotherapy alone vs, radiation therapy alone.
3. Radiation therapy alone vs. chemotherapy plus radiation therapy.

B. Endpoint of time to recurrence (or survival)
1. Chemotherapy + cystectomy vs. cystectomy alone.
2. Radiation therapy + cystectomy vs. cystectomy alone.
3. Chemotherapy + radiation therapy vs. radiation therapy.
4. Chemotherapy + radiation therapy vs. chemotherapy alone.
5. Chemotherapy + radiation therapy + cystectomy vs. cystectomy alone.

An outline of some possible study questions based on endpoints of local control within the bladder, response duration and survival are listed in Table 6.9. An estimate of the number of patients needed to evaluate endpoints in this type of trial is provided by the experience of the National Bladder Clinical Cooperative Group A (NBCCGA) (Einstein et al. 1985). The trial addressed the question of whether cisplatin, given in the adjuvant setting, would delay the time to

Table 6.10. Current studies of invasive bladder tumours

Group	Eligibility	Design	Targeted difference	Projected number of patients
MSKCC	$T_{2-4}N_0$	M–VAC+RT → SURGERY M–VAC ——→ SURGERY	20%	200
NCI Canada	$T_{2-4}N_{0-3}$	60 Gy+DDP 60 Gy 40 Gy+DDP → CYST 40 Gy——→ CYST	25%	160
Australia	$T_{2-4}N_{0-3}$	45–50 Gy ——→ 10–15 Gy DDP ——→ 45–50 Gy ——→ 10–15 Gy		160
LA County/USC	$T_{2-4}N_{0-3}$	Cystectomy ——→ CAP observation		150
SWOG–ECOG	$T_{2-4}N_{0-3}$	MVAC × 3 ——→ Cystectomy cystectomy		

MSKCC: Memorial Sloan-Kettering Cancer Center
SWOG: Southwest Oncology Group
ECOG: Eastern Cooperative Oncology Group
USC: University of Southern California

recurrence and subsequently improve survival in patients with muscle infiltrating urothelial tumours treated by a combination of radiation therapy and cystectomy. Postoperatively, patients were randomised to therapy with cisplatin or "no therapy". Of 475 considered, 220 were entered, 180 completed radiation therapy and radical cystectomy, 83 were randomised, 43 received cisplatin but only 9 (0.02%) completed the planned therapy. The conclusion that cisplatin was ineffective was based on a very select population. Careful planning to ensure adequate numbers of patients, with adequate follow-up, using a fixed and well tolerated treatment regimen is crucial prior to embarking on such studies. Table 6.10 highlights some of the ongoing randomised trials at various centres along with the estimated differences in response rates between the two treatment arms. A review will show the large number of evaluable cases required to estimate a statistically significant difference.

Conclusions

The clinical management of patients with muscle-invasive transitional cell carcinoma of the bladder has been substantially influenced by improvements in surgical technique, perioperative care, radiotherapeutic achievements and progress in the last decade in the use of combination chemotherapy. Growth factors such as G-CSF may provide an adjunct to chemotherapy by ameliorating the myelosuppression and mucositis often associated with chemotherapy (Gabrilove et al. 1988). This may permit safe administration of higher doses of chemotherapy and increase the dose intensity of the treatment programme (Hryniuk and Bush 1985). Data from the radiation therapy literature and the observation of complete responses to chemotherapy alone or with aggressive transurethral resection now make bladder preservation a realistic therapeutic goal. Further investigations utilising the combined expertise of the urologist, medical oncologist, radiotherapist and pathologist will be required to integrate most beneficially the available treatment options. More study of the interaction of chemotherapy and radiation will be of interest, as pilot studies suggest synergy in vitro and in vivo (Steel 1983; Marks et al. 1987). Most important will be investigations on the biology of bladder cancer, aimed at defining the malignant and metastatic potential of an individual tumour at the start of therapy, so that more rational treatments can be designed. Toward this aim, immunohistochemistry of cell surface antigens (Fradet et al. 1986; Cordon-Carbo et al. 1986; Bander 1987; Biedler et al. 1988) and molecular probes to define drug resistance (Fojo et al. 1987), and any genes associated with metastases and invasiveness will clearly be of value.

Finally, while bladder preservation is a desirable therapeutic goal, it is unclear whether the presently available staging techniques allow proper selection of patients without jeopardising survival (Scher et al. 1988; Zincke et al. 1988). Only large, prospective randomised trials will be able to define the role of a particular treatment strategy.

Acknowledgement. This work was supported in part by National Cancer Institute Contracts CA-05826 and CM-57732.

References

Al-Sarraf M, Frank J, Smith JA et al. (1984) Phase II trial of cyclosphosphamide, doxorubicin, and cisplatin (CAP) versus amsacrine in patients with transitional cell carcinoma of the urinary bladder: A Southwest Oncology Group Study. Cancer Treat Rep 69: 189

Bander NH (1987) Monoclonal antibodies in urologic oncology. Cancer 60 [Suppl 4a]: 514–520

Batata MA, Chu FCH, Hilaris BS et al. (1981) Factors of prognostic and therapeutic significance in patients with bladder cancer. Int J Radiat Oncol Biol Phys 7: 575–579

Bell DR, Gerlach JH, Kartner N et al. (1986) Detection of p-glycoprotein in ovarian cancer: a molecular marker associated with multidrug resistance. J Clin Oncol 3: 311–315

Biedler JL, Meyers MB, Spengler BA (1988) Cellular concomitants of multidrug resistance. In: Mechanisms of Drug Resistance in Neoplastic Cells. Bristol–Myers Symposium. Academic Press, New York

Blandy JP, England HR, Evans SJW et al. (1980) T3 bladder cancer – the case for salvage cystectomy. Br J Urol 52: 506–510

Bloom HCG, Hendry WR, Wallace DM et al. (1982) Treatment of T3 bladder cancer: A controlled trial of preoperative radiotherapy and radical cystectomy versus radical radiotherapy; second report and review. Br J Urol 43: 136–151

Boileau MA, Johnson DE, Chan RC, Gonzales MO (1980) Bladder carcinoma: results with preoperative radiation therapy and radical cystectomy. Urology 16: 569–576

Bredael JJ, Croker BP, Glen JF (1980) The curability of invasive bladder cancer treated by radical cystectomy. Eur Urol 6: 206–210

Camey M (1985) Bladder replacement by ileocystoplasty following radical cystectomy. World J Urol 3: 161–168

Camey M, Le Duc A (1979) L'enterocystoplastie avec cystoprostatectomie totale pour cancer de la vessie. Ann Urol 13: 114–122

Carmichael J, Cornbleet M, MacDougall S et al. (1985) Cisplatin and methotrexate in the treatment of transitional cell carcinoma of the urinary tract. Br J Urol 57: 299–302

College of American Pathologists (1986) Guidelines for data to be included in consultation reports on breast cancer, bladder cancer, and Hodgkin's disease. Pathologist 40: 18–23

Coppin C, Brown L, The GU Tumor Group (1986) Concurrent cisplatin with radiation for locally advanced bladder cancer: A pilot study suggesting improved survival. Proc Am Soc Clin Oncol 5: 99

Cordon-Cardo C, Lloyd KO, Finstad CL et al. (1986) Immunoanatomic distribution of blood group antigens in the human urinary tract: influence of secretor status. Lab Invest 55: 444–454

Dershaw D, Scher H (1987) Sonography in the evaluation of carcinoma of the bladder. Urology 39: 454–457

Einstein AB, Coombs J, Pearse H et al. (1985) Cisplatin (CP) adjuvant therapy following pre-operative radiotherapy plus radical cystectomy (RT+RCy) for invasive bladder carcinoma: A randomized trial of the National Bladder Cancer Group (NBCG). American Urol Assoc 133: 222 (Abstract no. 433)

Feinstein AR, Sossin DM, Wells CR (1985): The Will Rogers phenomenon: stage migration and new diagnostic techniques as a source of misleading statistics for survival in cancer. New Engl J Med 312: 1604–1608

Fojo AT, Ueda K, Slamon DJ et al. (1987) Expression of a multidrug-resistance gene in human tumors and tissues. Proc Natl Acad Sci USA 84: 265–269

Fosså SD, Dingson E, Johannsen NB et al. (1987) Pre-cystectomy chemotherapy in patients with muscle infiltrating bladder tumors. Scand. J Urol Nephrol 21: 39–42

Fradet Y, Cordon-Cardo C, Whitmore WF et al. (1986) Cell surface antigens of human bladder tumors: Definition of tumor subsets by monoclonal antibodies and correlation with growth characteristics. Cancer Res 46: 5183–5188

Friedell GH (1987) Urinary bladder cancer: selecting initial therapy. Cancer 60: 496–501

Gabrilove J, Jakubowski A, Scher H et al. (1988) A study of recombinant human granulocyte colony stimulating factor in cancer patients at risk for chemotherapy-induced neutropenia. New Engl J Med 318: 1414–1422

Goffinet DR, Schneider NJ, Glatstein EJ et al. (1975) Bladder cancer: results of radiation therapy in 384 patients. Radiology 11: 149–153

Goodman GB, Hislop DG, Bellwood JM et al. (1981) Conservation of bladder function in patients with invasive bladder cancer treated by definitive irradiation and selective cystectomy. Int J Radiat Oncol Biol Phys 7: 559–573

Greiner R, Skaleric KC, Veraguth P (1977) The prognostic significance of ureteral obstruction in carcinoma of the bladder. Int J Radiat Oncol Biol Phys 2: 1095–1100

Hall RR (1985) Chemotherapy of invasive carcinoma of the bladder. Aust NZ J Surg 55: 249–252

Hall RR (1986) Transurethral resection and systemic chemotherapy as primary treatment for T_3 bladder cancer. In: Yagoda A (ed) Bladder cancer: future directions for treatment. John Wiley and Sons, New York, pp 117–122

Hall RR (1987) Is cystectomy necessary for invasive bladder carcinoma? Presented at the Second Heinrich Warner Stiftung Symposium. November 5, 1987, Hamburg, Germany

Hall RR, Newling DWW, Ramsden PD et al. (1984) Treatment of invasive bladder cancer by local resection and a high dose methotrexate. Br J Urol 56: 668–672

Harker WG, Meyers FJ, Freiha FS et al. (1985) Cisplatin, methotrexate, and vinblastine (CMV): An effective chemotherapy regimen for metastatic transitional cell carcinoma of the urinary tract. A Northern California Oncology Group Study. J Clin Oncol 3: 1463–1470

Herr H (1985) Preoperative irradiation with and without chemotherapy as adjunct to radical cystectomy. Urology 131: 127–134

Herr H (1987) Conservative management of muscle-infiltrating bladder cancer: Prospective experience. J Urol 138: 1162–1163

Hill DE, Ford KS, Soloway MS (1985) Radical cystectomy and adjuvant chemotherapy. Urology 25: 151–154

Hillcoat BL, Raghavan D (1986) The Australian Bladder Cancer Study Group: A randomized comparison of cisplatin (C) versus cisplatin and methotrexate (C+M) in advanced bladder cancer. Proc Am Soc Clin Onc 5: 110 (Abst 426)

Hricak H (1987) Urologic cancer: methods of early detection and future developments. Cancer 60 [Suppl 4a]: 677–685

Hryniuk W, Bush H (1984) The importance of dose intensity in chemotherapy of metastatic breast cancer. J Clin Oncol 2: 1281–1288

Jacobs SC, McClellan SL, Maher C, Lawson RK (1984) Pre-cystectomy intra-arterial cis-diammine-dichloroplatinum II with local bladder hyperthermia for bladder cancer. J Urol 131: 473–476

Jakse G, Fritsch E, Frommhold H (1987) Treatment of locally advanced bladder cancer by combined chemotherapy and irradiation. In: Hubner W, Porpaczy P, Schramek P, Studler G (eds) 10th international symposium of the Ludwig Boltzman Institute for research on infections and tumours in the urinary tract. Gildesdruck, Vienna, pp 115–122

Jewett HJ, Strong GH (1946) Infiltrating carcinoma of the bladder: relation of depth of penetration of bladder wall to incidence of local extension and metastases. J Urol 55: 366–372

Khandekar JD, Elson PJ, DeWys WD et al. (1985) Comparative activity and toxicity of cis-diamminedichloroplatinum (DDP) and a combination of doxorubicin, cyclophosphamide, and DDP in disseminated transitional cell carcinomas of the urinary tract. J Clin Oncol 3: 539–545

Kock NG, Nilson AE, Norlen L et al. (1978) Urinary diversion via a continent ileum reservoir: clinical experience. Scand J Urol Nephrol [Suppl] 49: 23–31

Lieskovsky G, Skinner DG (1984) Role of lymphadenectomy in the treatment of bladder cancer. Urol Clin North Am 11: 709–716

Logothetis CJ, Samuels ML, Ogden S et al. (1985a) Cyclophosphamide, doxorubicin and cisplatin chemotherapy for patients with locally advanced urothelial tumors with or without nodal metastases. J Urol 134: 460–464

Logothetis CJ, Samuels ML, Selig DE et al. (1985b) Combined intravenous and intra-arterial cyclophosphamide, doxorubicin, and cisplatin (CISCA) in the management of select patients with invasive urothelial tumors. Cancer Treat Rep 69: 33–38

Maatman TJ, Montie JE, Bukowski RM et al. (1986) Intra-arterial chemotherapy as an adjuvant to surgery in transitional cell carcinoma of the bladder. J Urol 135: 256–260

Marks LB, Prout GR Kaufman SD et al. (1987) Invasive bladder cancer: MCV (methotrexate, cisplatin, vinblastine) followed by cisplatin plus pelvic irradiation and possible cystectomy: patient tolerance and local tumor response. Int J Radiat Oncol Biol Phys 13: 101 (Abst 32)

Marshall VF (1952) Relation of preoperative estimate to pathologic demonstration of extent of vesical neoplasms. J Urol 68: 714–723

Mathur VK, Krahn HP, Ramsey EW (1981) Total cystectomy for bladder cancer. J Urol 125: 784–786

Meyers FJ, Palmer JM, Freiha FS et al. (1985) The fate of the bladder in patients with metastatic bladder cancer treated with cisplatin, methotrexate and vinblastine: A Northern California Oncology Group Study. J Urol 134: 1118–1121

Miller LS, Johnson DE (1973) Megavoltage radiation for bladder carcinoma: None, postoperative, or preoperative. Seventh National Cancer Conference. Proceedings pp 771–782

Montie JE, Whitmore WF, Grabstald H, Yagoda A (1981) Unresectable carcinoma of the bladder. Cancer 51: 2351–2355

Montie JE, Pontes JE, Smyth EM (1987) Selection of the type of urinary diversion in conjunction with radical cystectomy. J Urol 137: 1154–1155

Morrison R (1975) The results of treatment of cancer of the bladder: a clinical contribution of radiobiology. Clin Radiol 76: 67–78

Mostofi FK (1979) Pathology in staging of bladder cancer. In: Wilkinson PM (ed) Clinical cancer – principal sites II. Pergamon Press, Elmsfor, New York, p 213 (Advances in medical oncology research and education, vol 11)

Mostofi FK, Ito N, Weinstein R (1985) Pathology. In: Denis L, Niijima T, Prout G, Schroder F (eds) Developments in bladder cancer. EORTC Genitourinary Group Monograph 3. Alan R. Liss, New York, pp 67–83

Mulder JH, Fossa SD, De Pauw M et al. (1982) Cyclophosphamide, adriamycin and cisplatin combination chemotherapy in advanced bladder carcinoma: an EORTC phase II study. Eur J Cancer Clin Oncol 18: 111–112

Neumann MP, Limas C (1986) Transitional cell carcinomas of the urinary bladder: Effects of preoperative irradiation on morphology. Cancer 58: 2758–2763

Novick AC, Stewart BH (1976) Partial cystectomy in the treatment of primary and secondary carcinoma of the bladder. J Urol 116: 570–574

Oliver RTD, Kowk HK, Highman WJ et al. (1986) Methotrexate, cisplatin and carboplatinum as single agents and in combination for metastatic bladder cancer. Br J Urol 58: 1–5

Pearse HD, Reed RR, Hodges CV (1978) Radical cystectomy for bladder cancer. J Urol 119: 216–218

Poole-Wilson DS, Barnard RJ (1971) Total cystectomy for bladder tumours. Br J Urol 43: 16–24

Prout GR (1976) The surgical management of bladder carcinoma. Urol Clin North Am 3: 149–175

Prout GR, Acosta A, Denis L et al. (1986) The TNM classification in clinical research. In: Denis L, Niijima T, Prout G, Schroder FH (eds) Developments in bladder cancer. Alan R. Liss, New York, pp 295–300

Raghavan D (1987) Neo-adjuvant chemotherapy for invasive high-risk bladder cancer. Presented at the 21st Annual clinical conference on recent advances in the systemic therapy of genitourinary malignancies. 11 November, Houston, Texas

Raghavan D, Pearson B, Duval P et al. (1985) Initial intravenous cis-platinum therapy: improved management for invasive high risk bladder cancer? J Urol 133: 399–403

Reid EC, Oliver JA, Fishman IJ (1976) Preoperative irradiation and cystectomy in 135 cases of bladder cancer, Urology 8: 247–250

Richie JP, Skinner DG, Kaufman JJ (1975) Radical cystectomy for carcinoma of the bladder: 16 years of experience. J Urol 113: 186–189

Ro JY, Ayala AG, El-Naggar A (1987) Muscularis mucosa of the urinary bladder: importance for staging and treatment. Am J Surg Pathol 11: 668–673

Scher HI, Sternberg CN (1985) Chemotherapy of urologic malignancies. Semin Urol 3: 239–280

Scher HI, Herr H, Yagoda A, et al. (1988a) Neoadjuvant M-VAC (methotrexate, vinblastine, adriamycin and cisplatin): the effect on primary bladder tumors. J Urol 139: 470–474

Scher HI, Herr H, Sternberg CN et al. (1988b) Neo-adjuvant M-VAC (methotrexate, vinblastine, adriamycin and cisplatin) for invasive bladder cancer. Proc Am Soc Clin Oncol 7: C-466

Scher HI, Herr H, Sternberg CN et al. (1989) Neo-adjuvant chemotherapy for invasive bladder cancer: experience with the M-VAC regimen. Br J Urol (in press)

Schilman CC, Wespes E, Delcour C, Struyven J (1985) Intra-arterial chemotherapy of infiltrative bladder carcinoma. Eur Urol 11: 220–223

Schwartz S, Yagoda A, Natale RB et al. (1983) Phase II trial of sequentially administered cisplatin cyclophosphamide and doxorubicin for urothelial tract tumors. J Urol 130: 681–684

Shipley WU, Rose MA (1985) Bladder cancer: the selection of patients for full-dose irradiation. Cancer 55: 2278–2284

Shipley WU, Coombs LH, Einstein AB et al. (1984) Cisplatin and full dose irradiation for patients with invasive bladder carcinoma: a preliminary report of tolerance and local response. J Urol 132: 899–903

Shipley WU, Rose MA, Perrone T et al. (1985) Full-dose irradiation for patients with invasive bladder carcinoma: clinical and histological factors prognostic of improved survival. J Urol 134: 679–683

Shipley WU, Kaufman, SD Prout GR (1986) Combined chemotherapy and full dose irradiation in the treatment of patients with locally advanced bladder cancer. In: Yagoda A (ed) Bladder cancer: future directions for treatment, John Wiley, New York, pp 123–131

Shipley WU, Prout GR, Kaufman D, Perrone TL (1987a) Invasive bladder carcinoma: the importance of initial transurethral surgery and other significant prognostic factors for improved survival with full-dose irradiation. Cancer 60 [Suppl 4a]: 514–520

Shipley WU, Prout GR, Einstein AB et al. (1987b) Treatment of invasive bladder cancer by cisplatin and radiation in patients unsuited for surgery. JAMA 258: 931–935

Silverberg E (1985) Cancer Statistics. Cancer 35: 19–32

Simon SD, Srougi M (1986) Systemic M-VAC chemotherapy for primary treatment of locally invasive transitional cell carcinoma of the bladder (TCCB): a pilot study. Proc Am Soc Clin Oncol 5: 111

Skinner DG, Lieskovsky G (1984) Contemporary cystectomy with pelvic node dissection compared to preoperative radiation therapy plus cystectomy in the management of invasive bladder cancer. J Urol 131: 1069–1072

Skinner DG, Lieskovsky G (1988) Management of invasive high-grade bladder cancer. In: Skinner DG, Lieskovsky G (eds) Diagnosis and management of genitourinary cancer. W. B. Saunders Co, Philadelphia pp 295–312

Skinner DG, Tift JP, Kaufman JJ (1982) High dose, short course preoperative radiation therapy and immediate single stage radical cystectomy with pelvic node dissection in the management of bladder cancer. J Urol 127: 671–674

Smith JA, Whitmore WF (1981) Regional lymph node metastasis from bladder cancer. J Urol 126: 591–595

Splinter TAW, Schroder FH, Denis L et al. (1987) A phase II study of neoadjuvant chemotherapy in T3-4N0M0 transitional cell carcinoma of the bladder: a preliminary analysis. Presented at the Second Herner Warner Stiftung Symposium. 5 November, Hamburg, Germany

Splinter TAW, Denis L, Scher HI et al. (1989) Neoadjuvant chemotherapy of invasive bladder cancer: the prognostic value of local tumor response. In: Murphy GP, Khoury D (eds) International symposium in the therapeutic progress in urologic cancers. Alan R Liss, New York (in press)

Steel GG (1983) The combination of radiotherapy and chemotherapy. Steel, Adams & Peckham (eds). The biological Basis of Radiotherapy. New York, Elsevier Science Publisher, 1983, pp 239–248

Sternberg C, Scher H (1987) Advances in the treatment of urothelial tract tumors. Urol Clin North Am 14: 373–387

Sternberg C, Yagoda A, Scher H et al. (1985) Preliminary results of methotrexate, vinblastine, adriamycin and cisplatin (M-VAC) in advanced urothelial tumors. J Urol 133: 403–407

Sternberg CN, Yagoda A, Scher HI et al. (1988) M-VAC (methotrexate, vinblastine, adriamycin and cisplatin) for advanced transitional cell carcinoma of the urothelium. J Urol 139: 462–469

Stoter G, Splinter TAW, Child JA et al. (1987) Combination chemotherapy with cisplatin and methotrexate in advanced transitional cell cancer of the bladder. J Urol 137: 663–667

Timmer PR, Hartlief HA, Hooijkaas JAP (1985) Bladder cancer: pattern of recurrence in 142 patients. Int J Rad Oncol Biol Phys 11: 899–905

Torti FM, Phillips TL, Lum BL et al. (1986) Effect of preoperative cisplatin (CDDP) and radiation therapy (XRT) on downstaging of invasive bladder cancer: A NCOG study. Proc Am Soc Clin Oncol 5: 103

Troner MB, Birch R, Omura GA, Williams S (1987) Phase III comparison of cisplatin alone versus cisplatin, doxorubicin and cyclophosphamide in the treatment of bladder (urothelial) cancer: A Southeastern Cancer Study Group Trial. J Urol 137: 660–662

Utz DC, Schmidtz SE, Fugelso PD, Farrow GM (1973) A clinicopathologic evaluation of partial cystectomy for carcinoma of the urinary bladder. Cancer 32: 1075–1077

Van der Werf-Messing B (1975) Carcinoma of the bladder T3NXM0 treated by preoperative irradiation followed by cystectomy. Third report of the Rotterdam Radiotherapy Institute. Cancer 36: 718–722

Van der Werf-Messing B (1984) Carcinoma of the urinary bladder treated by interstitial radiotherapy. Urol Clin North Am 11: 659–670

Van Oosterom AT, Akaza H, Hall R et al. (1986) Response criteria phase II/phase III invasive bladder cancer. In: Denis L, Niijima T, Prout G, Schroder FH (eds) Developments in bladder cancer. New York, Alan R. Liss, Inc. pp 301–310 (EORTC Genitourinary Group Monograph 3)

Wallace DH, Bloom HJG (1976) The management of deeply infiltrating (T3) bladder carcinoma: controlled trial of radical radiotherapy versus preoperative radiotherapy and radical cystectomy (first report). Br J Urol 48: 587–594

Whitmore WF (1979) Management of bladder cancer. Current Problems in Cancer 4: 1–44

Whitmore WF (1980) Integrated irradiation and cystectomy for bladder cancer. Br J Urol 52: 1–9

Whitmore WF (1983) Management of invasive bladder neoplasms. Semin Urol 1: 4–10

Whitmore WF (1986) Bladder cancer: future directions in management. In: Yagoda A (ed) Bladder
    cancer: future directions for treatment. John Wiley and Sons, New York, pp 159–163
Whitmore WF, Batata M (1984) Status of integrated irradiation and cystectomy for bladder cancer.
    Urol Clin North Am 11: 681–691
Whitmore WF, Batata MA, Ghoneim MA et al. (1977) Radical cystectomy with or without prior
    irradiation in the treatment of bladder cancer. J Urol 118: 184–187
Winfield HN, Reddy PK, Lange PH (1987) Coexisting adenocarcinoma of the prostate in patients
    undergoing cystoprostatectomy for bladder cancer. Urology 30: 100–102
Wolf H, Kakizoe T, Smith PH et al. (1986) Bladder tumors: treated natural history. In: Denis L,
    Niijima N, Prout G, Schroder F (eds) Developments in bladder cancer. Alan R. Liss, New York,
    pp 223–255 (EORTC Genitourinary Group Monograph 3)
Yagoda A (1985) Progress in treatment of advanced urothelial tract tumors. J Clin Oncol 3: 1448–
    1450
Yagoda A (1987) Chemotherapy of urothelial tract tumors. Cancer 60: 574–585
Zincke H, Sen SE, Hahn RG, Keating JP (1988) Neo-adjuvant chemotherapy (M-VAC) for locally
    advanced ($T_{2-4}N_0M_0$) transitional cell carcinoma (TCC) of the bladder: do local findings suggest a
    potential for bladder salvage. Mayo Clinic Proc 63: 16–22

Chapter 7

Carcinoma of the Prostate – Non-metastatic Disease

F.S. Freiha

Introduction

The prostate gland is the second most common site of cancer in American men and ranks third in several Western European countries (Segi et al. 1969). In 1988, approximately 99 000 new cases of prostate cancer will be diagnosed in the United States and approximately 28 000 men will die from it (Silverberg and Lubern 1988). It is a disease of ageing men and with the increasing age of the male population worldwide, prostate cancer is expected to become a major public health issue.

Before recommending treatment to a patient with clinically localised prostate cancer, the urologist must try to answer two questions:

1. How much cancer does the patient have
2. Which treatment, if any, will favourably influence survival with the least possible morbidity

We shall present evidence to show that tumour volume influences the behaviour of prostate cancer and that new imaging modalities and biochemical testing will help the urologist assess the extent of disease more accurately than is possible at present. We shall also present results of the different treatments available to the patient with localised disease and the morbidity associated with each in order to shed some light on the controversy surrounding the management of prostate cancer.

Natural History

It is a common belief that the natural history of prostate cancer is variable and unpredictable. Emerging knowledge is changing this belief. Volume distribution data and morphometric studies show that, unlike other carcinomas in which small tumours have the same histological features as their larger counterparts, adenocarcinoma of the prostate undergoes loss of differentiation as it increases in size (McNeal et al. 1986). If malignant behaviour can be measured by the capacity of a tumour to penetrate the capsule, invade the seminal vesicles and metastasise to regional lymph nodes, then as prostate cancer grows and dedifferentiates, its malignant potential increases.

Morphometric Studies in Prostate Cancer

Morphometric reconstructions of radical prostatectomy specimens show a correlation between cancer volume and grade and the malignant behaviour of prostate cancer.

One hundred and thirty consecutive radical prostatectomy specimens were studied by the step-section technique. After fixation in 37% formalin, the gland was serially sectioned at 3-mm intervals perpendicular to the rectal surface and separated into right and left halves. Sections were embedded into paraffin, cut 7 microns thick and stained with haematoxylin and eosin.

The grade of cancer was determined according to the Gleason Classification (Gleason 1977) and the percentage of each primary histological pattern in every tumour was recorded.

Capsular penetration, defined as the extension of tumour through the prostatic capsule into the periprostatic tissues, was quantitated by measuring the extent of tumour involvement along the prostatic capsule in linear centimetres.

Cancer volume was determined by outlining the tumour on every slide, calculating its surface area with the use of a Compaq computer and multiplying that by the section thickness. To correct for tissue shrinkage caused by fixation, the sum total was multiplied by a factor of 1.5.

Tumour Grade

As primary tumours increase in size the percentage of the more undifferentiated primary histological patterns, Gleason patterns 4 and 5, increases.

The mean cancer volume for 34 tumours without Gleason patterns 4 and 5 was 1.44 ml and for 96 tumours with any amount of Gleason patterns 4 or 5 was 7.36 ml. As tumours increase in volume the percentage of Gleason patterns 4 or 5 increases proportionately (Fig. 7.1). Moreover, tumour grade and percentage of the more undifferentiated patterns correlate very well with the malignant behaviour of prostate cancer (Table 7.1).

Capsular Penetration

The mean cancer volume for 64 cases without capsular penetration was 2.48 ml

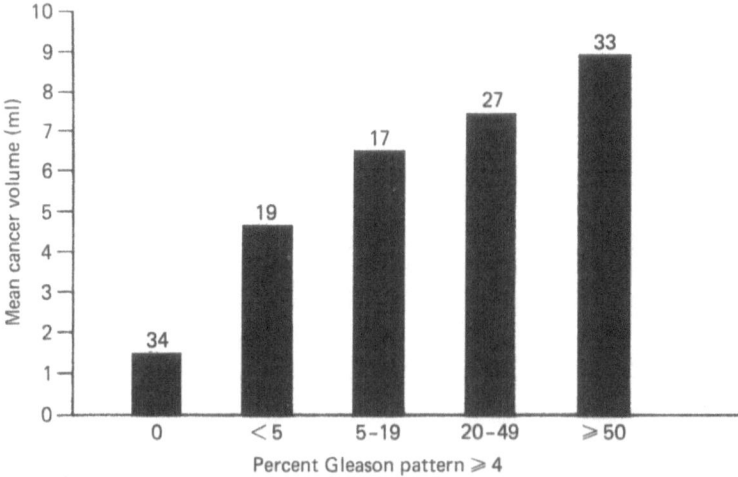

Fig. 7.1. Correlation between mean cancer volume and the percentage Gleason histological pattern 4 or more in 130 consecutive radical prostatectomy specimens. The number above each bar is the total number of cases in each category.

Table 7.1. Tumour grade and malignant behaviour of prostate cancer

Percentage Gleason pattern ≥ 4	No.	Capsular penetration		Seminal vesicle invasion		Lymph node metastasis	
		No.	%	No.	%	No.	%
0	34	4[a]	12	1	3	0	0
<5	19	6	32	1	5	0	0
5–19	17	9	53	2	12	0	0
20–49	27	18	67	9	33	4	15
≥50	33	29	88	14	42	13	39

[a] All less than 1 cm.

and for 66 cases with capsular penetration was 8.99 ml (Table 7.2). Capsular penetration and its extent also correlate well with the incidence of seminal vesicle invasion and lymph node metastasis. Of the 64 patients without capsular penetration only one had seminal vesicle invasion and none had lymph node metastasis. Of the 66 cases of capsular penetration, 14 had seminal vesicle invasion and 17 had lymph node metastasis (Table 7.3).

Table 7.2. Cancer volume and capsular penetration

Capsular penetration	No.	Mean cancer volume (ml)
Absent	64	2.48
		$P=0.0001$
Present	66	8.99

Table 7.3. Capsular penetration and incidence of seminal vesicle invasion and lymph node metastasis

Capsular penetration	No.	Seminal vesicle invasion	Lymph node metastasis
Absent	64	1 (1.5%)	0 (0%)
Present	66	14 (21%)	17 (26%)

Of the 66 cases of capsular penetration, 18 had less and 48 had more than 1 cm. Of the 18 with less than 1-cm capsular penetration, only one had seminal vesicle invasion and none had lymph node metastasis. Of the 48 with more than 1-cm capsular penetration 13 had seminal vesicle invasion and 17 had lymph node metastasis (Table 7.4).

Table 7.4. Extent of capsular penetration and incidence of seminal vesicle invasion and lymph node metastasis

Capsular penetration	No.	Seminal vesicle invasion	Lymph node metastasis
<1 cm	18	1 (6%)	0 (0%)
>1 cm	48	13 (27%)	17 (35%)

Cancer Volume, Lymph Node Metastasis and Seminal Vesicle Invasion

The mean cancer volume for 98 cases without seminal vesicle invasion or lymph node metastasis was 3.67 ml and, for 32 cases with seminal vesicle invasion and/or lymph node metastasis, 12.32 ml. The largest volumes were seen in patients with both seminal vesicle invasion and lymph node metastasis (Table 7.5). Thirty five of the 98 cases without seminal vesicle invasion or lymph node metastasis also had capsular penetration and their mean volume was 5.74 ml compared to 2.52 ml for the 63 cases without capsular penetration (Table 7.5).

Table 7.5. Cancer volume and malignant behaviour of prostate cancer

	No.	Mean cancer volume (ml)
Negative nodes Negative seminal vesicles No capsular penetration	63	2.52
Negative nodes' Negative seminal vesicles Capsular penetration	35	5.74
Negative nodes Negative seminal vesicles	98	3.67
Positive nodes Positive seminal vesicles	12	17.84
Positive nodes Negative seminal vesicles	5	9.08
Negative nodes Positive seminal vesicles	15	8.99

The results of these morphometric studies support the belief that poorly-differentiated prostate cancers evolve from well-differentiated cancers with the passage of time and increase in tumour volume. This loss of differentiation with growth and the correlation of that with malignant behaviour make prostate cancer and its natural history one of the most predictable of all human cancers.

Diagnosis and Staging

Patients with localised prostate cancer may be asymptomatic at the time of diagnosis or may have symptoms of bladder outlet obstruction. Diagnosis is suspected by rectal examination and confirmed by needle biopsy or aspiration cytology. Occasionally the diagnosis is incidentally made when tissue removed by transurethral or open prostatectomy, performed for obstruction symptoms, is found to have cancer.

Bone scans, chest and bone radiographs and serum phosphatase determinations detect or rule out metastasis and rectal examination has been, until recently, the only reliable method to assess the extent of local disease. Morphometric studies have taught us that tumour volume is a critical determinant of the malignant behaviour of prostate cancer and correlates well with tumour grade, extent of capsular penetration, seminal vesicle invasion and lymph node metastasis. Of all these variables, tumour volume is the only one that is potentially measurable preoperatively. Therefore, in order to measure volume and extent of local disease more accurately than is possible with rectal examination alone, imaging modalities and biochemical tests are being developed and their accuracy tested (Fig. 7.2).

Transrectal ultrasound

Transrectal sonography in the axial and sagittal projections allows for the complete assessment of the prostate gland and its relation to its capsule, the seminal vesicles and the bladder neck.

Cancer on sonograms is hypoechoic compared to normal or hypertrophied prostatic parenchyma. In a comparative study of preoperative transrectal ultrasound and histological reconstruction of 23 radical prostatectomy specimens performed at Stanford, transrectal ultrasound detected 15 of 23 cancers (65%). Of posteriorly located cancers 13 of 14 (93%) were detected and five of these (36%) showed an excellent match between the reconstructed volume of cancer and the volume of the hypoechoic areas. Only two of nine anteriorly and anterolaterally located cancers were detected.

Transrectal ultrasound cannot detect microscopic capsular penetration even when this extends for several centimetres along the capsule. Moreover, distortion, compression or obliteration of the seminal vesicles on ultrasound is seen only when the seminal vesicles are massively involved with tumour.

Transrectal ultrasound is an imaging modality which is still in its infancy. As we gather more experience with it and as the technology improves, its accuracy is apt

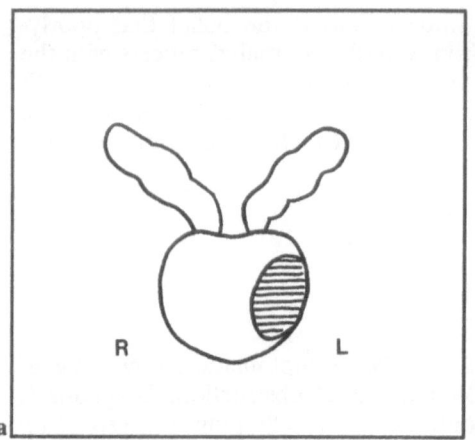
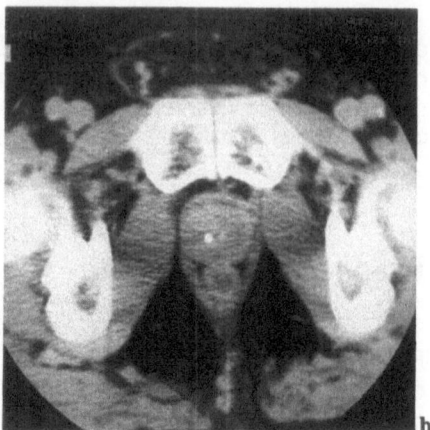

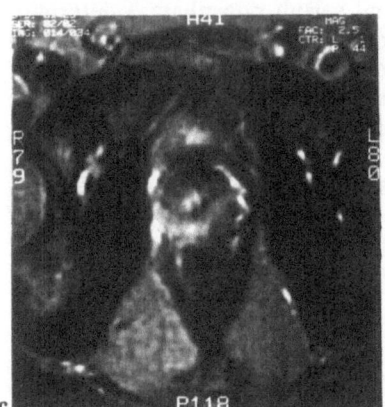
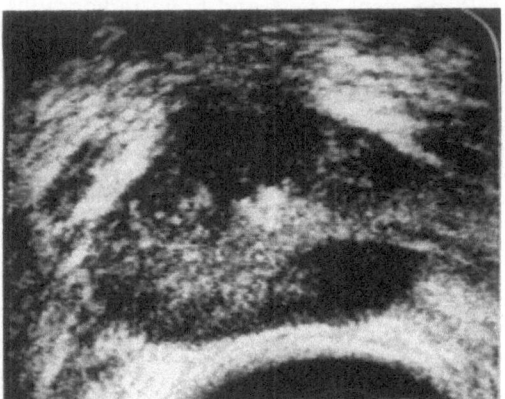

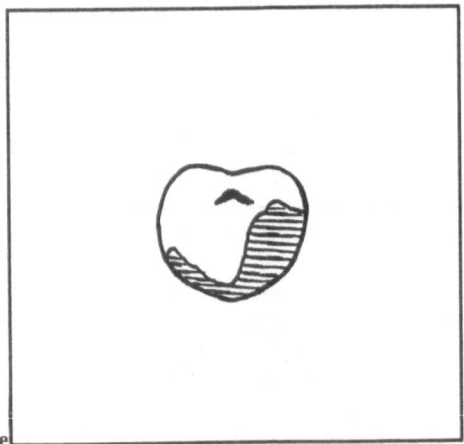

Fig. 7.2a–e. Findings on rectal examination, different imaging techniques and pathological reconstruction of a radical prostatectomy specimen. **a.** Findings on rectal examination. **b.** CT scan which fails to show any intraprostatic pathology. **c.** MRI showing a defect in the left peripheral prostate only. **d.** Transrectal ultrasound showing hypoechoic regions in both left and right peripheral zones which match the site of cancer shown on the pathological reconstruction, **e.**

to improve and its use as a screening test becomes more meaningful. At present, the sensitivity of transrectal ultrasound ranges between 62% and 65% (Hamper et al. 1986; Dahnert et al. 1986). Its specificity is even lower (Abu-Yousef and Narayan 1985; Pontes et al. 1985); however, it is an excellent modality for a guided biopsy when abnormalities are seen on sonogram.

Computed Axial Tomography (CT)

The value of computed tomography (CT) in staging prostate cancer is possibly to identify and measure the extent of tumour spread beyond the capsule, involvement of adjacent organs such as the bladder, and metastasis to pelvic and para-aortic lymph nodes. It has no value in confirming the presence or absence of disease or in volume measurement (Fig. 7.2).

CT criteria of lymphadenopathy are limited to size only. Carcinoma in normal-sized lymph nodes cannot be detected by CT because of its insufficient soft tissue resolution. Enlarged lymph nodes are suspected of harbouring metastatic carcinoma and confirmation by biopsy or fine needle aspiration remains necessary. The sensitivity of CT scans ranges between 50% and 75% and the specificity between 86% and 100% (Shankar et al. 1982; Golimbu et al. 1981; Morgan et al. 1981). Its accuracy is about 85%.

Magnetic Resonance Imaging (MRI)

Magnetic resonance imaging (MRI) exhibits excellent tissue contrast as compared to CT scans and is able to detect intraprostatic pathology and to show the different anatomical zones of the prostate. Its sensitivity in detecting cancer, however, is not very high. In a comparative study of preoperative MRI and histological reconstruction of 15 radical prostatectomy specimens, MRI detected 11 of 15 cancers (73%): all were posteriorly located. The correlation between the volume as measured by MRI and the reconstructed volume was poor. Its specificity is even lower, making it unsuitable for screening.

The ability of MRI to scan in three different planes, axial, sagittal and coronal makes it valuable for the assessment of extracapsular extension. Its accuracy in staging ranges between 83% and 89% (Ling et al. 1986; Biondetti et al. 1987; Hricak et al. 1987). Its ability to detect lymph node metastasis is similar to that of CT scans.

Prostate Specific Antigen (PSA)

Acid phosphatase is one of the first tumour markers ever described and, until recently, has been the only marker for prostate cancer. Methods of its determination, however, lack specificity and sensitivity.

Prostate specific antigen (PSA) is now the marker for prostate cancer. In a recent study conducted at Stanford University (Stamey et al. 1987), PSA and prostatic acid phosphatase (PAP), both determined by radioimmunoassay, were compared in 2000 serum samples from 600 patients, 240 of whom had prostate cancer. PSA was elevated in 122 of 127 (96%) prostate cancer patients including 58% of clinical stage A (T_0) patients and 100% of clinical stages B to D (T_1–T_4) patients. PAP was elevated in only 57 (45%) patients including none of the stage A patients, 9% of B1, 39% of B2, 40% of B3, 64% of C and 96% of patients with metastatic disease.

PSA correlates very well with tumour volume and its level drops to zero following radical prostatectomy when the disease is limited to the prostate and is completely excised. It is an excellent test for monitoring response to therapy and allows for adjuvant pelvic irradiation in patients with persistently elevated, or reappearance of detectable, levels of PSA.

PSA is organ-specific but not tumour-specific. Benign prostatic hyperplasia elevates serum PSA thereby preventing its use for screening.

Staging of the Lymphatic System

Imaging with CT scan and magnetic resonance rely upon nodal enlargement to detect adenopathy. Lymph node metastasis in patients with localised disease is often not macroscopic and does not change the size of nodes to make them detectable by CT scans and MRI.

Lymphangiography

Bipedal lymphograms display size, position and architecture of pelvic and para-aortic lymph nodes to the level of the renal hila. The advantage over CT scans and MRI is the ability to detect structural abnormalities in lymph nodes that are still normal in size.

The accuracy of lymphograms was studied in 132 patients who had complete and evaluable studies followed by lymph node biopsies (Table 7.6). The overall accuracy was 74%. The true-positive rate was 71%. The false-positive rate was 37% and the false-negative rate, 18%. These relatively high rates of false positives and false negatives limit the use of lymphangiography, an invasive test, in the routine evaluation of patients with localised prostate cancer.

Table 7.6. Correlation between lymphographic interpretations and results of lymph node biopsy in 132 patients with clinically localised prostate cancer

Lymphographic interpretation	Lymph node biopsy result		
	Negative	Positive	Total
Negative	64	14	78
Positive	20	34	54
Total	84	48	132

False-negative results are due either to microscopic metastasis or to total replacement of the node preventing it from taking up the contrast material. False-positive results are due to fatty replacements of nodal tissue, a common finding in older men, which causes a filling defect radiologically indistinguishable from metastatic disease.

Pelvic Lymphadenectomy

Pelvic lymphadenectomy is the most accurate method of detecting lymph node metastasis. It is a surgical staging procedure and has no therapeutic value. It is employed whenever a therapeutic decision will depend on the status of the lymph nodes and is routinely done prior to retropubic radical prostatectomy.

In 200 consecutive pelvic lymphadenectomies performed by the author prior to radical prostatectomy or radiation therapy where gross examination of the lymph nodes failed to reveal any abnormalities, and where frozen section examination was not done because the lymph nodes were felt to be normal, 11 patients were subsequently found, on permanent sections, to have lymph node metastasis, all microscopic and involving only 1 or 2 lymph nodes. This is a false-negative rate of 6%.

Is pelvic lymphadenectomy always necessary? By combining the clinical stage of the local tumour and its grade and the level of serum acid phosphatase, it is possible to identify groups of patients with low risk and groups with high risk for lymph node metastasis and spare them the procedure (Freiha et al. 1979). Table 7.7 shows that patients with localised disease (stages A, B1 and B2) and a Gleason pathological score of 8 or less and a normal acid phosphatase are at a very low risk of having lymph node metastasis. On the other hand, patients with bulky local disease (stages B3 and C), a Gleason score of 9 or 10 and an elevated serum acid phosphatase are at a very high risk of having lymph node metastasis. These two groups of patients can be spared pelvic lymphadenectomy. The majority of the patients, however, will fall in the intermediate risk category and may need pelvic lymphadenectomy prior to institution of therapy.

Table 7.7. Correlation between clinical stage, tumour grade, serum acid phosphatase and incidence of lymph node metastasis in 146 surgically staged patients with prostate cancer

Clinical stage	Gleason score	Serum acid phosphatase[1] levels in patients with positive nodes			
		Normal No.	%	Elevated No.	%
A, B1, B2	3–8	0/13	0	1/12	8
B3, C	3–5	0/5	0	0/1	0 LOW RISK
B3, C	6–8	10/28	36	32/65	49
B3, C	9–10	1/5	20	17/17	100 HIGH RISK

[1] Ratio indicates number of patients with positive nodes over total number of patients in subgroup

The serum PSA level is also helpful in predicting the likelihood of lymph node metastasis. Table 7.8 shows that patients with PSA levels of less than 15 ng/ml have a 2% chance of having lymph node metastasis compared to 63% of patients with PSA levels of more than 40 ng/ml.

Table 7.8. Serum prostate specific antigen (PSA) and incidence of lymph node metastasis in 68 patients undergoing radical prostatectomy

PSA (ng/ml)	No.	Lymph node metastasis	
		No.	%
<15	41	1	2
15–40	29	6	21
>40	8	5	63

Treatment

Hormonal therapy, radiation therapy and radical prostatectomy are accepted forms of therapy for patients with localised prostate cancer but the uncertainties surrounding their relative efficacy lead to controversy. The reasons for these uncertainties are many:

1. Prostate cancer occurs at an age when many different causes compete for the death of a patient. Many prostate cancer patients die with it rather than from it.
2. Randomised, controlled studies comparing the result of the various forms of therapy to each other and to no treatment are lacking.
3. The disease has a long natural evolution and it requires many years of follow-up before the efficacy of any form of therapy can be evaluated.
4. The available data from different treatment modalities are highly selective and inadequate for comparison because of lack of uniformity in staging, classification and response criteria.

External Beam Radiation Therapy

The Stanford University experience with surgically staged, uniformly treated patients with prostate cancer followed for from 9 to 16 years will serve as an excellent example of the value of extended-field radiation therapy in node-positive and node-negative patients. The Stanford method of treating patients with clinically localised prostate cancer is commonly employed all over the United States and the results of such treatment are uniform.

Between 1957 and 1977, 430 patients with prostate cancer were treated in the Division of Radiation Therapy at Stanford with irradiation to the prostate and the immediately adjacent periprostatic tissues. The 10-year disease-free survival for 230 men with disease limited to the prostate was 44% and for 200 men with extracapsular extension, 38%. To improve these results and to determine whether irradiation of known areas of lymph node metastasis will improve survival, an extended-field radiation therapy protocol was started in 1971.

The Stanford Protocol

Patients with clinically localised prostate cancer were surgically staged with pelvic lymphadenectomy and sampling of the low para-aortic lymph nodes and were assigned treatment in a randomised fashion according to the results of staging.

Patients with disease limited to the prostate were randomised to receive either prostatic irradiation only or prostatic and pelvic irradiation. When only the pelvic nodes were involved, patients were randomised to receive either prostatic and pelvic irradiation only or prostatic, pelvic and para-aortic irradiation. Patients with para-aortic lymphadenopathy received prostatic, pelvic and para-aortic irradiation. Radiation treatments were designed to deliver a total of 7000 rads to the prostate and 5000 rads to the regional lymph nodes over a period of seven weeks. Treatment was started 3 to 4 weeks following operation (Pistenma et al. 1979).

One hundred and forty-six patients were entered into the study. Table 7.9 shows the distribution according to the initial clinical stage based on digital rectal examination. The last patient finished treatment in August 1978. One hundred and forty patients were followed for 10 to 16 years or until death, and 6 have been followed for 9 years.

Table 7.9. Clinical stage based on digital rectal examination in 146 patients entered into the Stanford extended field radiation therpay protocol

Stage	Definition	No.
A1	No palpable tumour Incidental finding of cancer in surgical specimen Less than 5% of specimen involved by cancer	0
A2	Same as A1 except that more than 5% of specimen is involved by cancer	5
B1	Solitary nodule less than 1 cm in diameter surrounded by normal prostatic tissue (Jewett Nodule)	3
B2	Palpable tumour more than 1 cm in diameter but still confined to one lobe	17
B3	Palpable tumour in both lobes	50
C	Palpable tumour extending beyond the prostatic capsule and/or invading the seminal vesicles	71

Results

Survival. The overall incidence of lymph node metastasis was 42%. The more advanced the local disease, the higher the incidence of lymphatic spread (Table 7.10). Clinical stage and the status of lymph nodes were important determinants of disease-free survival.

Sixty of the 146 patients (41%) are alive, 41 (28%) without evidence of disease and 19 (13%) with disease (Table 7.11).

Of the 84 patients without lymphatic metastasis, 50 (60%) are alive, 40 (48%) without evidence of disease and 10 (12%) with disease. Only one patient (2%) of the 62 with positive nodes is alive without evidence of disease (Table 7.12). He finished treatment in June 1978. Nine patients with positive nodes are alive with disease, 45 died of prostatic cancer and seven died of unrelated causes, two of

Table 7.10. Clinical stage and incidence of lymph node metastasis in 146 surgically staged patients with prostate cancer

Clinical stage	No.	Lymph node metastasis	
		No.	%
A2	5	0	0
B1	3	0	0
B2	17	1	6
B3	50	21	42
C	71	40	56
Total	146	62	42

Table 7.11. Survival according to clinical stage

Clinical stage	No.	Alive without disease	Alive with disease
A2	5	3 (60%)	0 (0%)
B1	3	3 (100%)	0 (0%)
B2	17	9 (53%)	5 (29%)
B3	50	15 (30%)	5 (10%)
C	71	11 (15%)	9 (13%)
Total	146	41 (28%)	19 (13%)

whom had no clinical evidence of disease at the time of death. The average time-to-failure, defined as the time interval between end of therapy and first appearance of metastasis, of patients with positive nodes was 35 months with a range of one to 135 months. Twenty five patients failed within two years, 46 within five years and 11 after 5 years. The average time-to-failure of 30 patients without lymphatic metastasis was 60 months with a range of nine to 147 months. Four patients failed within 2 years, 15 within 5 years and 15 after 5 years.

Table 7.12. Survival according to lymph node status

Lymph nodes	No.	Alive without disease	Alive with disease
Negative	84	40 (48%)	10 (12%)
Positive	62	1 (2%)	9 (15%)

The fact that almost all patients with lymph node metastasis failed to survive free of disease indicates that irradiating regions of lymphatic involvement as well as irradiating the next group of uninvolved lymph nodes has no benefit.

Of the 25 patients with stages A2, B1 and B2 disease who would normally be candidates for radical prostatectomy, 15 (60%) are alive without evidence of disease 9 to 16 years after end of therapy. Patients with bulky local disease which is still confined to within the prostatic capsule (B3) have a 30% chance of surviving for 10 years without evidence of disease. For patients with any stage B disease the probability of surviving 10 years without evidence of disease is 40%.

Patients with extracapsular or seminal vesicle tumour extension (stage C) have a 15% 10-year disease-free survival.

Bagshaw (1987) recently updated the results of external beam radiation therapy in over 900 patients treated at Stanford since 1956. Approximately one-half of the patients had stage A or B disease and their actuarial survival according to the Kaplan–Meier calculations is as follows: 81% at 5 years, 60% at 10 years and 35% at 15 years. Of 204 patients at risk for 15 years, 11 were lost to follow-up and 55 were alive, making the observed, actual 15-year survival, 28%. The actuarial survival of patients with stage C disease is 61% at 5 years, 36% at 10 years and 18% at 15 years (Bagshaw 1987).

Recently, Shipley et al. (1987) reported on the Massachusetts General Hospital experience with radiation therapy in localised prostate cancer (1987). Twenty two per cent of 164 patients with stage B disease and 63% of 206 patients with stage C disease developed distant metastases within a period of 8 years after therapy.

Local Control. Histopathological information on the irradiated prostate is available in 77 of the 146 patients treated at Stanford: 68 specimens were obtained by perineal needle biopsy, six by transurethral resection and four at autopsy, all two or more years after the end of therapy. Fifty-two patients (68%) had positive biopsy and 25 (32%) had negative biopsy (Table 7.13).

Table 7.13. Results of postirradiation biopsy according to clinical stage of primary tumour

Clinical stage	No. patients biopsied	Positive biopsy	
		No.	%
A2	1	0	0
B1	2	1	50
B2	10	5	50
B3	23	14	61
C	41	32	78
Total	77	52	68

Ten patients (40%) with negative biopsy are alive without evidence of metastatic disease. Of the 8 patients with negative biopsy who died of prostate cancer, 5 had lymph node metastasis at initial staging.

Seven patients (13%) with positive biopsy are alive without metastatic disease. Two of the seven were treated with interstitial irradiation for local recurrence and are now 8 and 10 years after that therapy, respectively. They remain free of distant metastases. The remaining 5 patients are on diethylstilboestrol for local control. Thirty patients with positive biopsy died of prostatic cancer (Freiha and Bagshaw 1984).

Clinical local control was reported by Shipley who found tumour regrowth in 8% of stage B disease and 29% of stage C disease within a period of 8 years after therapy (Shipley et al. 1987).

Complications. The majority of the complications encountered in the Stanford series (146 patients) were due to the combination of lymphadenectomy followed by irradiation. Radiation enteritis requiring hospitalisation occurred in 17 patients, 9 of whom required operation. Fourteen of the 17 incidents of radiation enteritis and 8 of the 9 requiring operation occurred early in the course of the protocol when the intraperitoneal approach to the lymph nodes was used. After the intraperitoneal approach was abandoned and extraperitoneal lymphadenectomy adopted and performed in the last 100 patients, radiation enteritis occurred in 3 patients, one of whom required operation (Freiha and Salzman 1977).

Penile, scrotal or lower extremity lymphoedema, or any combination of these, occurred in half of the patients: however, it was transient in the majority. Permanent lymphoedema was observed in 4% of the patients.

Lymphocele requiring percutaneous drainage occurred in 6% of patients. Stricture disease was observed in 4 patients, all of whom had had transurethral resection prior to initiation of radiation therapy. Incontinence was observed in 3 patients, occurring many years after therapy secondary to local recurrence of tumour and involvement of the urogenital diaphragm.

Significant radiation cystitis with recurrent gross haematuria occurred in 4 patients.

Impotence was reported by 38% of the men who were potent prior to initiation of therapy.

Tolerance to external beam irradiation therapy without prior lymphadenectomy was analysed by Shipley et al. (1987) in 121 consecutively treated men in 1980 and 1981. These patients received 5040 cGy to the pelvic lymph nodes below the common iliac artery bifurcation and a total of 6480 cGy to 6840 cGy to the prostate. Intestinal and genitourinary complications occurred in 21% and 23% of patients, respectively and resolved in all except 7%. One patient developed severe radiation cystitis with bleeding necessitating cystectomy. Ten patients developed urethral strictures or bladder neck contracture and 9 were corrected by transurethral operation. The overall incidence of stricture disease was 8.3%. However, the incidence was 14% in patients who had transurethral prostatectomy prior to irradiation. The incidence of stricture in patients without prior resection was 1.7%. Impotence was reported in 37% of men who were potent at diagnosis.

Gastrointestinal complications manifested by diarrhoea persisting up to 4 months following radiation therapy or rectal bleeding occurred in 12% of men. An additional 9% of patients required treatment of these complications. They eventually subsided in all but 8 patients: 4 have persistent diarrhoea and 4 have infrequent episodes of rectal bleeding. No patient required operation for intestinal complications.

Interstitial Radiation

Interstitial radiation is among the oldest forms of therapy for prostate cancer. Initially developed in the early 1900s with the introduction of radium, interstitial therapy at that time competed only with radical prostatectomy as treatment for this disease. Enthusiasm for radiation waned in the 1940s and 1950s with the development of hormonal therapy. It was rekindled with the advent of megavoltage external beam therapy in the early 1960s. Since then, the relatively high incidence of rectal and bladder complications with external beam therapy coupled with reports of success with interstitial injection of radioactive gold, has led to investigation of other forms of radiation treatment. The three best studied isotopes are radioactive iodine (^{125}I), iridium (^{192}Ir), and gold (^{198}Au).

Current criteria for treatment require that the intraprostatic or extracapsular tumour burden be small, ideally less than 5 cm in largest diameter. When combined with external beam radiation therapy, the technique is applicable to stage B, C, or D1 tumours. The high recurrence rate and the technical difficulty in placing seeds limit its use for stage A2 cancer. All the methods of interstitial radiation share similar complications, the most severe being rectourethral fistula, proctitis and thromboembolism. All, however, have the expected advantage of delivering radiation to a field limited to the site of tumour, thereby reducing overall morbidity compared to radical surgery or external beam radiation.

Gold Radiotherapy

Although interstitial gold radiotherapy was the first form of high energy radiation treatment for prostate cancer (Flocks 1969) its use has been limited because of the difficulty in administering it safely. The first reports described injection of gold colloid. However, difficulty in dosimetry and distribution in the prostate led to the development of seeds (Flocks 1969; Guerriero et al. 1979; Scardino et al. 1982). ^{198}Au is a high energy beta and gamma emitter. Currently, seeds have a coating that blocks beta emission. Its half-value layer is 4.5 cm and half-life is only 2.7 days. Intraoperatively, six to ten seeds are placed in a cluster at the site of the tumour. They deliver 3000 rads to the prostatic and periprostatic tissues over 3 weeks. If the pelvic lymph nodes are positive at lymphadenectomy, supplemental external beam radiation is given to the pelvis.

The advantages of ^{198}Au therapy are that it involves fewer punctures of the prostate than ^{125}I, the half-life is short, allowing for safe and accurate dosing for supplemental external beam therapy, and transurethral resection of the prostate can be safely performed, if necessary, six weeks after treatment (Scardino et al. 1982). The greatest radiation risk is to the hands of the operating surgeon. Guerriero (1979) reports late complications including 12% mild and 4% severe proctitis; 14% mild and 3% severe cystitis; 2% rectal stenosis, and 3% impotence. There was no incontinence in 532 patients studied by Scardino (1982). Genital and leg oedema was 10% and lymphocele less than 2%. Disease-free survival at 10 years is 54% for stage B1 lesions, 26% for stage B2 lesions and 44% for stage C lesions. There was a 0% 10-year disease-free survival for stage A2 and D1 patients.

Iodine Radiotherapy

^{125}I has enjoyed great popularity in the treatment of localised prostate cancer and metastatic nodal disease when combined with external beam therapy. It has also been used as a form of salvage treatment for failures with external beam therapy (Goffinet et al. 1980). The isotope is low energy with a half-value layer of 1.7 cm. Its half-life is long, approximately 60 days, and over one year delivers a dose equivalent to 7000 rads external beam radiation. It is a safe isotope in the operating room owing to its low energy, and the incidence of complications compared to radical prostatectomy or external beam radiation therapy is low. Unfortunately, its therapeutic efficacy may also be relatively lower with a high rate of clinical progression within 10 years (Whitmore et al. 1987). It is appropriate for patients who have not had transurethral resection of the prostate and whose tumour volume is small.

The largest reported experience with ^{125}I therapy comes from Memorial Sloan–Kettering Hospital (Whitmore et al. 1987). Whitmore reports a progression rate for stages B1, B2, B3 and C lesions of 40%, 68%, 84% and 90% at 10 years, respectively. The complication rate of ^{125}I therapy when used alone is relatively low. However, when used as a salvage modality after previous external beam therapy, the complications increase dramatically. The overall incidence of early complications with interstitial therapy alone is related to surgical factors (Schellhammer and El-Mahdi 1983; Fowler et al. 1979). A 4.5% incidence of major complications in 200 patients included one pulmonary embolus, one myocardial infarction, and two abscesses. A 22% incidence of minor complications included superficial wound infections, obturator nerve injury, lymphocele and pedal oedema. Late complications (18%) were secondary to bowel and bladder damage. The incidence of impotence is approximately 7% with interstitial radiation alone, and 20%–30% in patients treated with combined therapy (Ross et al. 1982).

Iridium Radiotherapy

Removable ^{192}Ir wires or seeds have the advantage of more accurate placement at the site of the disease than ^{125}I seeds. Dosimetry is relatively more consistent, and because the radionuclide is removed after a short period of time (60 h–6 days) problems with migration of seeds do not occur. ^{192}Ir delivers a higher dose of radiation than ^{125}I (Court and Chassagne 1977). The tissue half-value layer is 6 cm. The half-life is 75 days. ^{192}Ir delivers 6000–7000 rad equivalent over 6 days, or 3000–4000 rad over 40 h. In this case it is usually followed by 3000–4000 rad of external beam radiation. It is safe for operating room personnel because the wires are afterloaded at the bedside postoperatively.

In a study of 43 patients treated with combined pelvic node dissection, ^{192}Ir and external beam radiation, there was 72% delayed morbidity consisting primarily of proctitis, cystitis and obstructive symptoms. Two patients developed rectourethral fistulae. Postoperative and early morbidity were 33% and 65% respectively. Fifteen of 29 patients who had needle biopsies at one year had evidence of residual tumour (Bosch et al. 1986).

Long-term follow-up of patients is needed in order to determine whether this form of interstitial therapy will significantly reduce the rate of progression of prostate cancer. There are insufficient data at this time to know which patients will achieve long-term remission.

Radical Prostatectomy

Total excision of the prostate gland, known as radical prostatectomy, can be accomplished equally well by a perineal or by a retropubic approach. Choice of the approach is a matter of training, familiarity and personal preference. The advantages of perineal radical prostatectomy include lower blood loss because there is no need to transect the dorsal vein complex, and a direct approach to the urethra which makes the urethro-vesical anastamosis easier to perform. Advantages of the retropubic radical prostatectomy include simultaneous access to the pelvic lymph nodes and a wider margin of resection than is possible with the perineal approach.

The ideal candidate for radical prostatectomy is a relatively young man with a small tumour confined within the prostate.

Until recently, the consensus was that patients with stage A1 disease needed no treatment. A recent report by Epstein et al. (1986) shows that 16% of patients with stage A1 disease followed for at least 8 years developed distant metastases, often without detectable changes in the primary tumour. These findings suggest that men with stage A1 prostate cancer who have a long life expectancy should be offered curative therapy because of their significantly longer period of risk for progression.

Patients with stage A2 prostate cancer have a much higher rate of progression than patients with stage A1 disease: 33% for stage A2 versus 2% for stage A1 during a follow-up period of at least 4 years (Cantrell et al. 1981). Moreover, recent data based on pathological examination in stage A2 disease reveal that the majority of patients have disease confined within the prostate and, therefore, should be considered excellent candidates for curative radical prostatectomy, especially if the operation is preceded by pelvic lymphadenectomy to identify those with lymph node metastases (Elder et al. 1985; Fowler and Mills 1985; Parfitt et al. 1983; Catalona et al. 1985).

Patients with stage B1 prostate cancer are, historically, the ideal candidates for radical prostatectomy. They usually have small volume disease, low grade tumours and less than 10% incidence of lymph node metastasis. Seminal vesicle invasion and capsular penetration are rare (Eggleston and Walsh 1985; Fowler and Mills 1985; Catalona and Scott 1985; Land and Narayan 1983). Moreover, the long-term disease-free survival of stage B1 patients treated by radical prostatectomy is unsurpassed by any other form of therapy (Gibbons et al. 1984; Walsh and Jewett 1980).

Morphometric reconstructions of radical prostatectomy specimens show that tumours less than 2.5 cm in volume have a low probability of penetrating the capsule, invading the seminal vesicles or metastasising to regional lymph nodes (Tables 7.2 and 7.5). Assuming tumours to be spherical, a 2.5-ml tumour would be a 1.7-cm diameter nodule which, according to the clinical staging described in Table 7.9, would be a stage B2 tumour. If capsular penetration alone without seminal vesicle invasion or lymph node metastasis is not considered a poor prognostic sign, then tumours with volumes up to 3.67 ml may be amenable to complete excision by radical prostatectomy. A 3.67-ml tumour would be a 1.9-cm diameter nodule which may include some stage B3 tumours.

There is no evidence that radical prostatectomy for stage C or for node-positive disease (D1) offers survival benefit over hormonal therapy alone and, therefore, it is not indicated except in very special circumstances such as for palliation or in clinical studies of adjuvant therapy.

Results

Survival. Most reported series of radical prostatectomy for stage A disease combine A1 and A2. The longterm disease-free survival is 90% and death from prostate cancer is 1% (Catalona and Scott 1986). Elder et al. (1985) recently reported on 25 patients with stage A2 disease treated by radical prostatectomy and followed-up for periods from 9 months to more than 10 years: one patient developed recurrent prostate cancer, one patient died of other causes without evidence of disease and 23 are alive without disease.

The most classical series of radical prostatectomy for stage B disease is the Johns Hopkins Hospital series reported on by Walsh and Jewett (1980). Of 57 patients with clinical stage B1 disease, 29 (51%) were alive and well 15 years after operation, 10 (17%) died of prostate cancer and 18 (32%) died of other causes within 15 years but had no clinical evidence of prostate cancer at the time of death. The 51% 15-year survival was similar to the expected survival in the general population.

The 15-year disease-free survival of men with clinical stage B2 treated by radical prostatectomy was 25% (Elder et al. 1982). Those who were found to have disease limited to the prostate on pathological examination had a 15 year disease-free survival of 50% compared to 13% for those who had extraprostatic extension.

In 1984, Gibbons et al. reported on the Mason Clinic experience with radical prostatectomy for stage B disease and found a disease-free survival of 90% at 5 years, 70% at 10 years and 50% at 15 years. Twenty-nine cases were at risk for 15-years. Gibbons (1987) recently updated this material and found an actual observed survival of 60% in 57 men followed for at least 15 years. Of these clinical stage B patients, 20% had pathological stage C disease. This actual observed disease-free survival exceeded the life expectancy of men of the same age, in the same region and during the same time interval. Forty-six patients (84%) are either alive and free of disease at 15 years following operation or were free of disease at the time of their death from other causes.

Local Control. Local recurrence of cancer following radical prostatectomy has been reported in 4% to 22% of patients, most of whom had stage C disease (Bass and Barrett 1980; Nichols et al. 1977; Schroeder and Belt 1975; Turner and Belt 1957). Local recurrences may arise from the intentional incomplete resection of the prostatic apex to facilitate the anastamosis of the urethra to the bladder and to prevent incontinence, or from residual extraprostatic disease. Radiation therapy is of benefit in local recurrence especially if given early. Of 32 such cases treated at Stanford, 13 were treated within 4 months after radical prostatectomy because of positive surgical margin and 19 were treated when local recurrence became palpable. The actuarial 5- and 10-year disease-free survival for the first group was 57%. For the second group, it was 40% at 5 years and 25% at 10 years (Ray et al. 1984).

Complications. Morbidity from radical prostatectomy is relatively minimal and mortality is less than 2% (Middleton 1977; Lieskowsky and Skinner 1983; Crawford and Kiker 1983). Intraoperative rectal injury occurs in up to 3% of patients. Thromboembolic disease, wound infection and lymphocele are seen in fewer than 5%. Late complications of bladder neck contracture or incontinence occur in 1% to 6% of patients. Table 7.14 lists the complications in 100 consecutive radical prostatectomies performed at Stanford. Three of the 4

Table 7.14. Complications in 100 consecutive radical prostatectomies

Complication	Rate
Mortality	0
Rectal Injury	0
Ureteral Injury	0
Thrombophlebitis	1
Pulmonary Embolus (not fatal)	1
Wound Infection	4
Pelvic Abscess	0
Lymphocele	1
Bladder Neck Contracture	2
Urethral Stricture	1
Incontinence	4
Impotence	50

incidents of incontinence occurred in patients with prior transurethral resection. All 4 needed correction with implantation of an artificial sphincter.

Impotence and Nerve-sparing Radical Prostatectomy. Until recently, impotence was a common and disturbing complication of radical prostatectomy occurring in more than 90% of men and influencing therapeutic decisions (often not in the best interest of the patient), by both patient and urologist. In 1982, Walsh and Donker suggested that impotence was caused by injury to the branches of the pelvic plexus which innervate the corpora cavernosa. Walsh then went on to describe the nerve-sparing technique for preservation of sexual function thus eliminating a major complication and renewing interest in the operation (Walsh et al. 1983). Of 60 patients who were potent preoperatively and who were followed-up for at least one year, 70% were potent. Postoperative potency correlated well with the extent of disease. In patients with lack of or with only microscopic capsular penetration, 84% were potent at one year compared to 43% with extensive involvement of the periprostatic tissues. Only 33% of patients with seminal vesicle invasion remained potent (Walsh and Lepor 1987). Careful pathological evaluation of radical prostatectomy specimens failed to reveal any evidence that the nerve-sparing technique compromised the radical nature of the operation (Eggleston and Walsh 1985). Unilateral preservation of the nerves does not seem to influence the potency rate.

The ideal candidate for the procedure is a sexually active man with stage A disease or with stage B disease localised to one lobe in whom the nerve-sparing will be done on the side opposite the tumour.

Hormonal Therapy

Clinical trials of hormonal therapy in localised prostate cancer are few and limited. Barnes (1981) reported a 27% 15-year survival for patients with stage A disease and a 28% for those with stage B disease. All patients had either immediate or delayed therapy or no treatment. The 15-year survival of patients who had immediate therapy was 24% and for those who had delayed therapy,

32%. Patients under 70 years of age survived longer with delayed therapy than with immediate therapy.

Summary of Facts

1. The evolution and natural history of prostate cancer is predictable: the tumour grows with the passage of time and as the tumour grows it dedifferentiates and as it dedifferentiates, its malignant potential increases
2. Of all imaging modalities, transrectal ultrasound is the most accurate. It is a promising modality for potential use in screening
3. The prostate specific antigen is more sensitive and more specific than the prostatic acid phosphatase. It is now the marker for prostate cancer
4. Cancer progression occurs at every stage of the disease and, therefore, potentially curative treatment should be offered to every man with a long life expectancy
5. It is now clear that patients with nodal metastases do not benefit from extended field irradiation
6. A positive post-irradiation biopsy indicates persistent or recurrent active disease and patients with a positive biopsy are at risk for progression
7. To try to compare results of the different modalities of treatment is wrong because randomised prospective studies with large numbers of patients followed for a long period of time are not available. However, careful analysis of the available results of the different therapies seems to indicate that longterm disease-free survival is better with radical prostatectomy than with external beam radiation therapy, interstitial irradiation or hormonal therapy

Avenues for Research

1. Since volume of cancer is an important determinant of the malignant behaviour of prostate cancer, imaging modalities are needed to measure volume accurately prior to institution of any therapy.
2. Agreement on a staging and a grading classification universally acceptable and applicable.
3. Prospective, randomised trials comparing treatment modalities to each other and to no treatment.
4. Clinical trials of adjuvant therapy with hormones, irradiation or cytotoxic agents in patients with locally advanced and/or nodal disease. These patients do not do well with the available modalities of therapy.
5. The search for tumour specific antigen and the diagnostic and therapeutic roles of monoclonal antibodies against such antigen.

6. Increased understanding of the basic processes regulating function and growth of the normal and the cancerous prostate

References

Abu-Yousef MM, Narayan AS (1985) Prostatic carcinoma: detection and staging using suprapubic ultrasound. Radiology 156: 175–180

Bagshaw MA (1987) Status of the radiation treatment of prostatic cancer at Stanford. In: NIH Consensus Development Conference on Management of Clinically Localized Prostate Cancer. National Institute of Health, Bethesda, Maryland, USA, 15–17 June

Barnes RW (1981) Endocrine therapy of prostatic carcinoma. In: Ablin RJ (ed) Prostatic cancer. Marcel Dekker, Inc., New York, pp 219–228

Bass RB Jr, Barrett DM (1980) Radical retropubic prostatectomy after transurethral prostatic resection. J Urol 124: 495–497

Biondetti PR, Lee JKT, Ling D, Catalona WJ (1987) Clinical stage B prostatic carcinoma: staging with MR Imaging. Radiology 162: 325–329

Bosch PC, Forbes KA, Prassvinichai S, Miller JB, Golji H, Martin DC (1986) Preliminary observation on the results of combined temporary 192-Iridium implantation and external beam irradiation for carcinoma of the prostate. J Urol 135: 722–725

Cantrell BB, DeKlerk DP, Eggleston JC, Boitnott JK, Walsh PC (1981) Pathological factors that influence prognosis in stage A prostatic cancer. The influence of extent versus grade. J Urol 125: 516–520

Catalona WJ, Dresner SM (1985) Nerve-sparing radical prostatectomy: extraprostatic tumor extension and preservation of erectile function. J Urol 134: 1149–1151

Catalona WJ, Scott WW (1986) Carcinoma of the prostate. In: Walsh PC, Gittes RF, Perlmutter AD, Stamey TA (eds) Campbell's urology, 5th edition. W. B. Saunders Company, Philadelphia, pp 1463–1534

Court B, Chassagne C (1977) Interstitial therapy of cancer of the prostate using Iridium-192 wires. Cancer Treat Rep 61: 329–332

Crawford ED, Kiker JD (1983) Radical retropubic prostatectomy. J Urol 129: 1145–1148

Dahnert WF, Hamper UM, Eggleston JC, Walsh PC, Sanders RC (1986) Prostatic evaluation by transrectal sonography with histopathologic correlation: the echogenic appearance of early carcinoma. Radiology 158: 97–102

Eggleston JC, Walsh PC (1985) Radical prostatectomy with preservation of sexual function: pathological findings in the first 100 cases. J Urol 134: 1146–1148

Elder JS, Jewett HJ, Walsh PC (1982) Radical prostatectomy for clinical stage B2 carcinoma of the prostate. J Urol 127: 704–706

Elder JS, Gibbons RP, Correa RJ Jr, Brannen GE (1985) Efficacy of radical prostatectomy for stage A2 carcinoma of the prostate. Cancer 56: 2151–2154

Epstein JI, Eggleston JC, Paull G, Walsh PC (1986) Prognosis of untreated stage A1 prostatic carcinoma: a study of 94 cases with extended follow-up. J Urol 136: 837–839

Flocks RH (1969) Present status of interstitial irradiation in managing prostatic cancer. JAMA 210: 328–330

Fowler JE, Barzell W, Hilaris BS, Whitmore WF (1979) Complications of 125-Iodine implantation and pelvic lymphadenectomy in the treatment of prostatic cancer. J Urol 121: 447–451

Fowler JE, Mills SE (1985) Operable prostatic carcinoma: correlations among clinical stage, pathologic stage, Gleason histologic score and early disease-free survival. J Urol 133: 49–52

Freiha FS, Bagshaw MA (1984) Carcinoma of the prostate: results of post-irradiation biopsy. Prostate 5: 19–25

Freiha FS, Salzman J (1977) Surgical staging of prostatic cancer: transperitoneal versus extraperitoneal lymphadenectomy. J Urol 118: 616–617

Freiha FS, Pistenma DA, Bagshaw MA (1979) Pelvic lymphadenectomy for staging prostate cancer: is it always necessary? J Urol 122: 176–177

Gibbons RP (1987) Total prostatectomy for localized prostatic cancer. Long term surgical results and current morbidity: The Virginia Mason Clinic experience. In: NIH Consensus Development Conference on Management of Clinically Localized Prostate Cancer. National Institute of Health, Bethesda, Maryland, USA, 15–17 June

Gibbons RP, Correa RJ, Brannen GE, Mason JT (1984) Total prostatectomy for localized prostate cancer. J Urol 131: 73–76

Gleason DF (1977) Histologic grading and clinical staging of prostatic carcinoma. In: Tannenbaum M
    (ed) Urologic Pathology: the prostate. Lea & Febiger, Philadelphia, pp 171–197
Goffinet DR, Martinez A, Freiha FS, Pooler DM, Pistenma DA, Cumes D, Bagshaw MA (1980) 125-
    Iodine prostate implants for recurrent carcinomas after external beam irradiation: preliminary
    results. Cancer 45: 2717–2724
Golimbu M, Morales P, Al-Askari S, Shulman Y (1981) CAT scanning in staging of prostatic cancer.
    Urology 19: 305–308
Guerriero WG, Barrett MT, Bartholomew T, Carlton CE, Hudgins PT (1979) Combined interstitial
    and external radiotherapy in the definitive management of carcinoma of the prostate. In: Johnson
    DE, Samuels ML (eds) Cancer of the genitourinary tract. Raven Press, New York, pp 207–216
Hamper JM, Dahnert WF, Eggleston JC, Walsh PC, Sanders RC (1986) Ultrasonography of prostatic
    carcinoma employing amplitude-envelop (AM) and frequency demodulated (FM) imaging. J
    Ultrasound Med 5: 557–562
Hricak H, Dooms GC, Jeffrey RB, Avallone A, Jacobs D, Benton WK, Narayan P, Tanagho EA
    (1987) Prostatic carcinoma: staging by clinical assessment, CT and MR imaging. Radiology 162:
    331–336
Jewett HJ (1969) The results of radical perineal prostatectomy. JAMA 210: 324–325
Lang PH, Narayan P (1983) Understaging and undergrading of prostate cancer. Urology 21: 113–118
Lieskovsky G, Skinner DC (1983) Technique of radical retropubic prostatectomy with limited pelvic
    node dissection. Urol Clin North Am 10: 187–198
Ling D, Lee JKT, Heiken JP, Balfe DM, Glazer HS, McClennan BL (1986) Prostatic carcinoma and
    benign prostatic hyperplasia: inability of MR imaging to distinguish between the two diseases.
    Radiology 158: 103–107
McNeal JE, Kindrachuk RA, Freiha FS, Bostwick DG, Redwine EA, Stamey TA (1986) Patterns of
    progression in prostate cancer. Lancet I: 60–63
Middleton AW Jr (1977) A comparison of the morbidity associated with radical retropubic
    prostatectomy with and without pubectomy. J Urol 117: 202–205
Morgan CL, Calkins RF, Cavalcanti EJ (1981) Computed tomography in the evaluation, staging and
    therapy of carcinoma of the bladder and prostate. Radiology 140: 751–761
Nichols RT, Barry JM, Hodges CV (1977) The morbidity of radical prostatectomy for multifocal stage
    1 prostatic carcinoma. J Urol 117: 83–84
Parfitt HE Jr, Smith JA Jr, Seaman JP, Middleton RG (1983) Surgical treatment of stage A2 prostatic
    carcinoma: significance of tumour grade and extent. J Urol 129: 763–765
Pistenma DA, Bagshaw MA, Freiha FS (1979) Extended-field radiation therapy for prostatic
    adenocarcinoma: status report of a limited prospective trial. In: Johnson DE, Samuels ML (eds)
    Cancer of the genitourinary tract. Raven Press, New York, pp 229–247
Pontes JE, Eisenkraft S, Watanabe H, Onc H, Saitoh M, Murphy GP (1985) Preoperative evaluation
    of localized prostatic carcinoma by transrectal ultrasonography. J Urol 134: 289–291
Ray GR, Bagshaw MA, Freiha FS (1984) External beam radiation salvage for residual or recurrent
    local tumor following radical prostatectomy. J Urol 132: 926–930
Ross G, Borkon WD, Landry LJ, Edwards FM, Weinstein SH, Abadir R (1982) Preliminary
    observations on the results of combined 125-Iodine seed implantation and external irradiation for
    carcinoma of the prostate. J Urol 127: 699–701
Scardino PT, Guerriero WG, Carlton CE (1982) Surgical staging and combined therapy with
    radioactive gold grain and external irradiation. In: Johnson DE, Bioleau MA (eds) Genitourinary
    tumors: fundamental principles and surgical techniques. Grune and Stratton, New York, pp 75–90
Schellhammer PF, El-Mahdi AM (1983) Pelvic complications after definitive treatment of prostate
    cancer by interstitial or external beam radiation. Urology 21: 451–457
Schroeder FH, Belt E (1975) Carcinoma of the prostate: a study of 213 patients with stage C tumors
    treated by total perineal prostatectomy. J Urol 114: 257–260
Segi M, Kurihara M, Matsuyama T (1969) Cancer mortality for selected sites in 24 countries.
    Department of Public Health, Tohoku University School of Medicine, Sendai, Japan, No. 5
    (1964–1965), p 120
Shanker Giri PG, Walsh JW, Hazra TA, Texter JH, Koontz WW (1982) Role of computed
    tomography in the evaluation and management of carcinoma of the prostate. Int J Radiat Oncol
    Biol Phys 8: 283–287
Shipley WU, Coachman NM, McNulty PA, Healy EA, Elman AJ, Prout GR Jr, Heney NM,
    Althansen AF, Suit HD (1987) Radiation therapy of men with localized prostatic carcinoma: The
    Massachusetts General Hospital experience. NIH Consensus Development Conference On
    Management of Clinically Localized Prostate Cancer, National Institute of Health, Bethesda,
    Maryland, USA, 15–17 June. NCI Monographs 7: 67–73

Silverberg E, Lubern JA (1988) Cancer statistics, 1988. Cancer 38: 5–22

Stamey TA, Yang N, Hay AR, McNeal JE, Freiha FS, Redwine E (1987) Prostate-specific antigen is the serum marker for adenocarcinoma of the prostate. N Engl J Med 317: 909–916

Turner RD, Belt E (1957) A study of 229 consecutive cases of total perineal prostatectomy for cancer of the prostate. J Urol 77: 62–77

Walsh PC, Donker PJ (1982) Impotence following radical prostatectomy: Insight into etiology and prevention. J Urol 128: 492–497

Walsh PC, Jewett HJ (1980) Radical surgery for prostatic cancer. Cancer. 45: 1906–1911

Walsh PC, Lepor H, Eggleston JC (1983) Radical prostatectomy with preservation of sexual function: anatomical and pathological considerations. Prostate 4: 473–485

Walsh PC, Lepor H (1987) The role of radical prostatectomy in the management of prostatic cancer. Cancer 60: 526–537

Whitmore WF Jr, Hilaris B, Sogani PC, Herr HW, Fair WR (1987) Interstitial irradiation with [125]I. In: NIH Consensus Development Conference on Management of Clinically Localized Prostate Cancer. National Institute of Health, Bethesda, Maryland, USA, 15–17 June

Chapter 8

Carcinoma of the Prostate – Metastatic Disease

M. Pavone-Macaluso

Introduction

The hormonal treatment of prostatic carcinoma has been widely employed for over 40 years since the classical paper by Huggins and Hodges in 1941. Many points still remain controversial and no standard hormonal therapy has been uniformly adopted throughout the world. The main controversies are listed in Table 8.1.

Table 8.1. Main controversies regarding hormonal treatment in prostate cancer

Choice of drug (or orchidectomy) in the untreated patient
Start of the treatment: early (at diagnosis) or delayed (at onset of symptoms)
Clinical value of the treatment (merely palliative or capable of improving survival)
Mechanism of action
Biological basis of primary resistance: the escape phenomenon
Predictability of clinical response: value of receptor assays and intracellular hormone determinations
The concept of "total androgenic blockade"
Choice of treatment and value of the hormones in the patient relapsing after initial response

While we know that there is no definitive solution to the controversies, we will try to discuss them to the best of our knowledge, stressing the results of randomised clinical trials, in the hope that their conclusions will lead closer to the truth than those resulting from uncontrolled studies. One is very unlikely to be fully exempt from personal inclinations and bias and, in particular, our present thinking has been greatly influenced by the studies and attitudes of the EORTC Urological Group. The choice of the references has favoured European contributions. A large bibliography from the American literature can be found in a recent review by J. A. Smith (1987).

Choice of Treatment

The first hormonal treatments were orchidectomy and oestrogens: other drugs were subsequently employed until, in recent years, rather expensive associations of an antiandrogen and a luteinising hormone releasing hormone (LH-RH) analogue have been suggested as the treatment of choice.

For many years the emphasis has been laid upon the reduction of circulating androgens to obtain useful clinical results. In recent years the role of intracellular androgens has been given even greater importance. If we consider prostatic cancer to be an androgen-dependent tumour, all treatments that effectively block intracellular androgenic activity will be able to affect the growth of the cells, and they will all show similar efficacy if given at sufficient doses. The clinician's choice will depend more on the side effects and on the patient's acceptance of a given treatment than on minor differences in efficacy. The side effects should be well known to the clinician and lead to a personalised treatment for every patient after considering the specific risk factors. If efficacy and side effects are expected to be similar, then the cost should play a role in selecting the best treatment to be adopted.

Orchidectomy

It is often stated that orchidectomy is poorly accepted by the patient, who is very unwilling to accept castration, viewed as an irreversible and mutilating operation with a dismal psychological impact. This may be the case for some patients, but orchidectomy is readily accepted by others, provided the situation is explained with tact, time and human understanding. The surgical trauma and the postoperative complications are minimal, and the implantation of testicular prostheses and even the use of subcapsular orchidectomy (instead of the complete emptying of the scrotal content) have made this operation more acceptable from the psychological standpoint. The hormonal effect of subcapsular orchidectomy, judged by plasma testosterone levels, is not inferior to that of a complete castration. Once orchidectomy has resulted in castrate levels of plasma testosterone, these remain unchanged for the years to come and do not require additional drug supplements. This is especially useful for senile, unreliable patients whose compliance to the prescribed treatment may be poor, as well as for those who have not been given full explanations regarding the nature of their disease and the side effects of the treatment. In our experience this is not uncommon in Southern Europe. Patients lacking understanding and motivation are likely to stop taking the drugs as soon as they feel better and wish to avoid the unpleasant effects, such as sexual impairment and gynaecomastia, which they correctly attribute to the

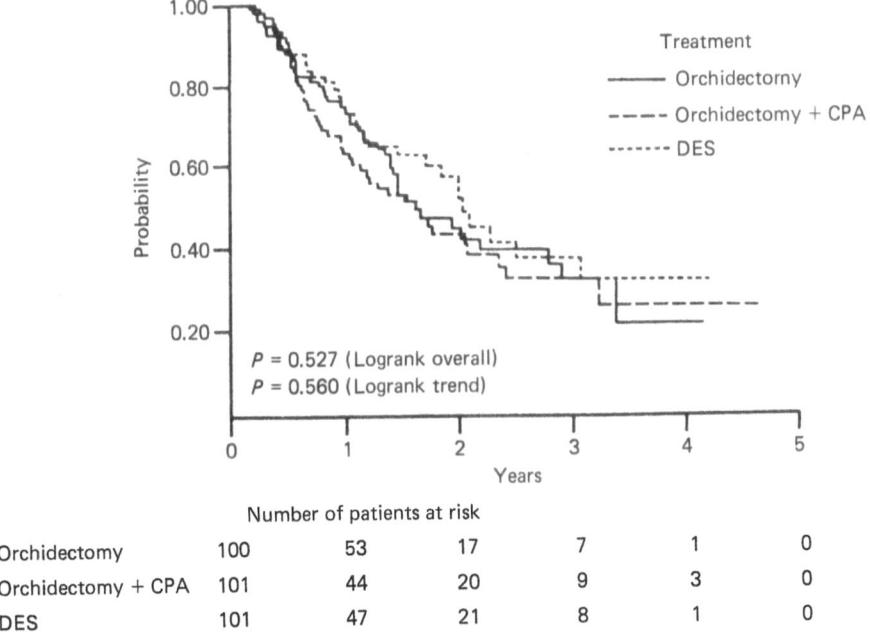

Fig. 8.1. Time to progression in EORTC trial 30805 (from Robinson 1987).

treatment. These patients and those who live in distant or remote areas, for whom problems with follow-up can be foreseen, may be good candidates for orchidectomy, a simple, definitive operation, with little cost and practically no side effects. Hot flushes rarely represent a problem. They occur in 20%–30% of all cases. Reduction of libido and impotence are very frequent, but not absolutely constant. They are also the result of all the other forms of androgen deprivation except pure antiandrogens. There is a minimal surgical risk but the patient is not obliged to take pills for the rest of his life. We will discuss later the issue of the so called "complete androgen blockade". According to its proponents, the clinical efficacy of orchidectomy will be greatly improved by subsequent antiandrogenic treatment. In our view, no convincing evidence has been presented so far to support this conclusion. Conversely, the updated results of EORTC trial 30805 (Robinson 1987) have failed to show any difference in survival and time to progression between orchidectomy alone and orchidectomy plus cyproterone acetate (CPA): (Figs. 8.1, 8.2). The results are still preliminary and CPA may be not as good as pure antiandrogens. Nevertheless, until the results of randomised trials disprove this assumption, orchidectomy has been prematurely put in the limbo of obsolete, old-fashioned procedures, to be rejected by modern science. It still remains the treatment of choice for selected patients.

Other Surgical Ablative Procedures

Adrenalectomy and hypophysectomy have been completely abandoned. Cryosurgical destruction of the pituitary gland or stereotaxic implantion of radio-

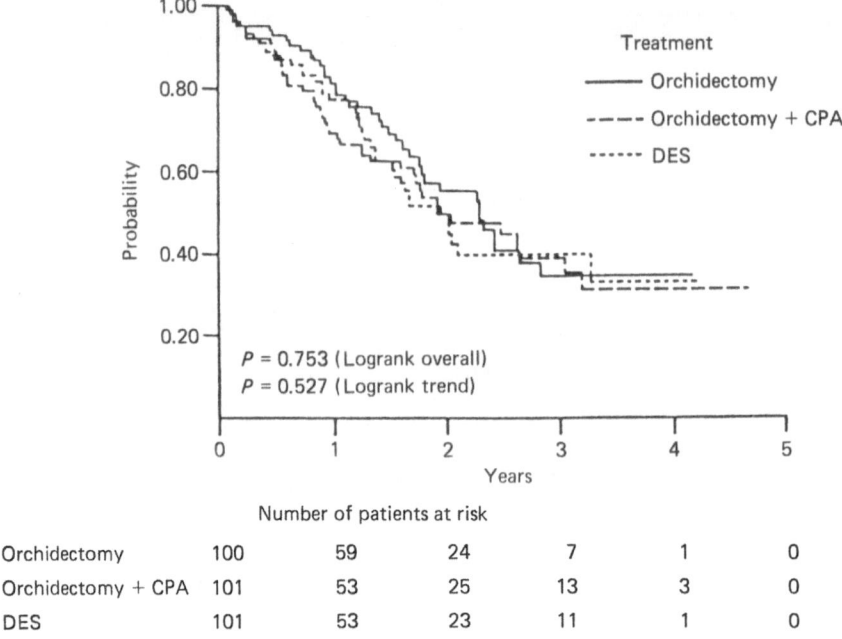

Fig. 8.2. Duration of survival in EORTC trial 30805 (from Robinson 1987).

isotopes may still remain an heroic palliative procedure for patients with severe pain, refractory to less invasive treatments.

Oestrogens

Oestrogens have fallen into progressive disrepute since VACURG study 1 disclosed the cardiovascular (CV) toxicity of diethylstilboestrol (DES) 5 mg daily. A subsequent study by the same group concluded that 1 mg DES is as effective as 5 mg, but devoid of the CV toxicity associated with the higher dose (Byar 1973). A recent study by the EORTC urological group has shown that the clinical efficacy of 1 mg DES is comparable to that of orchidectomy, with or without CPA, but the side effects, especially hypertension and deep vein thrombosis, are not negligible (Robinson 1987). This low dose of DES (1 mg daily) has been criticised on the ground that it does not produce a stable fall in plasma testosterone levels. Therefore, the dose of 3 mg DES daily (1 mg t.d.s.) became common practice, but its CV toxicity had never been fully evaluated until EORTC trials 30761 and 30762 gave evidence that it is rather severe (De Voogt et al. 1986) (Table 8.2). Severe and lethal side effects were more frequent in study 30762, which recruited patients almost exclusively from Britain, than in 30761, (Table 8.3), in which most patients were from Italy, France, Spain and Portugal, suggesting racial or dietary influences. CV toxicity usually occurred within the first 6 months from start of treatment (Fig. 8.3). These studies also demonstrated that patients above 75 years of age, above 75 kilos of weight and with a previous history of CV disease were especially at risk. The obvious conclusion is that DES

Table 8.2. The type of CV toxicity during the 30762 study according to treatment

	Estracyt	Diethylstilboestrol (DES)
Fluid retention	21	18
ECG changes	4	4
Infarct	3	12
Hypertension	0	2
Thrombo-embolic disease	9	7
Any combination	1	2
Total	38	45

Table 8.3. The type of CV toxicity during the 30761 study according to treatment

	CPA	MPA	DES
Fluid retention	2	5	8
ECG changes	1	5	6
Infarct	3	0	1
Hypertension	0	0	4
Thrombo-embolic disease	2	5	6
Total	8	15	25

is to be avoided at least in these high risk patients. It is likely that the same conclusion should be applied to oestrogens different from DES. In the Scandinavian countries, a long-acting, i.m. form of polyoestradiol phosphate (Estradurin R) in association with oral ethynyloestradiol (Etivex R) has represented the standard form of oestrogen treatment for many years. It has also been associated with a high incidence of CV complications. The use of other oestrogens in

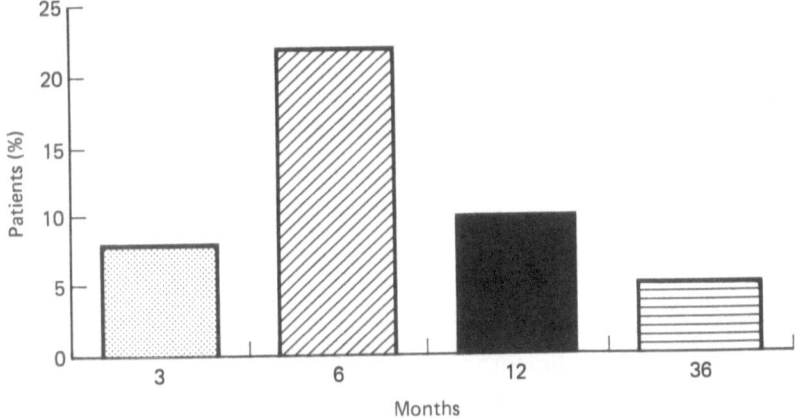

Fig. 8.3. Time intervals at which cardiovascular complications were detected, cumulatively for all treatment arms, in EORTC trials 30761 and 30762.

prostatic cancer has been limited to a few series with low numbers of patients, and their optimal therapeutic dose is yet to be defined. There is, however, sufficient evidence from other fields of medicine that CV toxicity is a feature of all compounds with oestrogenic properties which are metabolised in the liver. The only possible exception is natural oestradiol administered by the subcutaneous route. The addition of diuretics and inhibitors of platelet aggregation may prevent some of the untoward effects of oestrogens, but adds to the complexity of the treatment and increases the number of possible side effects. In short, 1 mg DES may still be an acceptable therapeutic option for low risk patients. In countries (including Italy) where DES has disappeared from the market, it is probably better to withhold oestrogens altogether, in favour of other less toxic and widely accepted treatments.

Oestrogens also cause gynaecomastia, which can be painful and cumbersome, stimulate the release of adrenal androgens and increase the circulating levels of prolactin. Prolactin itself does not stimulate growth of prostate cancer cells, but can potentiate the effects of androgens. Therefore, the antiprolactins bromocryptine or lisuride have been routinely administered to patients receiving oestrogens to counteract any effect deriving from excessive release of prolactin. Side effects can be produced by bromocryptine but there is no convincing evidence of its clinical efficacy in these circumstances (Jacobi 1982).

The mechanism of action of oestrogens is commonly held to be due exclusively to the fact that they block luteinising hormone (LH) release by the pituitary, thereby decreasing production of testosterone from the testis and producing a fall of circulating testosterone to castrate levels. There are, however, other mechanisms. In the first place, oestrogens stimulate the production of sex-hormone-binding-globulin (SHBG), which reduces free testosterone and renders it unavailable to the prostate. Oestrogens can also act directly on the Leydig cells, so reducing testosterone production. In addition, a direct cytotoxic action on the prostatic cancer cell has been postulated, according to several investigations (reviewed by Altwein in 1983). This has received further confirmation recently (Schulz et al. 1987). Such observations have renewed the interest of clinicians in the use of oestrogens, especially in high doses in the form of DES-diphosphate (fosfestrol); this compound appears to be of special interest in the treatment of prostate cancer when there is a relapse after initial response to hormones. It may also be useful in inducing a rapid androgen deprivation even in the untreated patients if a prompt effect is required. If fosfestrol is administered intravenously at the dose of 1 g daily (dissolved in 300 ml 5% dextrose in water) for 5 days, plasma testosterone is reduced to castrate levels within 12 hours after infusion (Maatman et al. 1985).

Pure antiandrogens

Flutamide

Flutamide is a well known antiandrogen, which acts by a peripheral blockade of intranuclear androgen receptors. It has been recently advocated as a necessary supplement to orchidectomy or chemical castration by the LH-RH analogues in order to achieve "complete androgen blockade", to which we will refer later in this chapter. However, one of the unique features of flutamide is that it does not necessarily abolish libido and potency in sexually active patients. Results from phase III studies show that flutamide, administered alone, is at least as effective as DES in the treatment of advanced prostate cancer (Neri 1987). In a Danish randomised study, flutamide (750 mg daily) was compared with DES (3 mg). At 12 months either an objective response or stabilisation was seen in 13 of 20 patients treated with flutamide compared to 8 of 20 patients treated with DES (Lund and Rasmussen 1987). The difference was not statistically significant, but DES caused more frequent and more severe side effects than flutamide. Gynaecomastia was prevented by irradiating the breasts before treatment. No significant alteration of libido or potency was observed in patients treated with flutamide, while all those treated with DES became impotent. In the flutamide group, rise in plasma testosterone was moderate and inconstant, with a very large standard deviation. After 12 months, plasma testosterone concentrations had reverted to normal levels (Fig. 8.4).

Clinical results have been very encouraging in previously untreated patients (Sogani and Whitmore 1979). In a randomised study comparing flutamide (750 or 1500 mg daily) with DES (1 mg daily) there were no apparent differences in response between patients on flutamide and those receiving DES (Jacobo et al. 1976). In Italy, a large cooperative group has treated patients with either stage C

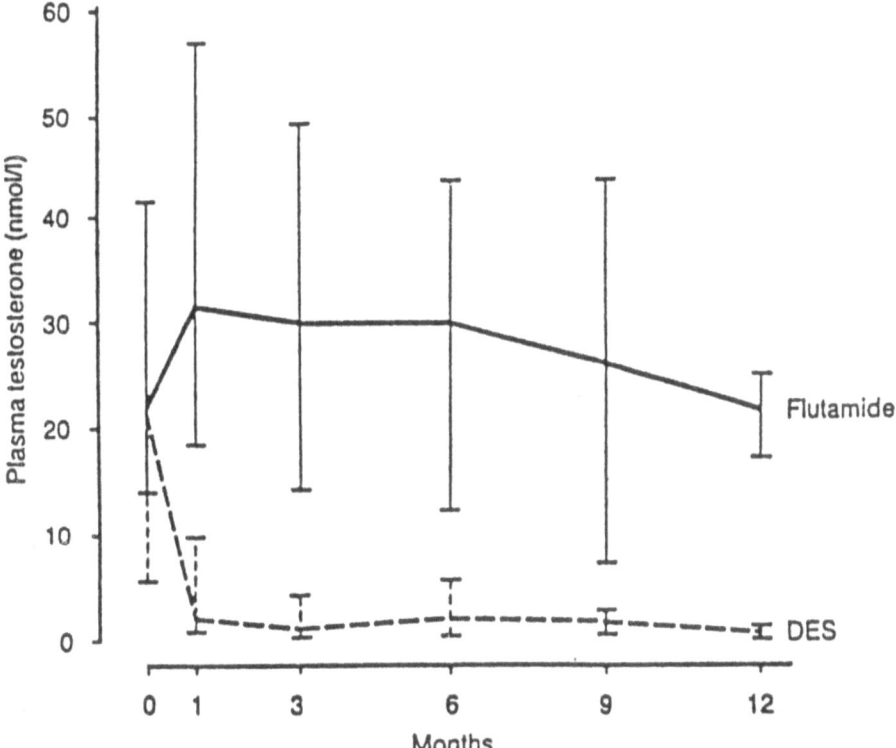

Fig. 8.4. Mean plasma testosterone levels in patients receiving flutamide and DES (from Lund and Rasmussen 1987).

or stage D prostate cancer with flutamide (Consoli et al. 1987). Other patients were treated with a combination of flutamide and the LHRH superagonist, Zoladex. Not only was it impossible to detect any difference in response rate, but there was even a trend in favour of flutamide. This was not a randomised trial and thus the results must be taken with caution.

In our experience (Daricello et al. 1987), response rate, time to progression and survival were not different, stage by stage, from those reported in historical series, where "classical" drugs, such as DES (3 mg), CPA, or estramustine were employed.

A direct comparison is impossible but the conclusion can be drawn that some patients benefit from flutamide and remain potent, if they so wish. The use of pure antiandrogens in prostate cancer has been criticised on the ground that they produce a marked rise in plasma testosterone levels in intact experimental animals. On the other hand, it is uncertain to what extent flutamide is capable of producing a total blockade of the androgen receptors in the nuclei of the androgen-sensitive cells. It is feared, therefore, that a rise in circulating (and, possibly, intracellular) androgens, not associated with a complete inhibition of their intracellular activity, may result in excessive androgenic stimulation. The rise in plasma testosterone is very marked in rats but its extent does not seem to be as great in other animal species and in particular, in man. In young adults flutamide brings about a rise in circulating LH, testosterone and oestradiol, but this effect is of much lower magnitude than in rats (Knuth et al. 1984). In older subjects, namely in patients with prostate cancer treated with flutamide, the rise in plasma testosterone has been inconstant and quite moderate (Prout et al. 1975).

No correlation between testosterone fluctuations and clinical response has been observed so far. No data have been reported on intracellular levels of DHT and no Leydig cell hyperplasia has been observed in patients treated with flutamide. It is our feeling that, unless the data reported by ourselves and by other authors can be disproved, the theoretical objections are of insufficient value. It is hoped that randomised clinical trials comparing flutamide alone with flutamide and castration (or LH-RH analogues) will be performed in the near future. The only randomised study reported so far compared flutamide with estramustine phosphate (Johansson et al. 1987). The preliminary results seem to indicate that these two drugs produce a similar initial response, but that its duration is more prolonged in the estramustine-treated group. However, the numbers are small and these results await confirmation. Meanwhile, it is our present view that flutamide is a legitimate therapeutic option in informed patients with a strong motivation to maintain their sexual activity. It is relatively well tolerated, but it must be administered with caution in patients with borderline liver insufficiency, because its side effects may occasionally be rather severe (MacFarlane and Tolley 1985). Subjective and objective responses may also occur in patients progressing after initial response to castration (Kaisary et al. 1987; Di Silverio et al. 1987).

Nilutamide (Anandron)

Nilutamide is given usually in association with LH-RH agonists (Labrie et al. 1983; Navratil 1987) or as a complement to orchidectomy (Beland et al. 1987; Brisset et al. 1987). Its use in monotherapy is still preliminary, and no results have been published so far, although a preliminary evaluation (P. Periti, personal communication and PONCAP Cooperative Group 1988) showed results that were not inferior to those obtainable with conventional hormonal therapy of untreated patients. Of 37 patients (36 with metastases) evaluable for response at 3 months from start of therapy, 23 were previously untreated. Partial responses were found in 39% of patients and 61% remained with stable disease. Pain decreased in 62% of patients including those in relapse after previous treatments, and pain completely disappeared in 52% of all cases. A marked decrease in serum prostatic acid phosphatase to almost normal values was also observed in some patients with stabilisation and progression. Increase in plasma testosterone was moderate and never rose above normal values. It is unknown whether niluta-mide-treated patients maintain potency if they are sexually active. The side effects were moderate, although emeralopia was a disturbing phenomenon in 23.1% of cases. Other side effects were: hot flushes (54%), nausea or vomiting (48%), gynaecomastia (39%), gastralgia (9%), diarrhoea (9%), antabuse effect (8%), skin rash (6%). The advantages over flutamide consist of more favourable pharmacokinetics enabling a lower daily dose, usually 300 mg. However, Brisset et al. (1987) reported that 150 mg yielded identical results in castrated patients, with regard to progression rate and survival. The experience is still limited and further data are needed. The role of nilutamide in association with either chemical or surgical castration will be further discussed in the paragraph devoted to "complete androgen blockade".

Progestins and Progestational Antiandrogens

Synthetic Progestational Agents without Significant Antiandrogenic Activity

The first favourable results with progesterone compounds were reported more than 30 years ago, as shown in a recent review (Denis and Bouffioux 1983). Subsequent reports, dealing with hydroxyprogesterone caproate, chlormadinone acetate and megestrol acetate have also yielded favourable results, but reports were based on small numbers of patients. Chlormadinone acetate (CMA) is still widely used in Japan (Kitajima et al. 1985). CMA, 100 mg/day orally, was as effective as diethylstilboestrol 3 mg/day and other oestrogens at equivalent doses, if the 5-year survival was used as an endpoint. In Europe, another progestational compound, medroxyprogesterone acetate (MPA), has been widely used in hormone-dependent tumours, especially in breast cancer.

Low doses of MPA (30 mg daily by month) were used in VACURG study III and compared with DES 1 mg, Premarin (conjugated equine oestrogens) 2.5 mg and DES + MPA. MPA at this dose had no effect on the size of the primary tumour, while 1 mg of DES produced a 30% decrease in the palpable area of the tumour. MPA was also less effective than oestrogens in other ways (Byar 1977a). Higher doses were used in subsequent studies (Pavone-Macaluso et al. 1978; Bouffioux 1980) which showed that MPA could produce objective and subjective responses in about 40% of cases, including patients pretreated with oestrogens. This prompted a further evaluation of MPA, which was compared with a standard dose of oestrogens (DES 3 mg) and with cyproterone acetate, in a prospective randomised trial conducted by the EORTC Urological Group in trial 30761

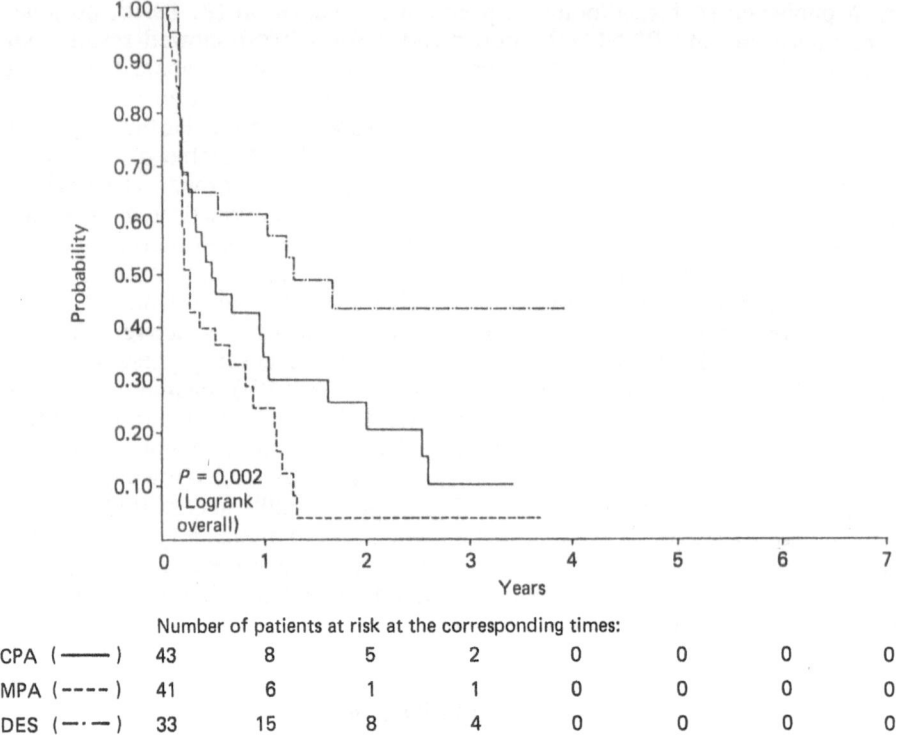

Fig. 8.5. Time to progression in EORTC trial 30761 (from Pavone-Macaluso et al. 1986).

(Pavone-Macaluso et al. 1986). As shown in Figs. 8.5 and 8.6, MPA was significantly less effective than either DES or CPA in influencing the progression-free interval and survival. There were also less local and distant responses in patients treated with MPA than in the other treatment groups (Tables 8.4 and 8.5). It was still possible to show that some responses could be attributed to MPA. The metastatic lesions improved in only 3% of patients but stabilisation occurred in 40%. A greater than 50% objective response of the local tumour, as palpable by the finger, was reported in 26% of cases. It was described as a complete response in one case. In another 55% the disease remained stable during the treatment.

Table 8.4. The best local response by treatment group in EORTC trial 30761

Treatment	Number of patients	Assessment of response (%)				"Objective response" (%)
		CR	PR	NC	PROG	CR + PR
CPA	60	15.0	25.0	46.7	13.3	40
MPA	58	1.7	24.1	55.2	19.0	25.8
DES	57	15.8	38.6	42.1	3.5	54.4

MPA vs DES P=0.003
CPA vs DES P=0.17
CPA vs MPA P=0.15

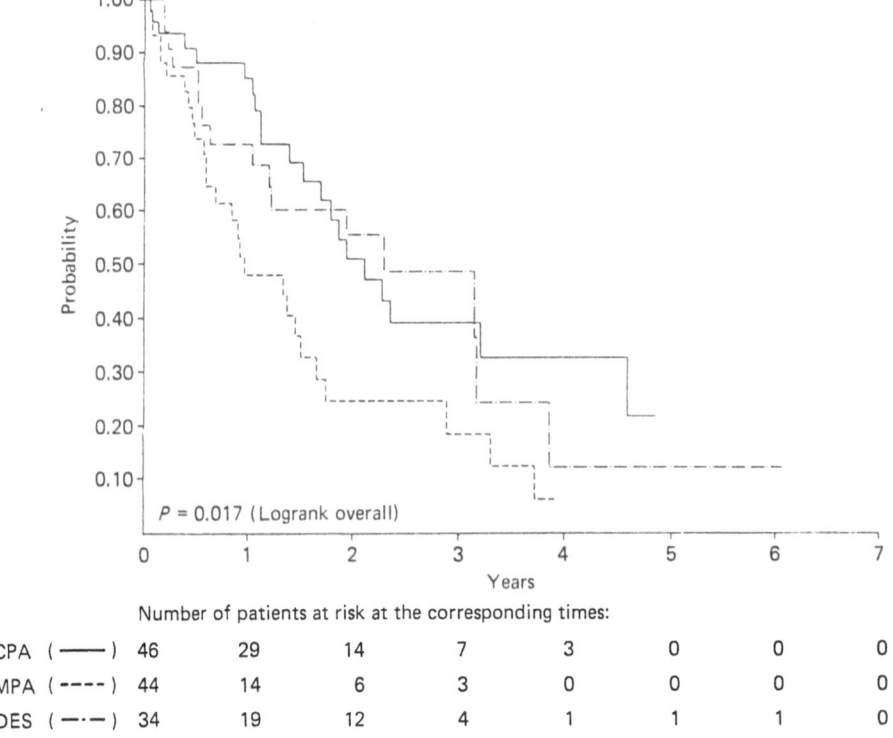

Fig. 8.6. Duration of survival in EORTC trial 30761 (from Pavone-Macaluso et al. 1986).

Number of patients at risk at the corresponding times:

CPA (——)	46	29	14	7	3	0	0	0
MPA (----)	44	14	6	3	0	0	0	0
DES (—·—)	34	19	12	4	1	1	1	0

Cardiovascular toxicity was much lower than in patients treated with DES. When toxicity was evaluated by combining the results of trial 30761 with those of a parallel EORTC study (30762 in which DES 3 mg was compared with estramustine phosphate), it was quite clear that MPA was slightly more toxic than CPA, but CV toxicity was significantly less in MPA-treated patients than in those receiving either DES or estramustine (Figs. 8.7 and 8.8). As discussed in our original paper (Pavone-Macaluso et al. 1986), various considerations can be put forward to account for the inferior results observed in the MPA-treated patients:

Table 8.5. The best distant response by treatment group. Response of bony metastases in EORTC trial 30761

Treatment	Number of patients	Assessment of response (%)				"Objective response" (%)
		CR	PR	NC	PROG	CR + PR
CPA	38	5.3	7.9	39.5	47.4	13.2
MPA	35	0	2.9	40.0	57.1	2.9
DES	28	3.6	14.3	42.9	39.3	17.9

MPA vs DES $P=0.11$
CPA vs DES $P=0.86$
CPA vs MPA $P=0.24$

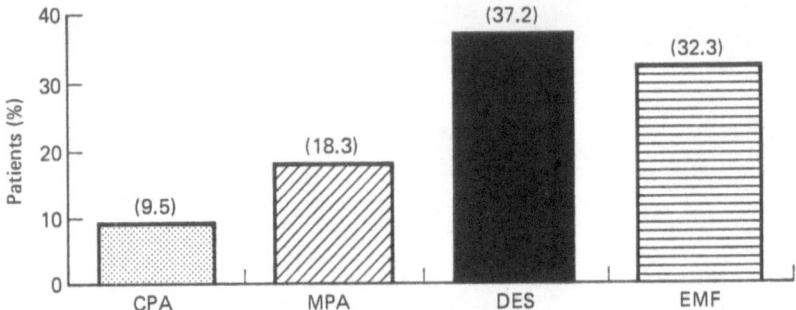

Fig. 8.7. Overall incidence of CV toxicity by treatment in EORTC trials 30761 and 30762 (CPA, cyproterone acetate; MPA, medroxyprogesterone acetate; DES, diethylstilboestrol; EMF, estramustine phosphate).

1. It cannot be excluded that the dose used in this study was too low and that higher doses, between 500 and 2000 mg daily, such as those employed by other workers (Pannuti et al. 1980) in breast and prostate cancer, might yield better results
2. In our series, the MPA-treated patients presented a higher percentage of unfavourable prognostic factors than patients in the other treatment groups. However, despite adjustment for the most important prognostic factors, MPA still remained less effective than the other drugs
3. MPA may present an androgenic effect per se, apart from its action in decreasing serum LH levels, reducing the testicular production and perhaps

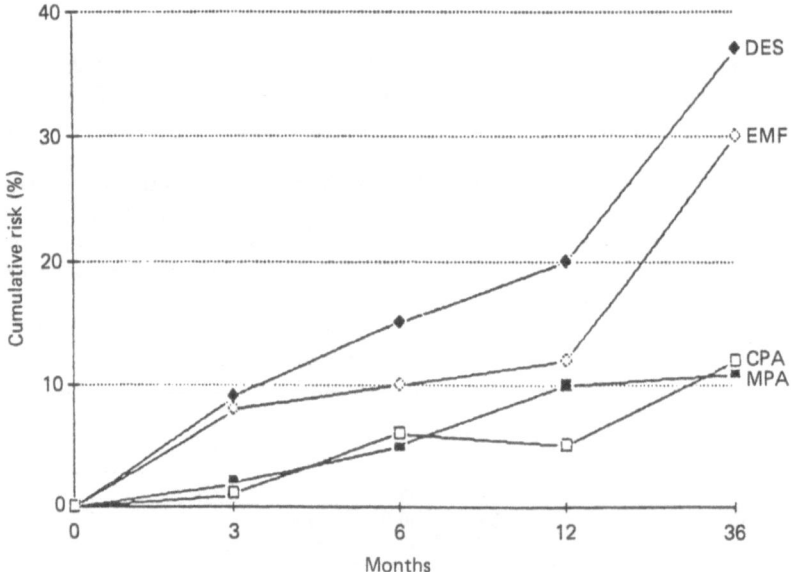

Fig. 8.8. Cumulative risk of CV toxicity in EORTC trials 30761 and 30762 (for abbreviations see Fig. 8.7).

the peripheral activation of testosterone. Fosså et al. (1984) demonstrated in a randomised study that the palliative effect of MPA in relapsing prostatic cancer is greater than that of prednisolone. However, a transient exacerbation of pain and even recovery of sexual potency in individual patients while on MPA was attributed to a possible androgenic effect of this compound

Cyproterone Acetate

Cyproterone acetate (CPA) is a steroid molecule, which displays antiandrogenic, progestational and antigonadotrophic effects. Because of its antiandrogenic properties, CPA blocks the binding of dihydrotestosterone to the specific receptors in the prostatic cells. In addition, it exerts a central inhibitory effect, reducing the secretion of LH and in turn the release of testosterone from the testes. It has been reported that CPA has a marked suppressive effect on the ACTH–adrenal function, probably owing to a cortisol-like action and, in rats, inhibits the growth of the ventral prostate induced by adrenal androgens (Isurugi et al. 1980). Bracci and Di Silverio (1979) pioneered its clinical use and reported large numbers of patients treated with CPA, administered in most cases after orchidectomy, introducing the concept of "complete androgenic blockade". A similar approach was subsequently followed by Giuliani et al. (1980) who reported a better 5-year crude survival rate in patients treated with orchidectomy and CPA than in patients treated with orchidectomy and DES.

In other centres CPA was given as the only treatment, either orally, at doses ranging between 100 and 300 mg daily, or intramuscularly, using a depot preparation (Jacobi et al. 1980). This treatment appeared to be at least as good as oestradiol undecylate, but caused significantly fewer and milder side effects than the oestrogen.

The results of a phase III randomised trial performed by the EORTC Urological Group confirmed that with regard to clinical efficacy CPA (250 mg daily, per os) was similar to DES and better than MPA (Pavone-Macaluso et al. 1986) but there were fewer side effects. The fact that a few patients died from CV disease during treatment, or more frequently, after the treatment was stopped, is to be considered merely coincidental and cannot be attributed to the treatment. In theory, CPA (which reduces plasma testosterone to castrate levels, acts peripherally as an anti-androgen and decreases production of adrenal androgens) should produce an optimal "complete androgen blockade". It has been claimed that CPA cannot be compared to pure antiandrogens, because it can produce androgen-like effects under certain experimental circumstances. In particular, if pregnant guinea pigs are treated with CPA, female foetuses present persistence of Wolffian ducts, partial development of prostate and epididymis and other "virilising" manifestations. However, this has not been confirmed in other animal species and in different experimental conditions. On the contrary, an androgen-like action of CPA is contradicted by the following facts:

1. It produces feminisation of male foetuses in all species
2. It is devoid of proliferative effect on the prostate of juvenile castrated rats
3. It shows experimental and clinical antiandrogenic effects under all conditions of endogenous hyperandrogenism (Habenicht et al. 1988).

Furthermore, if dogs are treated with androgens, the prostate show a castration-like appearance if sufficient CPA is added (Tunn et al. 1979).

In conclusion, CPA provides excellent androgenic deprivation, even in monotherapy. It has minimal if any, CV toxicity. Its main side effects are: impotence and occasional depression of mood. It produces a moderate increase of prolactin which is significantly lower than that produced by oestrogens.

LH-RH analogues

A recent alternative modality for reducing testosterone concentration is the use of the analogues of luteinising hormone releasing hormone (LH-RH). Super-agonists, rather than antagonists, have been employed for clinical use. Adminis-tration of LH-RH agonists, which are more powerful than the natural hormone, initially promotes gonadotrophin release and produces a rise in testosterone secretion but chronic administration ultimately produces a fall in LH secretion and plasma testosterone concentration falls to castrate levels. Various formula-tions are currently available: Buserelin (Suprefact R) is usually administered by daily i.m. injection for a few days and then by nasal spray 6 times daily. More recently, the same analogue has been prepared in a depot form. Other super-agonists in clinical use are: goserelin (Zoladex R), leuprolide, triptorelin (Decapeptyl R) and nafarelin. Goserelin and triptorelin have been extensively tested in Europe (Robinson et al. 1987; Boccardo et al. 1987). Goserelin is given subcutaneously, at the dose of 3.6 mg at monthly intervals. All the existing analogues show excellent tolerance and produce practically no side effects, except hot flushes, which may be rather disturbing, but tend to disappear with time. Decrease of libido and erectile potency is a very frequent phenomenon, as expected. Since the LH-RH analogues produce a kind of chemical castration, the clinical efficacy is anticipated to be as good as that of surgical orchidectomy, but not superior to it. In fact, randomised studies have confirmed that buserelin and castration obtain identical clinical results (Kaisary et al. 1988). The only advantage of the analogue is that it avoids the psychological trauma and the minor postoperative complications of castration. Furthermore, leuprolide (daily subcu-taneous injections of 1 mg aliquots) and DES (3 mg daily) showed identical response rates in a prospective randomised trial (Garnick 1986). Time to disease progression and death rate were identical for the two groups. However, 13% of the DES patients discontinued treatment because of side effects, compared to only 3% of those receiving leuprolide (Smith 1985). Identical conclusions were reached by another study in which Goserelin depot was compared with DES 3 mg/day (Emtage et al. 1987).

It should be kept in mind that the initial rise in plasma testosterone, if the analogues are given as the only treatment, can produce a "flare phenomenon". This occurs in about 5%–10% of cases, often producing an exacerbation of pain from metastatic bony lesions. Its complications may sometimes be life-threaten-ing, resulting in paraplegia due to spinal cord compression, ureteric obstruction and other severe side effects due to accelerated cancer growth. Therefore, many authors favour the administration of an oestrogen (DES 3 mg daily) or an anti-androgen for 2–4 weeks, to be started before or at the same time as the LH-RH analogue, in order to prevent the flare phenomenon (Bouffioux et al. 1987).

The main problem with the LH-RH analogues is their high cost, which may prevent their adoption as a routine treatment for extended periods of time. A useful suggestion is to test the response to antiandrogenic treatment by a short course of an analogue, so that only the responding patients will be submitted to castration (Newling 1987).

Estramustine phosphate

Estramustine phosphate (Estracyt) is a molecule in which oestradiol is chemically bound to the alkylating agent, nitrogen mustard. The rationale is to carry the cytostatic compound to the target organ by mediation of the hormone moiety, which is presumed to bind to a specific receptor in the cancer organ. Strangely enough, estramustine accumulates in the prostate because of binding not with oestrogen receptors, but with a specific receptor protein that binds estramustine and is contained in the prostate in high amounts. This is not the only unexpected phenomenon, for it has been shown that the cytotoxic action of this compound is not that of the alkylating agents, but is similar to that of the vinca alkaloids inducing mitotic arrest. It has been demonstrated that 10%–15% of estramustine administered is metabolised into oestrogens (oestradiol and oestrone) which enter the circulation. Therefore, it is thought that Estracyt has a double action: both oestrogenic and cytotoxic (Khoury 1986). Estracyt has been used both in patients relapsing after failure of primary treatment and in those previously untreated. In the latter, conflicting results have been reported. The EORTC urological group (Smith et al. 1986) compared low dose Estracyt (280 mg twice daily for 8 weeks and 140 mg twice daily thereafter) with DES (3 mg daily) in previously untreated patients with stages C and D prostate cancer. This randomised phase III trial showed no significant difference between treatments for response rate of metastases, interval to progression and overall survival. Estracyt was associated with cardiovascular toxicity in 38 of 115 patients (33%). Although the overall incidence of CV toxicity was similar in both arms of the trial, the incidence of severe and lethal events was more than twice as high in patients receiving DES than in those treated with Estracyt. CV deaths were 16% and 7% respectively.

Similar results were obtained in another randomised study in which Estracyt (840 mg daily) was compared with a combination of two different oestrogens: polyoestradiol phosphate (80 mg monthly i.m.) and 17-α-ethinyloestradiol (2 mg daily for 2 weeks followed by a reduced maintenance dose). No difference was observed between the two groups with regard to any of the response criteria investigated (Anderson et al. 1980). However, Benson et al. (1983), comparing high dose Estracyt (1000 mg/day) with DES (3 mg/day) concluded that Estracyt was slightly, but significantly, better than DES in non-castrated patients, whereas this difference was not apparent in patients who had undergone orchidectomy prior to the treatment. At this dose schedule, cardiovascular side effects were similar in the two groups (43% and 45% respectively). Such CV side effects were mainly due to water and sodium retention, while those depending on alterations of blood clotting were more marked in the group receiving DES. In all series, the main side effect of Estracyt was poor gastrointestinal tolerance especially at high doses, requiring interruption of the treatment in 10%–15% of cases. No marrow toxicity is seen when Estracyt is given orally but patients may develop an increase in the number of circulating platelets. Hepatic toxicity and neurotoxicity are usually mild. The suggestion that Estracyt is better than other hormonal treatments in poorly differentiated cancer (G3) has not been confirmed in the EORTC trial (Smith et al. 1986). The efficacy and side effects of estramustine were compared with flutamide in a recent study (Johansson et al. 1987). The initial response rate was similar in both groups and no difference in survival was seen but the objective response obtained with estramustine appeared to be of relatively longer duration. However, there were only 30 patients in both groups and the significance of these findings remains uncertain. All the estramustine-treated patients lost their libido, whereas only 20% of those treated with flutamide did so.

In conclusion, Estracyt is a useful treatment for advanced prostate cancer. For various reasons, including its relatively high cost, especially in comparison with oestrogens (Smith 1985), most workers favour an alternative therapy in previously untreated patients, while there is agreement on its value as a second-line endocrine management. It appears to be especially useful in patients relapsing after radiotherapy as, under these circumstances, its toxicity is much lower than that of cyclophosphamide or other chemotherapeutic agents.

Complete Androgen Blockade

The theory of complete androgen blockade is based on the following assumption: the cells composing a prostatic tumour that fail to respond to adequate androgen deprivation are not androgen-insensitive cells, but rather they are hypersensitive to androgens. Thus, they continue to grow after castration because they are stimulated by the low amounts of androgens left after orchidectomy or other treatments which reduce the circulating androgens to castrate levels. Such remaining androgens are basically of adrenal origin, as suggested by the remissions observed after adrenalectomy or hypophysectomy in patients having relapsed following previous endocrine therapy. As pointed out in various papers by a group of Canadian workers (Labrie et al. 1988), although orchidectomy is followed by a 90% reduction in circulating androgens, the intracellular levels of DHT are only reduced by 50% and unless intracellular androgens are blocked by antiandrogens they may exert a stimulatory effect on hypersensitive prostate cancer cells. To support this assumption, the belief that adrenal androgens play a major role is essential. Although they are considered as "weak androgens", they may indeed stimulate the prostatic cells if they are converted into active androgens, such as DHT. To what extent and consistency this metabolic step takes place in man is uncertain. The weak androgenic properties of the adrenal precursors are compensated by the large amounts in which they are produced by human males whose plasma levels of dihydroepiandrosterone sulphate are 834 ng/ml, while normal testosterone levels are only 4–6 ng/ml.

Furthermore, Bélanger et al. (1984) reported that the antiandrogen nilutamide induced a decrease of adrenal androgens in the plasma of treated subjects. Although the mechanism of this fall was not elucidated (decreased synthesis, enhanced catabolism or increased elimination) it was suggested that it could add to the value of the antiandrogenic properties of the drug, in particular after castration.

The problem is further confused by the fact that apparently only the human being produces large amounts of adrenal androgens. Therefore the role of adrenal androgens cannot be tested in the common laboratory animals; no other substitute providing an appropriate experimental model is available.

In addition, there is no clearcut evidence that adrenal androgens can stimulate the normal prostate in man: the prostate is consistently atrophic in eunuchs (Wu and Gu 1987) and in patients with hypopituitarism (Oesterling et al. 1986). Nonetheless, it is clear that patients die of prostatic carcinoma even without testes and adrenals. Many authorities still hold the view that such patients do not die because of residual androgens in the serum or within the prostate, but because of the emergence of totally androgen-independent cells (Schulze et al. 1987). Another assumption has been that antiandrogens completely block the intracellular androgens, irrespective of the origin of the latter hormones. If this is the case, the antiandrogen alone is all that is needed. Since the proponents of the new concept have not been in favour of the latter therapeutic alternative, it has been necessary to conclude that "complete androgen blockade" is a utopian idea and that the term itself is a misnomer. Therefore, "combination therapy" has been used in recent papers from the Quebec group, instead of "complete androgen blockade". A recent review has been made by Schroeder (1985), to whom the reader is referred for more information on the basic controversies about this issue. The clinical results still deserve confirmation. Much expectation followed the reports by Labrie et al. (1983) who claimed that castration (by LH-RH analogues or by orchidectomy) supplemented by a pure antiandrogen (nilutamide or flutamide) produced results that were much better than those described in historical and even in contemporary series. In particular, three points were stressed and advertised:

1. The high percentage of very early complete responses – as high as 29.2% compared to an average of only 4.6% in patients treated with the LH-RH analogues alone. However, if patients had received combination therapy for 2 years, 45% of them were reported to have achieved a complete response (Labrie et al. 1988)
2. A four-fold decrease in progression
3. A very striking improvement in survival rate.

These data refer to previously untreated patients with D2 prostatic cancer, but even for patients in relapse from previous therapies the probability of surviving was reported to be more than doubled if they were given the combined therapy. The same effect upon survival was also inferred for earlier stages (Fig. 8.9), leading to the statement that "combination therapy with flutamide should be started early in the disease", at least in stage C (Labrie et al. 1987).

These results are so greatly superior to those seen after conventional treatments that it was unanimously felt that they deserved confirmation, especially as these data did not stem from a prospective randomised trial, since the controls were taken from old historical series or from the recent literature.

It has already been quoted that the EORTC study 30805 has so far failed to show that the combined treatment, orchidectomy + CPA, is better than castration alone. It was argued that CPA is a different antiandrogen and not a "pure antiandrogen", and that results could not therefore be compared with those of the Canadian group.

The initial results of randomised studies using either nilutamide (Béland et al. 1987; Navratil 1987; Brisset et al. 1987) or flutamide (Delaere et al. 1987;

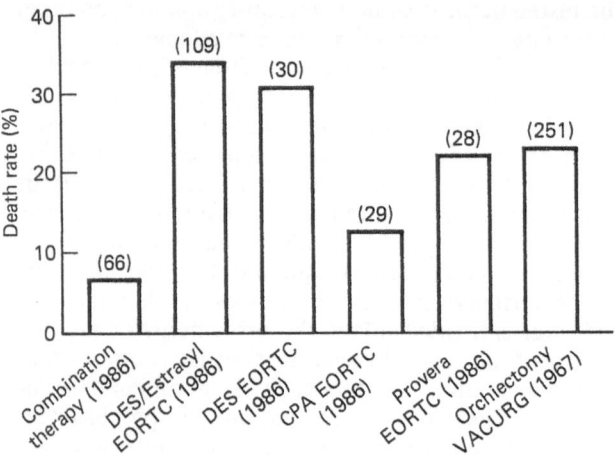

Fig. 8.9. Comparison of the probability of death in patients with clinical Stage C prostate cancer who received the combination therapy with flutamide and the LH-RH agonist (D-Trp), LH-RH ethylamide, Estracyt, DES, cyproterone acetate (CPA), medroxyprogesterone acetate (Provera) or orchidectomy.

Crawford et al. 1987b) have failed to show any benefit in survival in patients receiving the combination therapy versus those treated with orchidectomy or the LH-RH analogues only. Complete responses were observed by Delaere et al. (1987) in only one of 87 patients (i.e. 1.3%) treated with castration and flutamide. In some reports, there was a trend towards a shorter time to response in the antiandrogen group compared to the placebo group but this was of variable significance. In the NCI study (Crawford et al. 1987b) the time advantage was about one month (Eisenberger, personal communication) but it is not surprising that this should occur if the control group is treated with the LH-RH analogues. In the latter group, the androgenic deprivation only occurs after 2–3 weeks, during which there is androgenic overstimulation. Brisset et al. (1987) observed that the anandron-treated patients had a slower progression at 6 months, although all patients were castrated. However this difference was not statistically significant and was not maintained at 12 and 18 months.

   In conclusion, the initial hope that combination therapy represents a dramatic improvement in the treatment of advanced prostatic cancer has not been fostered by results from other groups, raising the possibility of selection bias in the previous reports. Differences in response criteria may be another explanation. The concept is attractive and perhaps a few patients can benefit from this approach. Unfortunately, combined therapy entails a greater cost and involves a greater incidence of side effects than surgical or chemical castration only. Therefore, in our view, its use cannot be routinely recommended at the present time until its superiority over conventional treatment is clearly proved.

Aminoglutethimide (AG)

A "medical adrenalectomy" can be produced by AG. AG inhibits the enzymatic conversion of cholesterol to delta-5-pregnenolone thereby blocking adrenal steroidogenesis. As a result, it reduces the synthesis of glucocorticoids, mineralo-corticoids and sex steroids (Crawford et al. 1987a).

AG is derived from the hypnotic drug glutethimide. It also causes a temporary reduction of thyroxine which can be compensated by increased TSH production. To block the production of adrenal androgens, AG is usually given at doses (500–1000 mg daily) which also block glucocorticoids, so that hydrocortisone replacement must also be given, and mineralocorticoid replacement may also be useful at least in some patients.

Preliminary experience in breast cancer has shown that if AG is given at lower doses, glucocorticoids may not be necessary but there is insufficient experience with this practice in prostatic cancer. The toxicity is considerable, so that AG has been employed only for patients in relapse and not as a primary therapy for untreated patients. The main side effect, as expected, is somnolence which may be rather severe and progress to lethargy. Other possible side effects are fever, rash, nausea, ataxia, nystagmus, neutropenia, let alone the side effects due to the administration of cortisone.

In patients with progression after initial treatment, AG therapy can be followed by 10% partial responses, while 40% of the patients show stable disease and 50% continue to progress (Crawford et al. 1987b). Subjective response was reported in 60% of patients. It is unclear to what extent the latter effect is attributable to the glucoactive steroid administered together with AG.

Ketoconazole (KC)

KC is a well known antimycotic imidazole-derivative which at relatively low doses (200 mg daily per os) leads to destruction of *Candida albicans* and other fungi, by inhibiting the cytochrome P-450 enzyme-dependent synthesis of ergosterol in the fungine body. At higher doses (1200 mg), it reduces testosterone production in both adrenals and testes, by inhibition of two cytochrome P-450-dependent enzymes: 17-hydroxylase and 17-20 lyase (Trachtenberg 1984). In man, testosterone values reach castration levels within a few hours (Mahler et al. 1987). KC may thus produce a real "complete androgen blockade" and be of great value in the treatment of advanced prostate cancer. Unfortunately, its toxicity is quite severe and the drug does not lend itself to generalised use, apart from cases refractory to conventional treatments. The most common side effect is gastro-intestinal intolerance, which can be rather severe in the form of gastric discomfort, anorexia and vomiting. Other side effects include hepatic toxicity, weakness and fatigue. Complete blockade of adrenal steroidogenesis may lead to acute, potentially lethal, addisonian crises. In conclusion, KC may delay progression, induce objective responses and symptomatic palliation even in patients relapsing after previous therapy, but it must be handled with the utmost caution.

Other Hormones and Drugs

Antioestrogens (Tamoxifen) have induced a few responses (De Voogt 1985). Corticosteroids may be of benefit either for the "medical adrenalectomy" they produce (Robinson 1983) or for their intrinsic anti-inflammatory action and their effect in improving the patient's feeling of well being. However, high-dose MPA proved to be better than prednisolone in this regard (Fosså et al. 1984). Parathyroid hormone may improve the action of radioactive phosphorus. Calcitonin may bring about symptomatic relief in painful osteolytic metastases. Spironolactone may decrease the production of adrenal androgens. Prednimustine is still in the investigational stage.

Finally, androgens can be used to stimulate cells to enter the proliferation cycle thereby rendering them susceptible to cycle-specific cytotoxic chemotherapy (Manni et al. 1987). Some patients may experience a transient benefit, but others do worse. From published reports androgen priming did not appear to potentiate the efficacy of chemotherapy but was actually associated with a worse outcome.

Cytotoxic Chemotherapy

Cytotoxic chemotherapy has not yet offered significant survival advantage in prostate cancer and its real value has been questioned (Tannock 1985).

When the world's literature was reviewed in the early years of this decade (Pavone-Macaluso 1982), the following conclusions emerged:

1. In metastatic patients relapsing after failure of endocrine manipulation, chemotherapy may produce temporary objective response where alternative forms of androgen deprivation fail
2. The best single agent or combinations of agents have yet to be identified
3. There is no evidence that treatment with multiple drug combinations is better than therapy with a single drug
4. The multiple drug cocktails may show an increased toxicity
5. Clinical response to cytotoxic chemotherapy is statistically associated with increased survival
6. Patients with progressive disease who have received irradiation to the pelvis should be treated with drugs having little myelotoxicity, such as streptozotocin, estramustine, prednimustine or vincristine
7. The association of oestrogens and cytotoxic chemotherapeutic agents as the first step in "virgin" cases rests on stimulating theoretical grounds, but no clinical results are available which show improved results while addition of toxicity is to be feared.
8. The objective remissions are difficult to assess and response criteria must be very stringent for possible comparison of results
9. Systemic chemotherapy has not been shown to cure any patient with prostatic cancer, and no permanent and complete objective regression has been documented

Therefore if the aim of the therapy is merely that of obtaining palliation (with or without prolongation of acceptable life) it is imperative that the treatment must not lead to side effects that are more distressing for the patient than the disease itself. In other words, the quality of life should be given priority in the planning of treatment.

What significant changes or additions to these conclusions need to be made to these statements from the experience of the last 6 years? Not much appears from recent reports (Soloway 1985; Stoter and Jones 1988). However, it has been shown that weekly low dose doxorubicin (20 mg/m^2) is devoid of severe side effects, shows the same range of activity as the large dose monthly schedule and often improves the patients' quality of life (Robinson et al. 1983). Following this report, it was hoped that epirubicin, a less cardiotoxic derivative of doxorubicin might be even more helpful; however, it has had little success when used in very low, perhaps insufficient doses (12 mg/m^2). In addition, encouraging results have been obtained with mitomycin C, 15 mg/m^2 i.v. every 6 weeks (Jones et al. 1986). A partial response for a median duration of 6 months was achieved in 9 of 31 patients (29%). The median duration of survival was 8 months, there was significant improvement of symptoms and the drug was subjectively very well tolerated. Thus, at least two new schedules have emerged that can be of practical benefit to the patients with refractory disease and severe symptoms.

Choice of Hormonal Treatment in the Previously Untreated Patient

The detailed review of the various possibilities confirms that there is no universal panacea for all patients. In our view, at the present state of our knowledge, no single treatment producing effective androgen deprivation has been proved to be superior in efficacy to other therapies in previously untreated patients. Thus, insofar as the clinical efficacy of the various forms of hormonal manipulation is likely to be roughly equivalent, the choice of the most appropriate treatment for every single patient should rest, as the main determinant, on its tolerability to and acceptance by the patient (Pavone-Macaluso et al. 1987). When no specific risk factors leading to expected toxicity or influencing acceptance can be identified, cost should play a role in making the choice. Flutamide appears to be a reasonable choice in patients who wish to maintain an active sexual life. Combination of drugs may be more efficacious, at least in some patients, but their value still requires definitive confirmation. Hopefully, this will emerge from the ongoing studies of the EORTC urological group. Trial 30843, coordinated by H. J. de Voogt (Amsterdam) aims to compare the therapeutic effect of orchidectomy versus LH-RH-analogue (Buserelin) supplemented by an anti-androgen (CPA). Trial 30853, coordinated by L. Denis (Antwerp), is another randomised study to compare orchidectomy versus Goserelin plus flutamide.

Choice of the Treatment in the Unresponsive Patients or after Failure of the Primary Treatment

Unresponsiveness to the hormone therapy may by primary or secondary, when progression occurs during the treatment. In both cases the prognosis is poor. A secondary treatment is usually instituted, but the median survival in the patients showing progression after an initial response is of the order of 6 months only. In some cases, it is possible that progression is due to insufficient or inadequate treatment, as in the case of poor patient compliance. If serum testosterone has not been adequately suppressed, there is a chance of a secondary response after orchidectomy. In the opposite situation, orchidectomy is unlikely to be of any value.

If we believe that resistance is mainly due to selection of hormone-resistant cells, it would be logical to use chemotherapeutic agents rather than trying to employ a different form of hormonal treatment.

No rule can be established at the present time. Most urologists tend to employ second-line hormonal treatment: orchidectomy if plasma testosterone is not sufficiently reduced or one of following: estramustine phosphate, high dose fosfestrol (with or without antiprolactins), MPA, flutamide, ketoconazole, aminoglutethimide, CPA (Klijn et al. 1985; de Voogt 1985). It has been shown, when discussing the action of these various drugs, that each can produce objective responses (usually in no more than in 20% of cases) rarely exceeding 6 months in duration. Symptomatic relief can be good in a greater percentage of patients. The choice of the treatment depends more on the personal preference of the clinician than on objective data. Specific risk factors must be taken into consideration. Although cytotoxic chemotherapy is usually started after failure of second-line endocrine treatment, some authorities think it should be used earlier. It is certainly true that the poor results and the excessive toxicity of cytotoxic chemotherapy in prostatic cancer can be attributed, in part, to the fact that patients are treated when their performance status is poor and every treatment is doomed to fail.

Results of the Hormonal Treatment

The results of hormonal treatment have been the object of diverging interpretations. Although many papers and chapters in textbooks state that 80% responses can be achieved, this rate is over-optimistic and mainly based on the investigator's evaluation of symptomatic improvement.

A more realistic assessment can be reached if standard response criteria are adopted (Schroeder and EORTC Urological Group 1984). In spite of this, it is well known that it is extremely difficult to evaluate objective responses in prostate cancer, especially as far as the most common metastatic site, i.e. bone, is concerned. Palpable masses such as soft tissue lesions or superficial lymph nodes can be accurately measured but they are relatively rare and their prognosis is usually severe. If the EORTC response criteria are adopted, a standard hormonal treatment, such as DES 3 mg daily, determines objective responses in 51.5% and 31.4% (Smith et al. 1986) respectively of the primary tumours and the metastatic lesions. These figures were 55% and 18% in another EORTC study (Pavone-Macaluso et al. 1986).

Even the exact incidence of subjective improvement is difficult to assess, not only because of the intrinsic difficulty in obtaining accurate information, but also because of lack of uniformity in the selection of patients submitted to treatment. Only statistics emanating from centres where hormonal treatment is administered exclusively to patients with symptoms (usually pain), can give a reasonable assessment of how often palliation is achieved. In such cases significant relief of symptoms is believed to occur in about one-half of cases but this requires further evaluation. The effect of hormonal treatment upon survival is even more controversial. Although comparison of mortality rates of patients with prostate cancer shows a definite improvement in survival after the introduction of hormonal treatment in the early 1940s, such a comparison is based on historical controls. It is likely that the better survival depends more on collateral factors – which greatly improved in the years that immediately followed the second World War – than on the effect of hormonal therapy as such (Lepor et al. 1982). The VACURG studies (Byar 1977b) are often quoted to show that there is no evidence that treatment increases survival. In fact there is no difference between placebo and treatment with either orchidectomy or oestrogens. In this context, placebo is only the initial approach, but practically all the patients received secondary treatment in the case of progression or when they developed symptoms, so that these studies actually compared immediate versus delayed treatment. Therefore, the conclusion can be rephrased as "there is no evidence that immediate treatment improves survival". It should be noted, however, that if we only look at cancer-related survival, patients treated with oestrogens did better than those given placebo. In other words, the data can be interpreted as indicative of the fact that placebo and oestrogens are associated with the same survival, but oestrogens are responsible for cardiovascular mortality. It ensues that the other forms of hormone therapy which are exempt from such a toxicity, should not only reduce cancer-related death rate, but also improve overall survival.

A recent study of the EORTC urological group (Pavone-Macaluso et al. 1986) has shown that an effective form of hormonal treatment (such as CPA or DES) is correlated with a better survival than another form of treatment, MPA, which is inferior also in terms of local and distant responses. The interpretation of this observation can vary according to a priori opinions (Fair 1986) but many fields of general oncology show that treatments producing a higher objective response rate are also correlated with a better survival. In any case, even if we admit that androgen deprivation therapy does improve survival – at least in responding patients – the overall magnitude of this event is relatively minor, and the outcome depends more on prognostic factors (such as performance status, stage and grade) than on the treatment given. It should be stressed, however, that effective hormonal treatment is effective in delaying progression.

The same VACURG studies had clearly shown that progression from stage III to IV, i.e. the appearance of metastases, is significantly reduced when patients are treated with either castration or DES as compared to the group given placebo. The EORTC studies (Smith et al. 1986; Pavone-Macaluso et al. 1986) have confirmed that active forms of hormonal treatment (DES, CPA, Estracyt) are more efficacious than a less active drug such as MPA, whose effect is supposed to stand at an intermediate level between active treatment, such as DES, and placebo. It is likely that the most logical way of assessing results is that of taking primarily into account the quality of life of the patients given – or not given – a treatment (Calais da Silva and Aaronson 1988).

Indications for Hormonal Treatment in Prostatic Cancer

Although this chapter discusses primarily the treatment of metastatic prostate cancer, indications for hormonal treatment in the early stages of the disease should be mentioned. In general, hormonal treatment is useless and even contraindicated in patients with prostatic cancer To pT1–2, T1 and T2, No, Mo. With regard to category T3, preoperative oestrogens have been reported to be capable of reducing the local tumour mass thereby facilitating its surgical extirpation. Orchidectomy is routinely used in a few centres in the United States whenever radical prostatectomy is performed for category T3 (stage C) prostatic cancer. It is thought to be indicated in pN+ cancers. The value of the latter procedure is still to be established. In patients with locally advanced prostate cancer (T3 NxMo) treated with external beam radiation (7000 rads in 7 weeks) the addition of oestrogens was associated with a worse survival (Van der Werf-Messing 1977). In conclusion, the indications for hormonal treatment in the early stages, whenever a radical treatment can be employed with a curative aim, are rare and not fully established. The question is more debatable when we consider patients with advanced stage C (T3-T4, No or Nx, Mo) prostatic cancer. When the tumour is responsible for obstructive symptoms, many authorities prefer to use medical treatment rather than to perform a palliative TUR. Other urologists are in favour of early hormonal treatment even in asymptomatic patients whose cancer is not metastatic, but locally too extensive to be amenable to surgery or to irradiation. The rationale for this attitude lies in the fact that hormonal treatment can delay progression from stage C (Mo) to stage D (M1). Perhaps survival will not be affected, but it seems worthwhile to try to prevent (or delay) metastatic spread. Quality of life is likely to be better without than with metastases. Furthermore, there can be no serious doubt that it is better to treat a tumour while it is small rather than when it is large and it can also be argued that hormone therapy should be started early to prevent complications from uncontrolled tumour growth. These statements are supported by experimental studies (Isaacs 1985), but unfortunately there is no factual support from them which is based on experience with human carcinoma of the prostate (Chisholm 1986).

For sexually active patients who wish to maintain potency, flutamide rather than orchidectomy or drugs that reduce libido and potency can be employed as this form of treatment will not impair their quality of life. Two opposite views are held: Labrie et al. (1988) believe that treatment of patients with stage C prostatic cancer is mandatory as it will markedly improve survival, and other workers such as Newling et al. (1985) suggest that hormonal treatment should be delayed and obstructive symptoms treated, if needed, by transurethral resection. The reasons for not giving patients the hormonal treatment are the following:

1. No benefit in survival
2. Possible side effects of drugs, especially oestrogens
3. Loss of sexual function
4. Possibility that early treatment might favour the selection of hormone-resistant clones, thereby rendering the hormonal treatment ineffective when needed at the time of objective or symptomatic progression.

There is, however, no proof that the last event does occur in clinical practice. The same arguments have been put forward to favour a no-treatment policy even in patients with metastases but without symptoms. The issue has not yet been solved and, whenever the question is raised in meetings or workshops, a show of hands indicates that the room is equally divided (Blandy and Pavone-Macaluso 1983). In the absence of hard evidence the problem must be solved by controlled clinical trials. Unfortunately, the question still remains open as a phase III trial of the Medical Research Council in the United Kingdom comparing immediate and deferred orchidectomy has not yet been completed (Kirk 1988).

When metastatic prostatic cancer becomes symptomatic, the indications for hormonal treatment are universally accepted. Even for high grade (G3) cancer, hormonal treatment is indicated, since 20% of patients will respond. On the other hand, there is no possibility of predicting which patients will respond. The initial hope that determination of androgen receptors in the cytosol or even in the nuclei of neoplastic prostatic cells may discriminate responders from nonresponders has not been fulfilled. Perhaps the determination of intracellular dihydrotestosterone may be more helpful, but no large series have confirmed this assumption. Patients with high levels of plasma testosterone are more likely to respond than those presenting low levels. There are other observations and new techniques to predict hormonal responsiveness of human prostatic cancer (Barrack et al. 1987), but there is still no easy and reproducible way to predict the quality and duration of response to endocrine manipulation. The obvious conclusion is that hormonal treatment still remains the standard initial therapy for metastatic prostatic cancer. Clinical response will be the only guide to indicate whether a second-line therapy will be needed.

Palliative Treatment

Patients with locally advanced or metastatic prostatic cancer may require palliative treatments in addition to hormonal therapy. Outflow obstruction may require TUR although some centres prefer cryosurgical procedures. Anaemia may require correction and in the case of bilateral ureteric obstruction there may be a need for percutaneous nephrostomies and for indwelling ureteral stents. Refractory pain may require analgesics, irradiation of the painful lesion, administration of radioactive phosphorus, or lower and upper half-body irradiation. The latter procedure is dangerous and requires sophisticated haematological support, in view of the high risk of severe thrombocytopenia (Van der Werf-Messing 1983). In addition to its palliative benefit, it is hoped that half-body irradiation may have some curative qualities, to be exploited at least in patients with poorly differentiated lesions.

The terminal patient will require active and competent support. His pain must be relieved and his other physical and psychological problems must be given proper aid. The family should be kept informed and be helped in every possible way. To quote Whelan (1988) "the surgeon, as he strives to do during the phase of active treatment, must ensure that only the best treatment is available for his patients during their terminal illness. The surgeon who first diagnosed and who initiated treatment should not relinquish all responsibilities for them. . . . To be available finally may be all he has to offer."

Conclusion

This review of the possible therapies for patients with metastatic prostatic cancer demonstrates the many possibilities and highlights again the pre-eminence of hormonal treatment including orchidectomy.

Such information as is available on the use of cytotoxic chemotherapy does not yet suggest that this form of treatment is justified at the time of initial diagnosis though it can be of help in those who have failed on primary hormonal therapy.

The interesting concept of complete androgen blockade by the use of orchidectomy or oestrogenic therapy in association with antiandrogen treatment has yet to be shown to be superior to standard hormonal therapy alone or orchidectomy for newly diagnosed patients with metastatic disease.

Clearly, further work is needed to improve the management of these patients both at the time of diagnosis and when relapse occurs as so commonly it does.

References

Altwein J (1983) Estrogens in the treatment of prostatic cancer. In: Pavone-Macaluso M, Smith PH (eds) Cancer of the prostate and kidney. Plenum Press, New York, pp 317–328

Andersson L, Berlin T, Boman J, Collste L, Edsmyr F, Esposti PL, Gustafsson H, Hedlund PO, Hultgren L, Leander G, Nordle O, Norlen H, Tillegard P (1980) Estramustine versus conventional estrogen hormones in the initial treatment of highly or moderately differentiated prostatic carcinoma. A randomized study. Scand J Urol Nephrol [Suppl] 55 143–145

Barràck ER, Brendler CB, Walsh PC (1987) Steroid receptors and biochemical profiles in prostatic cancer: correlation with response to hormonal treatment. In: Murphy GP, Khoury S, Kuss R, Chatelain C, Denis L (eds) Prostate cancer. Part A: Research, endocrine treatment and histopathology. Alan R Liss, New York, pp 79–97

Béland G, Elhilali M, Fradet Y, Laroch B, Ramsey EW, Benner PM, Tewar HD (1987) Total androgen blockade vs orchiectomy in stage D2 prostate cancer. In: Murphy GP, Khoury S, Küss R, Chatelain C, Denis L (eds) Prostate cancer. Part A: Research, endocrine treatment and histopathology. Alan R Liss, New York, pp 391–400

Bélanger A, Dupont A, Labrie F (1984) Inhibition of basal and adrenocorticotropin-stimulated plasma levels of adrenal androgens after treatment with an antiandrogen in castrated patients with prostatic cancer. J Clin Endocrinol Metab 59: 422–426

Benson RC, Gill GM, Cummings KB (1983) Randomized double blind crossover trial diethyl stilbestrol (DES) and estramustine phosphate (Emcyt) for stage D prostatic carcinoma. Semin Oncol 10: suppl 3, 43–45

Blandy JP, Pavone-Macaluso M (1983) Strategy of treatment in the advanced stages. Round table report. In: Pavone-Macaluso M, Smith PH (eds) Cancer of the prostate and kidney. Plenum Press, New York, pp 413–416

Boccardo F, Décensi A, Guarneri D, Rubagotti A, Massa T, Martorana G, Giberti C, Cerruti GB, Tani F, Zanollo A, Germinale T, Bozzone C, Perri F, Usai E, Santi L, Giuliani L (1987) Long term results with a long-acting formulation of D-TRP-6-LH-RH in patients with prostate cancer: an Italian Prostatic Cancer Project (PONCAP) study: Prostate 11: 243–255

Bouffioux C (1980) Treatment of prostatic cancer with medroxyprogesterone acetate. In: Pavone-Macaluso M, Smith PH, Edsmyr F (eds): Bladder tumours and other topics in urological oncology. Plenum Press, New York, pp 463–465

Bouffioux C, Denis L, Mahler C, de Leval J (1987) Treatment of advanced prostatic cancer with LHRH analogues. Prevention of flare-up phenomenon. In: Murphy GP, Khoury S, Küss R, Chatelain C, Denis L (eds) Prostate Cancer. Part A: Research, endocrine treatment and histopathology. Alan R. Liss, New York, pp 255–260

Bracci U, Di Silverio F (1979) Terapia chirurgica ed ormonale del carcinoma prostatico. In: Bracci U, Di Silverio F (eds) Terapia dei tumori ormonodipendenti. Acta Medica, Rome, pp 173–201

Brisset JM, Boccon-Gibod L, Botto H, Camey M, Criou G, Duclos JM, Duval F, Gontiés D, Jorest R, Lamy L, Le Duc A, Mouton A, Petit M, Prawerman A, Richard F, Savatovsky I, Vallancien G (1987) Anandron (RU 23908) associated to surgical castration in previously untreated stage D prostate cancer: A multicenter comparative study of two doses of the drug and of a placebo. In: Murphy GP, Khoury S, Küss R, Chatelain C, Denis L (eds) Prostate cancer. Part A: Research endocrine treatment and histopathology. Alan R Liss, New York, pp 401–410

Byar DP (1973) The Veterans Administration Cooperative Urological Research Group's studies of cancer of the prostate. Cancer 32: 1126–1130

Byar DP (1977a) Preliminary experience with 30 mg daily of medroxyprogesterone in a large randomized clinical trial (abstract). In: Pavone-Macaluso M (ed) The tumours of genito-urinary apparatus. COFESE, Palermo, p 275

Byar DP (1977b) VACURG studies on prostate cancer and its treatment. In: Tannenbaum M (ed) Urologic pathology. The Prostate. Lea & Febiger, Philadelphia, pp 251–267

Calais da Silva F, Aaronson N (1988) Quality of life assessment in prostatic cancer. In: Smith PH, Pavone-Macaluso M (eds) Management of advanced cancer of the prostate and bladder. Alan R Liss, New York, pp 119–121

Chisholm GD (1986) Hormone therapy as palliative treatment for carcinoma of the prostate. In: Pagano F, Zattoni F (eds) Progress in prostatic cancer. CED RIM, Milano pp 85–90

Consoli C, Corrado F, Di Silverio F, Fontana D, Lotti T, Micali F, Pavone-Macaluso M, Piccinno A, Pisani F, Usai E, Recchia M, Granata P, Pintus C (1987) Risultati preliminari di uno studio multicentrico sul trattamento del carcinoma della prostata con flutamide. Proc. 60th Congress Italian Urological Society (Abstract) Acta Urol Ital 1: 231

Crawford ED, Ahmann FR, Davis MA, Levasseur YJ (1987a) Aminoglutethimide in metastatic adenocarcinoma of the prostate. In: Murphy GP, Khoury S, Küss R, Chatelain C, Denis L (eds): Prostate cancer. Part A: Research, endocrine treatment and histopathology. Alan R Liss, New York, pp 283–289

Crawford DE, McLeod D, Dorr A, Spaulding J, Benson R, Eisenberger M, Blumenstein B (1987b) A comparison of leuprolide with flutamide and leuprolide in previously untreated patients with clinical stage D2 cancer of the prostate, phase III, intergroup study–0036. J Urol 610 256A

Daricello G, Serretta V, Pavone-Macaluso M (1987) Flutamide in the treatment of advanced prostate cancer J Drug Dev [suppl 1] 1: 17–22

De Bruyne F, Witjes FA and the Dutch South Eastern Urological Cooperative Group (1987) In: Murphy GP, Khoury S, Küss R, Chatelain C, Denis L (eds): Prostate cancer. Part A: Research, endocrine treatment and histopathology. Alan R Liss, New York, pp 301–313

Delaere KP, Boccon-Gibod L, Corrado F, Dubernard JM, Frick J, Ghirlanda JM, Johansson JE, Khoury S, Lardennois B, Lobel B, Mangin E, Mazeman E, Pagano F, Schulman C, Scorticati CH, Serment G, Soret JY, Uson A, Zungri E (1987) Randomized, double-blind, parallel group study of flutamide and orchiectomy vs placebo and orchiectomy in men with D2 adenocarcinoma of the prostate. Poster presented at the 4th European Conference on Clinical Oncology, Madrid

Denis L, Bouffioux C (1983) Progestins in prostatic cancer. In: Pavone-Macaluso M, Smith PH (eds): Cancer of the prostate and kidney, Plenum Press, New York, pp 339–343

De Voogt HJ (1985) Second-line endocrine management: anti-androgens and anti-estrogens. In: Schroeder FH, Richards B (eds): Therapeutic principles in metastatic prostate cancer. Alan R Liss, New York, pp 351–357

De Voogt HJ, Smith PH, Pavone-Macaluso M, de Pauw M, Suciu S and members of the EORTC (European Organization for Research on Treatment of Cancer) Urological Group (1986). Cardiovascular side effect of diethylstilbestrol, cyproterone acetate, medroxyprogesterone acetate and estramustine phosphate, used for the treatment of advanced prostatic cancer. Results from EORTC trials 30761 and 30762. J Urol 135: 303–307

Di Silverio F, Tenaglia R, Bizzarri M, Biggio A, Saragnano R (1987) Experience with flutamide in advanced prostatic cancer patients refractory to previous endocrine therapy. J Drug Dev [Suppl 1] 1: 10–16

Emtage LA, Thethowan C, Hilton C, Arkell DG, Wallace DMA, Hughes MA, Farrar DJ, Young C, Jones M, Hay AM, Blacklock ARE, Rowse AD, Blackledge GRP (1987) A randomized trial comparing Zoladex 3.6 mg depot with stilboestrol 3 mg/day in advanced prostate cancer: patient characteristics, response and treatment failures. Eur J Cancer Clin Oncol 23: 1239 (abstract 33)

Fair WR (1986) Hormonal therapy of advanced prostatic cancer. J Urol 136: 653–654

Fosså SD, Ogreid P, Karlsen S, Havelan H, Jensen J, Trovag A (1984): High dose medroxyprogesterone acetate (MPA) versus prednisolone (P) in hormone-resistant prostatic cancer. In: Bracci U, Di Silverio F (eds) Advances in urological oncology and endocrinology. Acta Medica, Rome, pp 433–437

Garnick MB (1986) Leuprolide versus diethystilbestrol for previously untreated stage D2 prostate cancer. Results of a prospective randomized trial. Urology [Suppl 1] 27: 21–26

Giuliani L, Pescatore D, Giberti C, Martorana G, Natta G (1980) Treatment of advanced prostatic carcinoma with cyproterone acetate and orchiectomy – 5 year follow-up. Eur Urol 6: 145–148

Habenicht UF, Schroeder H, El Etreby F, Neumann F (1988) Advantages and disadvantages of pure antiandrogens and of antiandrogens of the cyproterone acetate-type in the treatment of prostatic cancer. In: Smith PH, Pavone-Macaluso M (eds): Mangement of advanced cancer of the prostate and bladder. Alan R. Liss, New York, pp 63–75

Huggins C, Hodges CV (1941) Studies on prostatic cancer. I. The effect of castration, of estrogen and of androgen injection on serum phosphatase in metastatic carcinoma of the prostate. Cancer Res 1: 293–297

Isaacs J (1985) The timing of androgen ablation therapy and/or chemotherapy in the treatment of prostatic cancer. Prostate 5: 1–18

Isurugi K, Fukutani K, Ishida H, Hosoi QY (1980) Endocrine effects of cyproterone acetate in patients with prostatic cancer. J Urol 123: 180–183

Jacobi GH (1982) Experimental rationale for the investigation of antiprolactins as palliative treatment for prostate cancer. In: Jacobi GH, Hohenfellner R (eds) Prostate cancer. Williams & Wilkins, Baltimore, pp 419–431

Jacobi GH, Altwein J, Kurth KH, Basting R, Hohenfellner R (1980) Treatment of advanced prostatic cancer with parenteral cyproterone acetate. A phase III randomised trial. Br J Urol 52: 208–215

Jacobo E, Schmidt JD, Weinstein SH, Flocks RH (1976) Comparison of flutamide (SCH–13521) and diethylstilbestrol in untreated advanced prostatic cancer. Urology 8: 231–234

Johansson JE, Andersson SO, Beckman KW, Lindgardh G, Zador G (1987) Clinical evaluation of flutamide and estramustine as initial treatment of metastatic carcinoma of prostate. Urology 29: 55–59

Jones WG, Fosså S, Bono AV, Croles JJ, Stoter G, de Pauw M, Sylvester R and members of the EORTC Genito-Urinary tract Cancer Cooperative Group (1986) Mitomycin-C in the treatment of metastatic prostate cancer: report on an EORTC phase II study. World J Urol 4: 182–185

Kaisary AV, Fellows GJ, Smith JC (1987) Antiandrogen (flutamide) therapy in management of relapsing metastatic prostatic carcinoma. J Urol 137: 256A

Kaisary AV, Ryan PG, Turkes A, Peeling WB, Griffiths K (1988) A comparison between surgical orchidectomy and LH-RH analogue (Zoladex ICI 118, 630) in the treatment of advanced prostatic carcinoma. A multicentre clinical study. In: Smith PH, Pavone-Macaluso M (eds) Management of advanced cancer of the prostate and bladder. Alan R Liss, New York, pp 89–100

Khoury S (1986) Estracyt: Update 1986. In: Pagano F, Zattoni F (eds) Progress in prostatic cancer. CEDRIM, Milano, pp 97–107

Kirk D (1988) Phase III trials of the Medical Research Council. In: Smith H, Pavone-Macaluso M (eds): Management of advanced cancer of the prostate and bladder. Alan R Liss, New York, pp 77–87

Kitajima N et al. (1985) Statistical evaluation on the significance of chlormadinone acetate as an endocrine therapy for prostatic cancer. Clin. Endocrinol (Horumon–To–Rinsho) 33: 157–163 (in Japanese)

Klijn JGM, Nielander AJM, Alexieva-Figusch J, Van Putten WLJ (1985) Orchidectomy and oestrogens as secondary forms of treatment for metastatic prostatic cancer. In: Schroeder FH, Richards B (eds) Therapeutic principles in metastatic prostatic cancer. Alan R. Liss, New York, pp 335–349

Knuth UA, Hano R, Nieschlag E (1984) Effect of flutamide or cyproterone acetate on pituitary and testicular hormones in normal men. J Clin Endocrinol Metab 59: 963–969

Labrie F, Dupont A, Bélanger A, Lacourcière Y, Raynaud JP, Husson JM, Gareau J, Fazekas ATA, Sandow J, Monfette G, Girard JG, Emond J, Houle JG (1983) New approach in the treatment of prostate cancer: complete instead of partial withdrawal of androgens. Prostate 4: 579–594

Labrie F, Dupont A, Cusan L, Giguère M, Manbés G, Bergeron N, Wegrzycki W (1987) Combinations therapy with flutamide and (D-Trp6 des Gly NH$_2$10) LHRH ethylamide in previously untreated C and D prostate cancer. Abstract presented at the 4th European Conference on Clinical Oncology, Madrid

Labrie F, Dupont A, Giguère M, Borsanyi JP, Lacourcière Y, Bélanger A, Lachance R, Emond J, Monfette G (1988) Combination therapy with flutamide and castration (orchidectomy or LHRH agonist): the minimal endocrine therapy in both untreated and previously treated patients with advanced prostate cancer of the prostate and bladder. In: Smith PH, Pavone-Macaluso M (eds) Management of advanced cancer of the prostate and bladder. Alan R Liss, New York, pp 41–62

Lepor H, Ross A, Walsh PC (1982) The influence of hormonal therapy on survival of men with advanced prostatic cancer. J Urol 128: 335–340

Lund F, Rasmussen F (1987) Flutamide versus stilboestrol in the treatment of advanced prostatic cancer: a randomized prospective study. Poster presented at the 4th European Conference on Clinical Oncology, Madrid.

Maatman TJ, Gupta MK, Montie JE (1985) Effectiveness of castration versus intravenous estrogen therapy in producing rapid endocrine control of metastatic cancer of the prostate. J Urol 133: 620–621

MacFarlane JR, Tolley DA (1985) Flutamide therapy for advanced prostatic cancer: a phase II study. Br J Urol 57· 172–174

Mahler C, Denis L, De Coster R (1987) The endocrine effect of ketoconazole high doses (KHD) In: Murphy GP, Khoury S, Küss R, Chatelain C, Denis L (eds) Prostate cancer. Part A: Research, endocrine treatment and histopathology. Alan R Liss, New York, pp 291–297

Manni A, Santen R, Boucher A, Lipton A, Harvey H, White D, Simmonds M, Gordon R, Rohner T, Drago J, Wettlaufer J, Glode L (1987) Androgen priming and chemotherapy in advanced prostate cancer (Abstract) J Endocrinol Invest 10 [Suppl 2]: 32

Navratil H (1987) Double blind study of anandron versus placebo in stage D2 prostate cancer patients receiving Buserelin. In: Murphy GP, Khoury S, Küss R, Chatelain C, Denis L (eds) Prostate cancer. Part A: Research, endocrine treatment and histopathology, Alan R Liss, New York, pp 401–410

Neri R (1987) Clinical utility of flutamide. J Drug Dev [suppl 1] 1: 5–9

Newling DWW, Hall RR, Richards B, Robinson MRG, Hetherington JW (1985) The natural history of prostatic cancer – The argument for a no treatment policy. In: Pavone-Macaluso M, Smith PH, Bagshaw MA (eds) Testicular cancers and other tumors of the genito-urinary tract. Plenum Press, New York, pp 443–448

Newling DWW (1987) The value of reversible androgen suppression as a diagnostic test. In: Murphy GP, Khoury S, Küss R, Chatelain C, Denis L (eds) Prostate cancer. Part A: Research, endocrine treatment and histopathology. Alan R Liss, New York, pp 261–265

Oesterling JE, Epstein JI, Walsh PC (1986) The inability of adrenal androgens to stimulate the adult human prostate: an autopsy evaluation of men with hypogonadotropic hypogonadism and panhypopituitarism. J Urol 136: 1030–1034

Pannuti F, Di Marco AR, Martoni A, Fruet F, Strocchi E, Burroni P, Rossi AP, Cricca A (1980) Medroxyprogesterone acetate in treatment of metastatic breast cancer: seven years of experience. In: Iacobelli S, Di Marco A (eds) Role of medroxyprogesterone in endocrine-related tumors. Raven Press, New York, pp 73–92

Pavone-Macaluso M (1982) Value of chemotherapy in prostate cancer management and present data on EORTC therapy trials. In: Jacobi GH, Hohenfellner R (eds) Prostate cancer. Williams & Wilkins, Baltimore, pp 321–339

Pavone-Macaluso M, Melloni D, La Piana E, Usai E, Oggianu F, Laudi M, Pagliano G, Cerati C (1978) La terapia del carcinoma della prostata con medrossiprogesterone acetato. Dati bibliografici e risultati preliminari. Urologia 45: 595–604

Pavone-Macaluso M, De Voogt HJ, Viggiano G, Barasolo E, Lardennois B, De Pauw M, Sylvester R (1986) Comparison of diethylstilbestrol, cyproterone acetate and medroxyprogesterone acetate in the treatment of advanced prostatic cancer: final analysis of a randomized phase III trial of the European Organization for Research on Treatment of Cancer Urological Group. J Urol 136: 624–631

Pavone-Macaluso M, Pavone C, Serretta V, Cacciatore M, Cavallo N, Romano C, Daricello G (1987) Side-effects of various modalities of hormonal treatment of prostatic carcinoma. (Abstract) J Endocrinol Invest 10 [suppl. 2]: 1987

Prout GR, Irwin RJ, Kliman B, Daly JJ, MacLaughlin RA, Griffin PP (1975) Prostatic cancer and SCH-13521. II: Histological alterations and the pituitary gonadal axis. J Urol 113: 834

Robinson MRG (1983) Carcinoma of the prostate: adrenal inhibors. In: Pavone-Macaluso M, Smith PH (eds) Cancer of the prostate and kidney. Plenum Press, New York, pp 349–354

Robinson MRG (1987) Complete androgen blockade: the EORTC experience comparing orchidectomy versus orchidectomy plus cyproterone acetate versus low-dose stilboestrol in the treatment of metastatic carcinoma of the prostate. In: Murphy GP, Khoury S, Küss R, Chatelain C, Denis L (eds) Prostate cancer. Part A: Research, endocrine treatment and histopathology. Alan R Liss, New York, pp 383–390

Robinson MRG (1988) EORTC protocol 30805: a phase III trial comparing orchidectomy versus orchidectomy and cyproterone acetate and low dose stilboestrol in the management of metastatic carcinoma of the prostate. In: Smith PH, Pavone-Macaluso M (eds) Management of advanced cancer of prostate and bladder. Alan R Liss, New York, pp 101–110

Robinson MRG, Denis L, Debruyne FMJ, Lunglmayr G, Mahler C, Newling DWW, Richards B, Smith PH, Whelan P (1987) The preliminary clinical evaluation of Zoladex depot injection in the management of carcinoma of the prostate. J Endocrinol Invest 10 [suppl 2]: 15

Schroeder FH, EORTC (European Organization for Research on Treatment of Cancer) Genito-Urological Group (1984) Treatment response criteria for prostatic cancer. Prostate 5: 181–191

Schroeder FH (1985) Total androgen suppression the management of prostatic cancer. A critical review. In: Schroeder FH, Richards B (eds) Therapeutic principles in metastatic prostatic cancer. Alan R Liss, New York, pp 307–317

Schulze H, Isaacs JT, Coffey DS (1987) A critical review of the concept of total androgen ablation in the treatment of prostate cancer. In: Murphy GP, Khoury S, Küss R, Chatelain C, Denis L (eds) Prostate cancer. Part A: Research, endocrine treatment and histopathology. Alan R Liss, New York, pp 1–19

Smith JA (1985) Treatment of metastatic carcinoma of the prostate with leuprolide, an LHRH analogue. In: Schroeder FH, Richards B (eds): Therapeutic principles in metastatic prostatic cancer. Alan R Liss, New York, pp 279–285

Smith JA (1987) Endocrine management of prostatic cancer. J Urol 137: 1–10

Smith PH (1985) Hormone therapy. In: Pavone-Macaluso M, Smith PH, Bagshaw MA (eds) Testicular cancer and other tumors of the genitourinary tract. Plenum Press, New York, pp 455–461

Smith PH, Suciu S, Robinson MRG, Richards B, Bastable JRG, Glashan RW, Bouffioux C, Lardennois B, Williams RE, De Puw M, Sylvester R (1986) A comparison of the effect of diethylstilbestrol and low dose estramustine phosphate in the treatment of advanced prostatic cancer: A phase III trial of the EORTC Urological Group. J Urol 136: 619–623

Sogani PC, Whitmore WF (1979) Experience with flutamide in previously untreated patients with advanced prostatic cancer. J Urol 122: 640–643

Soloway MS (1985) Chemotherapy for prostate cancer. The experience of the National Prostatic Cancer Project. In: Pavone-Macaluso M, Smith PH, Bagshaw MA (eds) Testicular cancer and other tumors of the genito-urinary tract. Plenum Press, New York, 467–474

Stoter G, Jones WG (1988) Chemotherapy of hormone refractory prostatic cancer. In: Smith PH, Pavone-Macaluso M (eds) Management of advanced cancer of the prostate and kidney. Alan R Liss, New York, pp 123–125

Tannock IF (1985) Is there evidence that chemotherapy is of benefit to patients with carcinoma of the prostate? J Clin Oncol 3: 1013–1021

Trachtenberg J (1984) Ketoconazole therapy in advanced prostatic cancer. J Urol 132: 61–63

Tunn U, Senge T, Schenck B, Neumann F (1979) Biochemical and histological studies of prostate in castrated dogs after treatment with androstanediol, oestradiol and cyproterone acetate. Acta Endocrinol 91: 373–384

Van der Werf-Messing B (1977) The experience of the Rotterdam Radiotherapy Institute (RRTI) in the treatment of urological tumours. In: Pavone-Macaluso M (ed) The tumours of genito-urinary apparatus. COFESE, Palermo, pp 93–99

Van der Werf-Messing B (1983): Renal cell carcinoma and carcinoma of the prostate: Achievements and challenges. In: Pavone-Macaluso M, Smith PH (eds): Cancer of the prostate and kidney. Plenum Press, New York, 1–16.

Whelan P (1988) Terminal care of patients with prostatic carcinoma. In: Smith PH, Pavone-Macaluso M (eds) Management of advanced cancer of the prostate and kidney. Alan R Liss, New York, pp 127–134

Wu J, Gu F (1987) The prostate 41–65 years post castration. Chin Med J 100: 271–272

Chapter 9

The Staging and Treatment of Testicular Cancer: Management of Stage I Disease

Sophie D. Fosså and A. Horwich

Introduction

A range of different clinical approaches is successful in curing patients with Stage I germ cell tumours of the testis. In non-seminoma these include retroperitoneal lymph node dissection (RLND) and deferred chemotherapy, RLND and routine adjuvant chemotherapy, radiotherapy with deferred chemotherapy and surveillance following orchidectomy. In seminoma, management policies have been more uniform with infradiaphragmatic lymph node irradiation following orchidectomy. However, a surveillance policy has recently been explored in this disease also in the management of these patients with minimum morbidity. This chapter will review this range of approaches, discussing their advantages and disadvantages.

Diagnosis

The incidence of testicular cancer has been rising over the past few decades and in many developed countries it is now the most common form of cancer in men aged 20–40 years. Patients with non-seminomatous tumours are generally 10 years younger than those with seminoma (Fig 9.1). The cancer usually presents with swelling of the testis. Although classically described as a painless mass, pain and

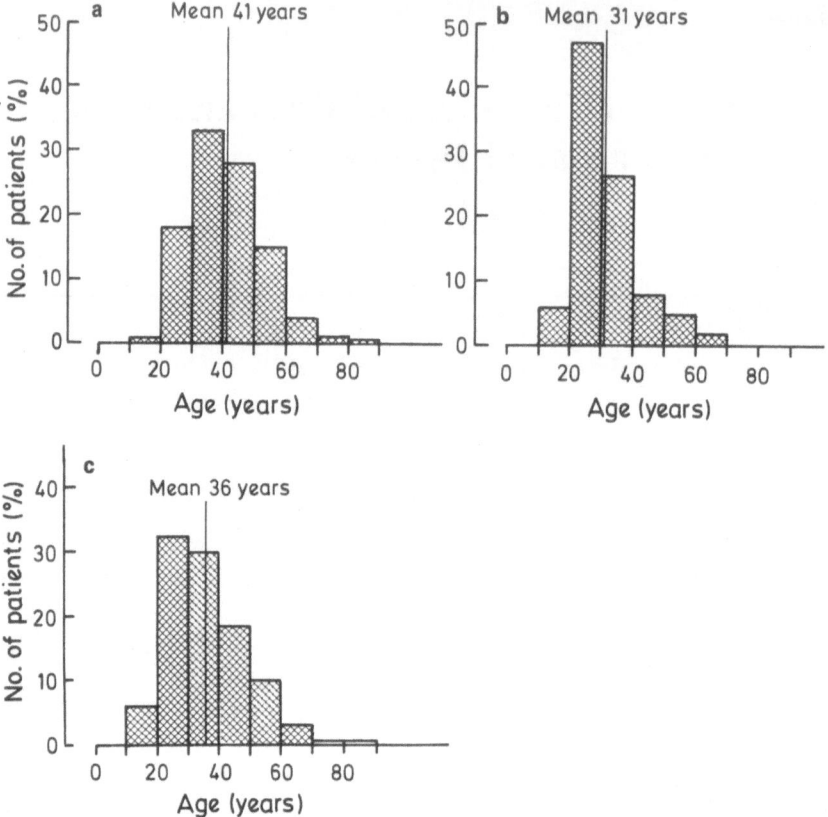

Fig. 9.1a–c. Age distribution in 1008 patients with testicular cancer (The Norwegian Radium Hospital 1970–1982). **a.** Seminoma (n=513); **b.** Non-seminoma (n=495); **c.** All patients (n=1008).

tenderness are also common (Table 9.1). The initial presentation is frequently misdiagnosed as epididymo-orchitis and treated with antibiotics though delay in diagnosis may also be due to the patient deferring a medical consultation. This underlines the need for public education about this disease and consideration of a policy of regular self-examination for men aged 15–45 years (Friman et al. 1986).

In difficult cases ultrasonography of the scrotal contents may be helpful to differentiate testicular tumours from epididymitis (Scott et al. 1986). Biopsy or needle aspiration through the scrotal skin is not recommended because of the risk of tumour implantation. However, this risk is probably very small (Kennedy et al. 1986). Additionally, patients may present with endocrine manifestations such as gynaecomastia or with the effects of metastatic disease e.g. back pain associated with retroperitoneal lymphadenopathy.

The diagnosis is established histopathologically following inguinal orchidectomy. The WHO and the Pugh histological classification systems are commonly used (Table 9.2) (Mostofi and Sobin 1977; Pugh 1976; Pugh and Cameron 1976).

If at the time of orchidectomy a biopsy of the contralateral testis is performed approximately 5% of cases will reveal carcinoma in situ (Von der Maase et al.

Table 9.1. Clinical signs of testicular cancer (Norwegian Radium Hospital 1985/86)

	No of patients		Total (89)
	Seminoma (46)	Non-seminoma (43)	
Testicular/scrotal swelling	41	42	83
Testicular/scrotal pain	24	32	56
Back pain	8	7	15
Gynaecomastia	2	5	7
Testicular maldescent	3	3	6
Patient's delay	8	4	12
(weeks; median and range)	(0–78)	(1–78)	(0–78)
Doctor's delay	2	3	5
(weeks; median and range)	(1–50)	(1–33)	(1–50)
Antibiotics ("epididymitis")	6	13	19

Table 9.2. Histological classification

WHO[a]	Pugh-Cameron
A *Tumours of one histological type*	Not used
Seminoma	Seminoma
Spermatocytic seminoma	Spermatocytic seminoma
Embryonal carcinoma	Malignant teratoma (undifferentiated) MTU, but this also includes yolk sac tumours in adults of WHO
Yolk sac tumour (infantile embryonic carcinoma)	Yolk sac tumour in children, MTU in adults
Polyembryoma	Not listed
Choriocarcinoma – pure	Not listed
Teratoma	Teratoma (includes WHO embryonal carcinoma, yolk sac tumour in adults, three types of teratoma, choriocarcinoma and epidermal cysts)
Mature	Teratoma differentiated – TD: includes epidermal cysts
Immature	Malignant Teratoma Intermediate – MTI
Teratoma with malignant transformation	Malignant Teratoma Intermediate – MTI
B *Tumours of more than one histological type*	Not used
Embryonal Ca and teratoma (Teratocarcinoma)	Malignant teratoma intermediate – MTI some MTU
Choriocarcinoma and any other type	Malignant teratoma trophoblastic, MTT
Other combinations, specify	MTI, MTU, combined tumours for those with seminoma

[a] Syncytiotrophoblasts alone and intratubular malignant germ cells are recorded separately. Syncytiotrophoblasts alone are not rcognised in Pugh-Cameron classification.

1986a), a change which appears to confer a high risk of subsequent malignancy of the order of 50% at 5 years. The incidence of carcinoma in situ is higher if the contralateral testis is atrophic or if there is a history of maldescent. Areas of current debate are which patients should have a biopsy of the contralateral testis at the time of orchidectomy for tumour and also whether carcinoma in situ of the contralateral testis should be managed by surveillance, second orchidectomy, or low dose irradiation (Von der Maase et al. 1986b).

Staging

The full staging description should mirror the extent of the malignant disease and help in prognostic classification. The major pattern of metastases of testicular germ cell tumours is to the retroperitoneal lymph nodes and for non-seminomatous tumours to the lung fields also. A small proportion of patients have metastases to supradiaphragmatic lymph nodes and rarely there are widespread haematological metastases in liver, bones and brain.

A major distinction in staging classification relates to whether the patients are assessed purely clinically, i.e. by physical examination, assay of serum tumour markers and radiological investigations (*Clinical stage: CS*) or whether the staging is additionally done by lymphadenectomy (*Pathological stage: PS*).

A number of staging systems are in use, amongst which the most widely used are the Royal Marsden Hospital classification (Table 9.3) and the Samuels classification (Samuels et al. 1976) or its subsequent modifications (Logothetis et al. 1986). As well as the extent of disease these classifications define the bulk and the bulk-number of deposits at different sites.

Table 9.3. The Royal Marsden Hospital staging classification. (Not based on lymphogram)

Stage I. No evidence of metastases

Stage II. Metastases confined to abdominal nodes, 3 sub-groups are recognised:
    A Maximum diameter of metastases <2 cm
    B Maximum diameter of metastases 2–5 cm
    C Maximum diameter of metastases >5 cm

Stage III. Involvement of supradiaphragmatic + or − infradiaphragmatic lymph nodes. No extralymphatic metastases
    Abdominal status: A, B, C as for Stage II.

Stage IV. Extralymphatic metastases. Suffixes as follows:
    0 – abdominal nodes negative; A, B, C as for Stage II.
    Lung status: L_1 ≤3 metastases; L_2 multiple <2 cm maximum diameter; L_3 multiple >2 cm diameter
    Liver status: H_+ = liver involvement

The stage distribution of seminoma is predominantly in Stage I and Stage II, in contrast to non-seminoma where 20%–25% of patients have Stage IV disease (Table 9.4).

Table 9.4. Stage distribution at the time of diagnosis (Royal Marsden classification system) (NRH: 1970–1982)

	Seminoma	Non-seminoma	Total
I	366	241	607
II	116	114	230
III	18	22	40
IV	13	118	131
Total	513	495	1008

Radiological Investigation

Assessment of patients with testicular tumours is done by chest radiography, computed tomographic scanning (CT) of the abdomen and thorax and/or by bipedal lymphography (Peckham 1981; Husband and Grimes 1985). Though the examinations are rarely discordant, lymphography has the advantage of demonstrating the internal architecture of normally sized lymph nodes revealing metastases in 1 of 7 CT-negative patients (Lien et al. 1983). CT scanning demonstrates nodes which do not opacify following pedal lymphography. Also abdominal ultrasound may reveal para-aortic lymphadenopathy and may be a useful adjunct in the very thin patient where CT definition is less good.

Today initial radiological staging of all patients should include a CT scan of the thorax and abdomen. Lymphography may be considered in equivocal and in CT-negative patients in whom surveillance is an option (vide infra).

Tumour Markers

Germ cell testicular tumours provide a model system in oncology for the use of serum markers. One or both of the tumour products, alphafetoprotein (AFP) and human chorionic gonadotropin (HCG) are produced in approximately 75% of patients with non-seminomatous germ cell tumours and may be helpful in diagnosis, prognostic classification (Horwich and Peckham 1984; Fosså et al. (1988), monitoring of response (Horwich et al. 1985) and diagnosis of relapse following treatment. The rate of change of serum marker levels following orchidectomy can be particularly helpful in the definition of Stage I disease. The physiological half-life of the beta subunit of HCG is 24–48 hours and that of AFP is 5–7 days. A rate of regression following orchidectomy which is significantly slower than these values may be indicative of metastatic disease and this may later be confirmed if the marker does not reach normal levels, or rises.

Before orchidectomy HCG is elevated beyond normal levels in approximately 40% of patients with seminoma CS I and normalises after removal of the primary tumour (Paus et al. 1987). However, the degree of abnormality is not as great as with non-seminomatous tumours. In seminoma CS I HCG production is probably of minor prognostic impact. Other tumour markers whose use has been explored in seminoma are lactate dehydrogenase (Von Eyben et al. 1983) and more recently placental-like alkaline phosphatase (Wahren et al. 1979; Horwich et al. 1985). These have yet to be shown to be more sensitive than the established biochemical and radiological investigations and their clinical role is not established.

Management

Management of Clinical Stage I Seminoma

Important clinical features of seminoma are its exquisite radiosensitivity and the rarity with which the illness progresses beyond the retroperitoneal lymph nodes.

These features have led to the adoption of orchidectomy and adjuvant nodal irradiation of Stage I testicular seminoma in most centres (Thomas et al. 1982; Hamilton et al. 1986).

The radiation dose needed to treat potential subclinical disease is very low (25–30 Gy when administered in 2 Gy fractions over 3 weeks). The irradiation field includes the para-aortic and ipsilateral iliac lymph nodes (Fig 9.2) and extends from the lower border of the vertebral body of D10 to the mid obturator region. The field is shaped by lead blocks and renal shielding is ensured by performing an intravenous urogram during the planning for radiotherapy. The contralateral testis can be shielded from scattered irradiation such that the total gonadal dose is of the order of 0.5 Gy. Some centres have routinely irradiated the entire scrotal

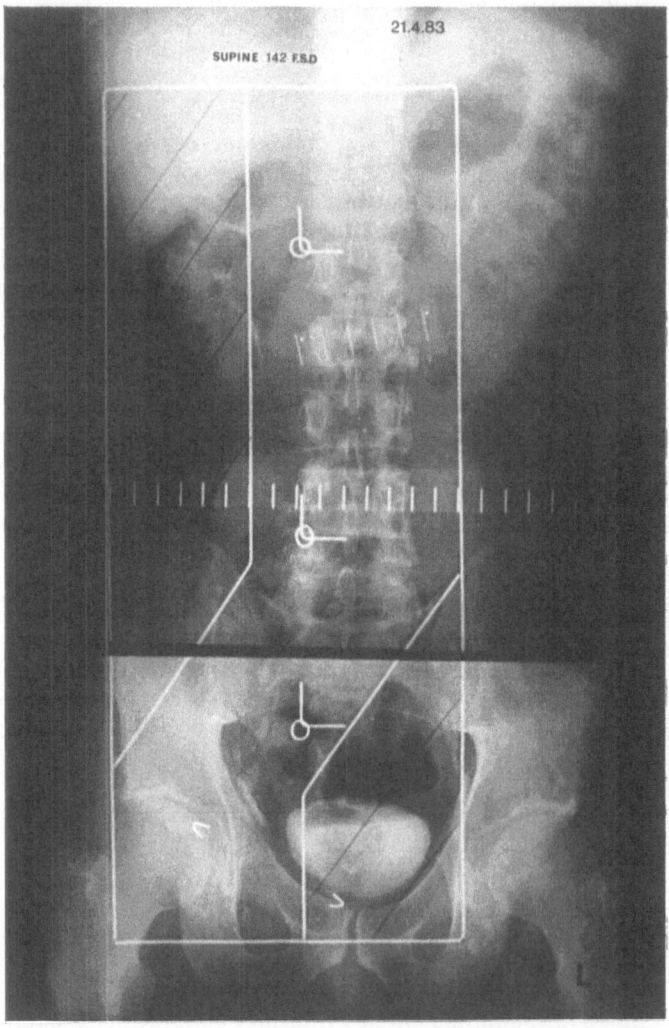

Fig. 9.2. Seminoma clinical Stage I: radiation field.

contents (Read et al. 1983). However, scrotal irradiation appears to be unnecessary even in patients with prior inguinal surgery or scrotal violation (Thomas et al. 1982; Kennedy et al. 1986).

The results of this approach are excellent (Table 9.5). Of a total of 597 patients treated at the Royal Marsden Hospital (RMH) and the Norwegian Radium Hospital (NRH) between 1963 and 1983 only 18 (3%) relapsed. Most of the relapsing patients can be cured today. Relapses occurred from 6 months to 110 months after radiotherapy and were sited in mediastinal nodes, left supraclavicular nodes, mediastinal and axillary nodes, lung, pleura and bones. Side effects of such adjuvant radiotherapy in seminoma CS I are very mild. There may be an increased incidence of peptic ulceration following this form of radiotherapy and in the Royal Marsden Hospital series 15 of 232 patients suffered this, typically 2–4 months after radiotherapy (Hamilton et al. 1987). Five patients in this series developed second non-testicular malignancies. In the series of 365 patients treated at the NRH, a second non-germ cell cancer occurred in 15 patients. The risk of developing lung cancer ánd malignant melanoma was almost significantly increased by multiples (Observed/Expected) of 2.1 and 4.8 respectively.

Table 9.5.   Results of radiotherapy of seminoma clinical stage I

	Royal Marsden Hospital 1963–1983	Norwegian Radium Hospital 1970–1982
No. of patients	232	365
No. of relapses	5	13
Relapse-free interval	21	11
(months; median and range)	(10–60)	(8–113)
Site of relapse		
Supraclav/Mediastinum	3	8
Lung	2	2
Markers only	0	1
Bone	0	2
Survival		
Alive NED	220	337
Dead of seminoma	0	4
Dead of intercurrent disease NED	12	24
Second non-germ cell cancer	5	15 (1 Jan 1987)
Peptic ulcer	15	9

In patients with testicular cancer spermatogenesis is frequently decreased after unilateral orchidectomy and before any further treatment (Fosså et al. 1984). Nevertheless, approximately two-thirds of patients irradiated for seminoma are fertile 3 years after radiotherapy. Theoretically there is a risk of radiation-induced genetic damage. However, no significant increase of malformations has been observed in children of fathers irradiated for testicular cancer (Senturia et al. 1985; Fosså et al. 1986b).

Surveillance for Stage I Seminoma

There are relatively few clinical data defining the incidence of subclinical abdominal node involvement in Stage I seminoma since most patients have been treated with adjuvant irradiation. In one series of patients staged predominantly by physical examination subsequent RLND suggested an incidence of occult metastatic disease of <10% (Maier et al. 1968). It therefore seems probable that adjuvant irradiation is unnecessary in the great majority of today's patients with Stage I seminoma defined more rigorously by lymphography or CT scanning. Due to the fact that effective chemotherapy is available for metastatic seminoma (Peckham et al. 1985; Fosså et al. 1987), it becomes possible to contemplate a management policy of surveillance after orchidectomy.

Table 9.6. Surveillance post orchidectomy for clinical Stage I seminoma of the testis (Royal Marsden Hospital 1983–1986)

Number of patients	Follow-up post orchidectomy (months)	Patients relapsing	Time to relapse (months)
90	4–40 (median 18)	10 (11%)	7–24 (median 11)

Table 9.6 illustrates the results from a surveillance study (Royal Marsden Hospital) of 90 seminoma patients followed from 4–40 months after orchidectomy (median 18 months). Ten patients relapsed 7–24 months post orchidectomy (median 11 months) and the risk of relapse was the same in the second as in the first year post orchidectomy (Fig. 9.3). The actuarial relapse-free rate was 90% at

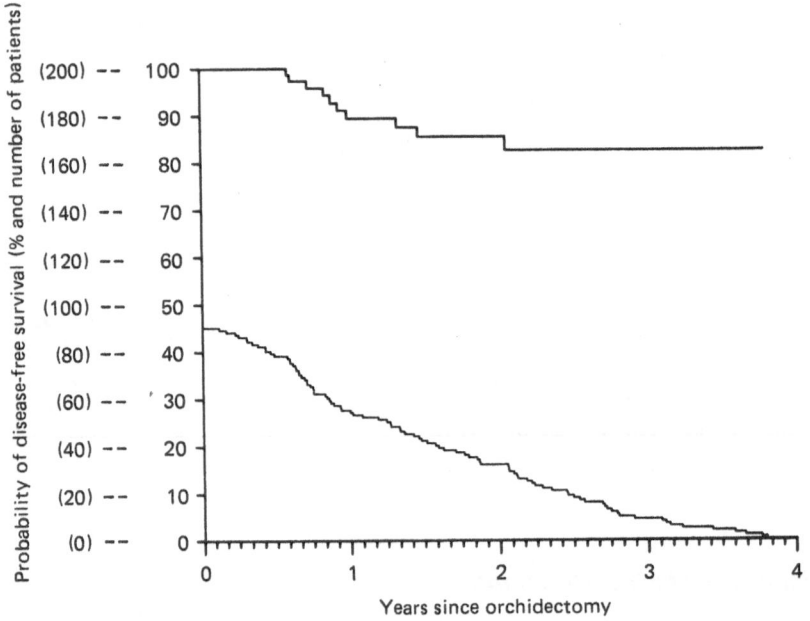

Fig. 9.3. Disease-free survival in clinical Stage I seminoma managed by surveillance post orchidectomy. The lower line indicates the number of patients at risk. (Royal Marsden Hospital 1983–1987)

one year and 85% at two years. Though most patients relapsed only within abdominal nodes, one relapsed with both abdominal lymphadenopathy and a single small lung metastasis. Of 9 patients treated for relapse with abdominal irradiation, 3 subsequently relapsed in supradiaphragmatic lymph nodes and were treated with chemotherapy. All the patients in this study are currently alive and disease-free. However, one patient who refused follow-up subsequently relapsed with high AFP levels and has died of progressive non-seminoma.

Discussion of Management of Clinical Stage I Seminoma

The results of treatment by orchidectomy and radiotherapy are excellent with minimal morbidity and with cure rates exceeding 90% (Earle et al. 1973; Maier and Sulak 1973; Schultz et al. 1984; Thomas et al. 1982; Hamilton et al. 1986). The policy of surveillance is still investigational. Surveillance is difficult in practice because of the protracted natural history of seminoma and because of the lack of a reliable serum marker although, more recently, an isoenzyme of placental alkaline phosphatase has been evaluated in metastatic seminoma and may prove useful as a component of surveillance (Horwich et al. 1985). Surveillance for Stage I seminoma should only be undertaken in the context of a formal prospective study and where reliable clinical follow-up can be assured. Adjuvant abdominal node irradiation remains the standard management.

Management of Stage I Non-Seminoma

The range of clinical approaches to non-seminoma clinical Stage I includes:

1. Abdominal node irradiation with chemotherapy for relapse
2. Abdominal node dissection either with adjuvant chemotherapy if nodes are involved, or with surveillance following excision of involved nodes reserving chemotherapy for relapse
3. Surveillance alone following orchidectomy

Radiotherapy

Lymph node metastases from non-seminomatous tumours require 45–50 Gy in daily 2 Gy fractions to cure small tumour deposits, and 40 Gy to cure microscopic levels of disease (Peckham 1979). The radiation field usually employed is similar to that described above for seminoma. Approximately 80% longterm survival is observed after radiotherapy of non-seminoma patients of stage CS I (Peckham 1979; Fosså et al. 1988).

Patients with subclinical disease at other sites than the retroperitoneum will relapse (predominantly in the lungs). Subsequent chemotherapy may be compromised by the prior irradiation partly because of impaired bone marrow reserve but also because of the additive effects of radiation and chemotherapeutic drugs on the bowel (Duchesne and Peckham 1984).

Retroperitoneal Lymph Node Dissection (RLND)

This approach predominates in American centres. The traditional approach resects lymph nodes around the inferior vena cava, the aorta and around the ipsilateral iliac vessels (Whitmore 1979). Some centres also resect lymph nodes above the renal vessels (Skinner 1978).

The procedure is felt to have both a diagnostic and a therapeutic role. Among non-seminoma patients with normal abdominal CT 20%–30% have retroperitoneal lymph node metastases (Donohue et al. 1978; Fosså et al. 1988). Pathological post-orchidectomy serum marker decrease and small vessel infiltration in the histological sections of the primary tumour represent independent parameters predictive for metastases (Fosså et al. 1988; Moriyama et al. 1985). In patients shown histologically to be free from lymph node metastases (PS I) there is a relapse rate of 10%–20% mainly in the lungs. These patients can be managed upon relapse with combination chemotherapy (Weissbach et al. 1987; Pizzocaro et al. 1985; Fosså et al. 1988). Of patients with histological evidence of abdominal node involvement, approximately 50% are cured by the surgical dissection alone, whereas the remainder will subsequently develop a recurrence, most often in the lungs. After lymphadenectomy, patients with PS II have been managed either by adjuvant chemotherapy or by surveillance, with chemotherapy for relapse. A recent cooperative group study in America has prospectively randomised patients with pathological Stage II, either to two cycles of cisplatin-based chemotherapy, or to surveillance after lymphadenectomy (Williams et al. 1986). Of the 195 evaluable patients the recurrence rate in the surveillance arm was 49% with three deaths from disease whereas in the adjuvant chemotherapy arm there were six recurrences (6%), but five of these did not receive their assigned adjuvant treatment. There was only one death from disease in this arm.

The major disadvantage of RLND is the possibility of long term side effects from the surgical procedure, in particular the high incidence of "dry" ejaculation after bilateral RLND (Whitmore 1979; Fosså et al. 1985: Fosså et al. 1986a). This is due to dissection of autonomic nerves responsible for semen emission. However, techniques for more limited RLND have been developed recently which preserve those nerves, critical for normal ejaculation (Fosså et al. 1985;

Table 9.7. Permanent "dry" ejaculation after unilateral (u) or modified (m) bilateral (nerve-sparing) RLND

Author	Type	No. of patients	"Dry" ejaculation (%)	No. of relapse (%)
Weissbach et al.	u	160	18	16
Pizzocaro et al.[a]	u	61	13	16
Fosså et al.[b]	u	105	13	8
Donohue et al.[c]	u	35	1	6
Javadpour	m	40	2	–

[a] Right: 4/33; Left: 4/28.
[b] Right: 0/55; Left: 14/50.
[c] Personal communication.

Weissbach et al. 1987; Lange et al. 1987; Pizzocaro et al. 1985; Javadpour 1988; Donohue et al. 1988) (Table 9.7, Fig. 9.4). During these surgical procedures care is taken to avoid the hypogastric nerve plexus below the inferior mesenteric artery. The modified bilateral (nerve-sparing) RLND represents a more or less bilateral lymph node dissection above the inferior mesenteric artery but a unilateral approach below this level. By the unilateral RLND the boundaries of the lymph node dissection are confined to one side of the patient. In preoperatively tumour-free patients, unilateral node dissection appears to be as sensitive a diagnostic technique as the more extensive procedures. Among the PS I patients 70%–85% maintain normal ejaculations after unilateral RLND. For patients with pathologically documented involvement of retroperitoneal lymph nodes, two (Williams et al. 1986; Weissbach et al. 1987) or three cycles (Fosså et al. 1988) of cisplatin-based regimens are effective in avoiding subsequent relapses. The toxicity of cisplatin-based regimes includes impairment of renal glomerular filtration rate in almost all patients, longterm mild Raynaud's phenomena in 30%–50% of patients and neurotoxicity and ototoxicity in a minority of patients (Fosså et al. 1988). The use of a reduced number of cycles of chemotherapy in an adjuvant setting is therefore of signficant benefit in reducing these complications. This may be true also for possible longterm consequences of treatment such as cardiovascular problems and chemotherapy-related second malignancies.

Surveillance for Clinical Stage I Non-Seminoma

This policy was introduced in the Royal Marsden Hospital in 1979. The eligibility criteria include a normal CT scan of thorax and abdomen, normal lymphogram, histological confirmation of non-seminomatous germ-cell tumour of the testis and either normal serum marker levels or rapid return of serum marker levels to normal values following orchidectomy. The surveillance policy comprises physical examination, chest radiography and assay of serum markers every month for the first year, every two months for the second year, every three months for the third year, and every four months for the fourth year. Initially, CT scans of thorax and abdomen were performed on alternate visits for the first two years but more recently the number of CT scans was reduced to a total of four scans during the first year and a further scan at the end of the second year.

Table 9.8. Surveillance post-orchidectomy for clinical Stage I non-seminoma of the testis. (Royal Marsden Hospital 1979–1985)

Total patients	Follow-up (months)	Relapses	% Relapse in			
			Only abdominal nodes[c]	Only lung[c]	Abdominal nodes and lung[c]	Serum markers only
132[a]	12–84	35[b]	47	17	13	23

[a] 131 alive and disease-free.
[b] Relapsing patients followed for 11–76 months post chemotherapy.
[c] With or without marker elevation.

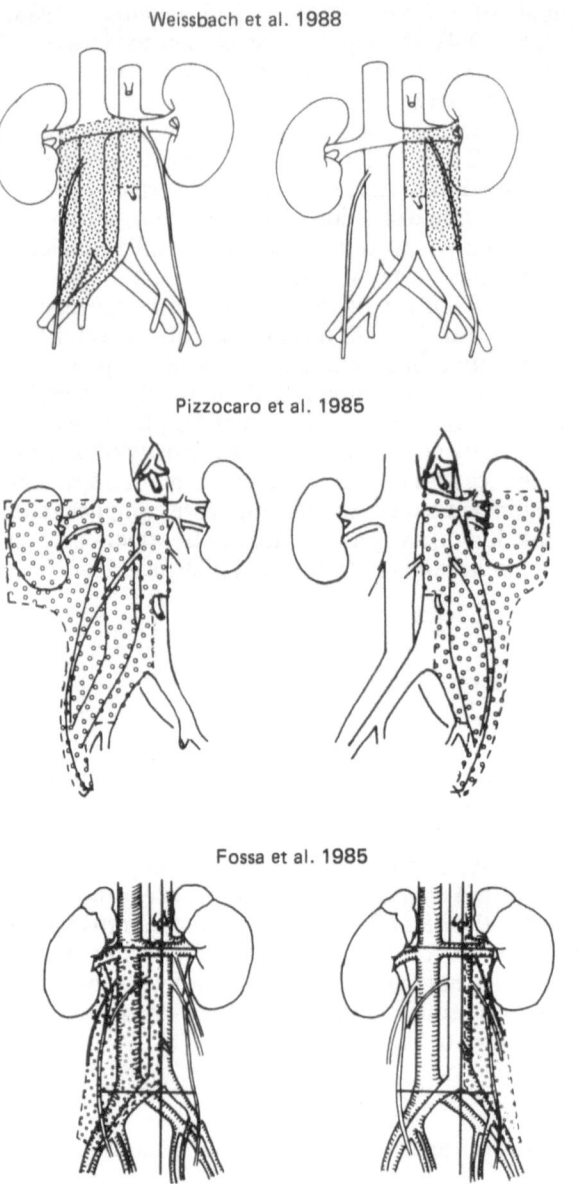

Fig. 9.4a, b. Extent of unilateral (**a**) and modified bilateral (nerve-sparing) (**b**) retroperitoneal lymph node dissection (RLND) in patients with non-seminoma clinical Stage I.

Table 9.8 illustrates the results of surveillance in patients followed from 12–84 months (median 43 months) from orchidectomy. Thirty-five patients (27%) relapsed and were then treated with combination chemotherapy consisting of bleomycin, etoposide and cisplatinum (Peckham et al. 1983). Ninety-seven percent are alive and disease-free with one patient dying in remission from

Lange et al. 1988

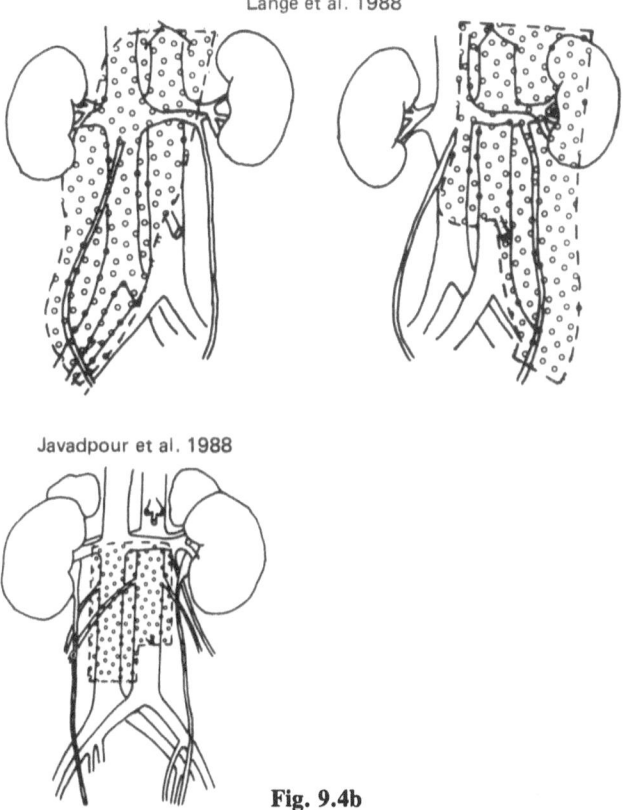

Javadpour et al. 1988

Fig. 9.4b

complications of renal failure. Of the relapses, 90% occurred within the first year after orchidectomy. The relapse was detected by rising serum marker levels in 74% of patients.

The presentation characteristics of relapsing patients were compared with non-relapsing patients in an attempt to identify factors predictive for relapse (Table 9.9). Risk factors for relapse include the histological subtype malignant teratoma undifferentiated (embyronal carcinoma), lymphatic and/or vascular invasion within the primary, and local extension involving the epididymis or the rete testis. A lower risk of relapse was associated with raised serum alphafetoprotein prior to orchidectomy. The risk of relapse was 12% in patients with malignant teratoma intermediate (teratocarcinoma) and no lymphatic invasion, 33% for malignant teratoma undifferentiated (embryonal carcinoma) with no lymphatic invasion, 40% for malignant teratoma intermediate (teratocarcinoma) with lymphatic invasion and 78% for malignant teratoma undifferentiated (embryonal carcinoma) with lymphatic invasion.

A recent study from the Medical Research Council identified the following independent risk factors as predictive for relapse in patients with non-seminoma CS I following the surveillance policy: Infiltration of lymphatic or blood vessels in the primary tumour, the presence of undifferentiated cells, the absence of yolk sac elements (Freedman et al. 1987).

Table 9.9. Prognostic factors in clinical Stage I non-seminoma (Royal Marsden Hospital 1979–1985; data from Hoskin et al. 1986)

	% relapse rate	Log rank P value
Epididymis/rete		
Involved	52	
Not involved	26	<0.05
Vascular invasion		
Present	46	
Absent	23	<0.01
Lymphatic invasion		
Present	57	
Absent	23	<0.005
Pre-orchidectomy serum AFP		
Raised	16	
Not raised	48	<0.01
Histology		
MTU (Embryonal Ca)	44	
MTI (Teratocarcinoma)	20	<0.005
MTT (Trophoblastic)	29	–

Discussion of Management of Clinical Stage I Non-Seminoma

This chapter describes a number of approaches to clinical Stage I non-seminoma. Most patients with clinical Stage I non-seminoma are cured today, and it is not clear that any individual approach is associated with a significantly higher overall survival rate. The appropriate issue to consider is therefore curability with a minimum of treatment-related morbidity. The disadvantages of adjuvant abdominal node irradiation are:

1. The acute and possible late side effects of radiotherapy. As target doses for non-seminoma have to be higher than in seminoma both the acute and longterm toxicity is more frequent and more pronounced

2. Subsequent chemotherapy in the 10%–20% of patients who relapse is often compromised

In an experienced centre the policy of limited node dissection is associated with few surgical side effects. Again, 10%–15% of patients will relapse even if the node dissection was histologically negative. However, subsequent chemotherapy has not been compromised. Node-positive patients may be treated with 2–3 courses of chemotherapy in an adjuvant setting. The preliminary results of surveillance are encouraging. However, this requires a high investment of medical health care resources and a reliable patient compliance over a 1–2 year period. Based on histopathological features of the primary tumour and the development of the post-orchidectomy serum markers it appears possible to define subgroups of clinical Stage I non-seminoma patients with either a low or a high risk of relapse.

Patients in the low risk group can probably be safely managed by surveillance, whereas a limited number of cycles of adjuvant chemotherapy seems to represent an adequate treatment in the high-risk patients.

The decision on appropriate management of clinical Stage I non-seminoma will depend upon the resources and expertise available at the centre managing the patients. In experienced hands and with recently developed reductions in toxicity the range of approaches described in this chapter are probably of equal validity. The clinical decision is based predominantly upon judgement of the risk of relapse and of the significance of particular toxicities in the individual patient.

References

Donohue JP, Einhorn LH, Periz JM (1978) Improved management of non-seminomatous testis tumours. Cancer 42: 2903–2908

Donohue JP, Rowland RG, Bihrle R (1988): Transabdominal retroperitoneal lymph node dissection. In: Skinner D, Lieskovsky G (eds). Textbook diagnosis and management of genitourinary cancer. W. B. Saunders, Philadelphia, pp. 802–816

Duchesne G, Peckham MJ (1984) Chemotherapy and radiotherapy in advanced testicular non-seminoma (2). Results of treatment. Radiother Oncol 1: 207–215

Earle JD, Bagshawe MA, Kaplan HS (1973) Supervoltage radiation therapy of testicular tumours. AJR 117: 653–661

Einhorn LH (1979) Chemotherapy of disseminated testicular cancer. West J Med 131: 1–3

Eyben FE von, Skude G, Fosså SD, Klepp O, Børmer O (1983) Serum lactate dehydrogenase (S-LDH) and S-LDH isoenzymes in patients with testicular germ cell tumors. MGG 189: 326–333

Fosså SD, Åbyholm T, Aakvaag A (1984) Spermatogenesis and hormonal status after orchidectomy for cancer and before supplementary treatment. Eur Urol 10: 173–177

Fosså SD, Ous S, Åbyholm T, Loeb M (1985) Post-treatment fertility in patients with testicular cancer. I. Influence of retroperitoneal lymph node dissection on ejaculatory potency. Br J Urol 57: 204–209

Fosså SD et al. (1986a) Fertility in patients with testicular cancer. In: Jones WG, Milford Ward A, Anderson CK (eds) Germ cell tumours II. Pergamon Press, Oxford, pp 461–466

Fosså SD, Almaas B, Jetne V, Bjerkedal T (1986b) Paternity after irradiation for testicular cancer. Acta Rad Oncol 25: 33–36

Fosså SD, Åbyholm T, Normann N, Jetne V (1986c): Post-treatment fertility in patients with testicular cancer. III. Influence of radiotherapy in seminoma patients. Br J Urol 58: 315–319

Fosså SD, Borge L, Aass N, Johannessen NB, Stenwig AE, Kaalhus O (1987) The treatment of advanced metastatic seminoma. Experience in 55 cases. J Clin Oncol 5: 1071–1077

Fosså SD, Aass N, Kaalhus O (1988) Testicular cancer in young Norwegians. J Surg Onc 39: 43–63

Freedman LS, Parkinson MC, Jones WG, Oliver RTD, Peckham MJ, Read G, Newlands ES, Williams CJ on behalf of the MRC Testicular Tumour Subgroup (Urological Working Party) (1987) Histopathology in the prediction of relapse of patients with Stage I testicular teratoma treated by orchiectomy alone: a Medical Research Council Collaborative Study. Lancet II: 294–298

Friman PC, Finney JW, Glasscock SG, Weigel JW, Christophersen ER (1986) Testicular self-examination: Validation of a training strategy for early cancer detection. J Appl Behav Anal 19: 87–92

Hamilton C, Horwich A, Easton D, Peckham MJ (1986) Radiotherapy for Stage I seminoma testis: Results of treatment and complications. Radiother Oncol 6: 115–120

Hamilton C, Horwich A, Bliss JM, Peckham MJ (1987) Gastro-intestinal morbidity of adjuvant radiotherapy in Stage I malignant teratoma of the testis. Radiother Oncol 10: 85–90

Hay JH, Duncan W,'Kerr GR (1984) Subsequent malignancies in patients irradiated for testicular tumours. Br J Radiol 57: 597–602

Horwich A, Peckham MJ (1984) Serum tumour marker regression rate following chemotherapy for malignant teratoma. Eur J Cancer Clin Oncol 20: 1463–1470

Horwich A, Tucker DF, Peckham MJ (1985) Placental alkaline phosphatase as a tumour marker in seminoma using the H17E monoclonal antibody assay. Br J Cancer 51: 625–629

Horwich A, Easton D, Husband J, Peckham MJ (1987) Prognosis following chemotherapy for metastatic malignant teratoma. Br J Urol 59: 578–583

Hoskin PJ, Dilly S, Easton D, Horwich A, Hendry WF, Peckham MJ (1986) Prognostic factors in Stage I non-seminomatous germ-cell testicular tumours managed by orchiectomy and surveillance: Implications for adjuvant chemotherapy. J Clin Oncol 4: 1031–1036

Husband J, Grimes DP (1985) Staging testicular tumours: The role of CT scanning. J Roy Soc Med [Suppl 6] 78: 25–31

Javadpour N (1986) Retroperitoneal lymphadenectomy with preservation of ejaculation. Proceedings of the AUA, May 1986: Los Angeles

Javadpour N (1988) Nerve sparing retroperitoneal lymphadenectomy for Stage I and II non-seminomatous testicular cancer. J Urol (in press).

Kennedy CL, Husband JE, Bellamy EA, Peckham MJ, Hendry WF (1985) The accuracy of CT scanning prior to para-aortic lymphadenectomy in patients with bulky metastases from testicular teratoma. Br J Urol 57: 755–758

Kennedy CL, Hendry WF, Peckham MJ (1986) The significance of scrotal interference in Stage I testicular cancer managed by orchiectomy and surveillance. Br J Urol 58: 705–708

Lange PH, Chang WY, Fraley EE (1987) Fertility issues in the therapy of testicular tumors. Urol Clin North Am 14: 731–747

Lien HH, Fosså SD, Ous S, Stenwig AE (1983) Lymphography in retroperitoneal metastases in non-seminoma testicular tumor patients with a normal CT-scan. Acta Radiol [Diagn] – (Stockh) 24: 319–322

Logothetis CJ, Samuels ML, Selig DE, Ogden S, Dexeus F, Swanson D, Johnson D, von Eschenbach A (1986) Cyclic chemotherapy with cyclophosphamide, doxorubin and cisplatin plus vinblastine and bleomycin in advanced germinal tumors. Am J Med 81: 219–228

Maase von der H et al. (1986a) Carcinoma in situ of contralateral testis in patients with testicular germ cell cancer: Study of 27 cases in 500 patients. Br Med J 283: 1398

Maase von der H, Giwercman A, Skakkebaek NE (1986b) Radiation treatment of carcinoma in situ of testis. Lancet I: 624–5

Maier JG, Sulak MH (1973) Radiation therapy in malignant testis tumours 1. Seminoma. Cancer 32: 1212–1216

Maier JG, Sulak MH, Mittemeyer BT (1968) Analysis of treatment success and failure. AJR 102: 596–602

Medical Research Council Working Party Report on Testicular Tumours (Chairman: MJ Peckham) (1985) Prognostic factors in advanced non-seminomatous germ-cell testicular tumours: results of a multicentre study. Lancet I: 8–11

Moriyama N, Daly JJ, Keating MA, Lin CW, Prout GR jr (1985) Vascular Invasion as a prognosticator of metastatic disease in nonseminomatous germ cell tumors of the testis. Cancer 56: 2492–2498

Mostofi FK, Sobin LH (1977) International histological typing of testis tumours (No. 16). WHO, Geneva

Paus E, Fosså SD, Risberg T, Nustad K (1987) The diagnostic value of human chorionic gonadotrophin in patients with testicular seminoma. Br J Urol 59: 572–577

Peckham MJ (1979) An appraisal of the role of radiation therapy in the management of non-seminomatous germ-cell tumours of the testis in the era of effective chemotherapy. Cancer Treat Rep 63: 1653–1658

Peckham MJ (1981) The role of CT scanning in oncology. In: Husband JE, Hobday PA (eds) Computed axial tomography in oncology. Proceedings 2nd European Seminar on Computerised Axial Tomography (ESCAT) held in London 4–7 February 1980. Churchill Livingstone, Edinburgh, pp 187–194

Peckham MJ, Barrett A, Horwich A, Hendry WF (1983) Orchiectomy alone for Stage I testicular non-seminoma. Br J Urol 55: 754–759

Peckham MJ, Horwich A, Hendry WF (1985) Advanced seminoma: Treatment with cis-platinum based chemotherapy or carboplatin (JM8). Br J Cancer 52: 7–13

Pizzocaro G, Salvioni R, Zanoni F (1985) Unilateral lymphadenectomy in intraoperative Stage I nonseminomatous germinal testis cancer. J Urol 134: 485–489

Pugh RCB (1976) Combined tumours. In: Pugh RCB (ed) Pathology of the testis. Blackwell, Oxford, pp 245–258

Pugh RCB, Cameron KM (1976) Teratoma. In: Pugh RCB (ed) Pathology of the testis. Blackwell, Oxford, pp 199–244

Read G, Robertson A, Blair V (1983) Radiotherapy in seminoma of the testis. Clin Radiol 34: 469–473

Samuels ML, Lanzotti VJ, Holoye PY, Boyle LE, Smith TL, Johnson DE (1976) Combination chemotherapy in germinal cell tumors. Cancer Treat Rev 3: 185–204

Scott RF, Bayliss AP, Calder JF, Garvie HH (1986) Indications for ultrasound in the evaluation of the pathological scrotum. Br J Urol 58: 178–182

Schultz HPM, Von der Maase H, Rorth M, Pedersen M, Sandber Nielsen E, Walbom-Jorgensen S and DATECA Study Group (1984) Testicular seminoma in Denmark 1976–1980: Results of treatment. Acta Radiol [Oncol] 23: 263–270

Senturia YD, Peckham CS, Peckham MJ (1985) Children fathered by men treated for testicular cancer. Lancet II: 766–769

Skinner DG (1978) Management of nonseminomatous tumors of the testis. In: Skinner DG, deKernion JB (eds) Genitourinary cancer. WB Saunders Company, Philadelphia, pp 470–493

Thomas GM, Rider WD, Dembo AJ, Cummings BJ, Gospodarowicz M, Hawkins NV, Herman JG, Keen CW (1982) Seminoma of the testis. Results of treatment and patterns of failure after radiation therapy. Int J Radiat Oncol Biol Phys 8: 165–174

Thomas PRM, Mansfield MD, Hendry WF, Peckham MJ (1977) The implications of scrotal interference for the preservation of spermatogenesis in the management of testicular tumours. Br J Surg 64: 352–354

Wahren B, Holmgren PA, Stigbrand T (1979) Placental alkaline phosphatase, alphafetoprotein and carcinoma embryonic antigens in testicular tumour tissue typing by means of cytologic smears. Int J Cancer 24: 749–753

Weissbach L, Hartlapp JH, Horstmann-Dubral B for Testicular Tumor Study Group (1988) Prospective multicentre trials on early stage nonseminomatous germ cell tumors of the testis. Progress report after 5 years. Rec Res Cancer Res. Springer-Verlag, Heidelberg

Whitmore jr WF (1982) Surgical treatment of clinical Stage I nonseminomatous germ cell tumors of the testis. Cancer Treat Rep 66: 55–10

Williams S, Muggia F, Einhorn L, Hahn R, Donohue J, Brunner K, Stablein D, De Wys W, Crawford D, Spaulding J for the Testicular Cancer Intergroup Study (1986) Resected Stage II testicular cancer: Immediate adjuvant chemotherapy. Proc ASCO Vol 5, Abstract No 380, p 98

Chapter 10

Chemotherapy in Disseminated Testicular Cancer

C.J. Rodenburg and G. Stoter

Introduction

Testicular germ cell tumours can be divided into seminomas and non-seminomas. Seminomas are radiosensitive and approximately 90% can be cured with radiotherapy since, in the majority of cases, the disease is limited to the testis with or without small metastases in the retroperitoneal lymph nodes.

In contrast, non-seminomatous tumours are not sensitive to radiotherapy. With the development of effective cisplatin combination chemotherapy, disseminated non-seminomatous testicular cancer has become a curable disease in about 70% of the patients. This is reflected in a 34% decrease in mortality in the USA over the period 1973 to 1978, despite an increasing incidence (Hubbard et al. 1982).

Non-Seminomatous Testicular Cancer

Historical Perspectives

In the early 1960s it became evident that testicular cancer was responsive to a variety of chemotherapeutic agents. Li et al. (1960) reported on 23 patients with disseminated non-seminomatous testicular cancer, 12 of whom responded to a regimen consisting of chlorambucil, actinomycin-D and methotrexate with 7 complete responses (CR). Other drugs were found to have anti-tumour activity, e.g. mithramycin, vinblastine, cyclophosphamide and bleomycin (Hainsworth and Greco 1983).

In the 1970s, Samuels improved the results with the use of vinblastine in combination with bleomycin. Nine of 23 (39%) patients achieved CR with a regimen consisting of bleomycin (30 mg given over 24 hours every day for 5 days) and vinblastine (0.2 mg/kg on days 1 and 2) for 1 to 5 courses (Samuels et al. 1975). In contrast to the relatively mild side effects seen with early regimens, the vinblastine–bleomycin regimen was very toxic. Myelosuppression was the major side effect, resulting in septicaemia in 3 patients. Two of the 23 patients died because of toxicity; of these, one developed bleomycin pneumonitis.

The most important step forward was made in 1974 with the introduction of cis-diammine-dichloroplatinum (cisplatin). Higby published a phase I study of cisplatin 20 mg/m^2/day, given intravenously for 5 consecutive days. Of 11 patients with testicular tumours refractory to conventional treatment, 9 responded including 3 CRs (Higby et al. 1974). Nausea and vomiting occurred invariably with the administration of cisplatin, while renal toxicity could be alleviated with forced diuresis by hyperhydration and mannitol.

These promising results prompted Einhorn and Donohue in 1974 to add cisplatin to the combination of vinblastine and bleomycin (PVB). In their first study (Einhorn and Donohue 1977), cisplatin 20 mg/m^2/day was given intravenously for 5 days, vinblastine 0.2 mg/kg/day for 2 days and bleomycin 30 mg intravenously on days 2, 9 and 16 of each cycle. Courses of cisplatin and vinblastine were repeated every 3 weeks for 3 to 4 cycles and bleomycin was given 12 times. The results in 47 evaluable patients were dramatic, with 33 of 47 (70%) CRs. Four patients died because of drug-induced toxicity. In addition, 5 patients with a partial response became disease-free after surgical removal of residual disease. After a minimum follow-up of 2 years 60% (28 of 47) were still free of disease. At the Memorial Sloan–Kettering Cancer Center cisplatin was added to vinblastine, bleomycin, actinomycin-D and chlorambucil, referred to as VAB-2; this resulted in only 24% longterm survival (Cheng et al. 1978). Subsequent alterations in the VAB regimens led to the ultimate choice of VAB-6 which yielded similar results to Einhorn's PVB regimen (Bosl et al. 1986).

In Europe, cisplatin was introduced in 1976. The first results were published in 1979 (Peckham et al. 1979; Stoter et al. 1979). Approximately 70% of patients achieved longterm complete responses, but about 5% of all treated patients died of acute toxicity, mainly sepsis and bleomycin-induced lung fibrosis.

Refinements with Respect to Side Effects

The severe toxicity of cisplatin combination chemotherapy posed a difficult problem. Cisplatin causes nausea and vomiting in all patients and is nephrotoxic, neurotoxic and ototoxic. Vinblastine causes myelosuppression with the risk of sepsis, and has neuromuscular side effects resulting in constipation or painful ileus, while adding to the peripheral neutoxicity of cisplatin. Bleomycin frequently produces fever with chills, and hyperpigmentation of the skin with hyperkeratosis. Lung fibrosis occurs in about 5%–10% of the patients, even below a cumulative dose of 360 mg, and causes death in 1%–3% of all treated patients. Therefore, after their original report, Einhorn et al. compared vinblastine 0.4 mg/kg with 0.3 mg/kg per cycle in a randomised study of PVB chemotherapy (Einhorn and Williams 1980). Identical treatment results were achieved, but the incidence of granulocytopenic fever episodes decreased from 35% to 15%. This was confirmed by a study of the EORTC, which in addition showed a decrease of mucositis from 53% to 37% of patients ($P=0.006$) (Stoter et al. 1986a). Bleomycin-induced lung toxicity, defined as a decrease of vital capacity of 20% or more, was observed in 60 (42%) of 144 patients, and 3 of 220 patients died of pneumonitis. These data show that bleomycin is a toxic drug.

Recently Published Studies

VP16–213 (etoposide) is an epipodophyllotoxin derivative active in testicular cancer (Cavalli et al. 1981). Since it lacks the neuromuscular toxicity of vinblastine, Einhorn et al. started a randomised study in which etoposide was substituted for vinblastine in the PVB regimen. Thus, patients were randomised to BEP (bleomycin, etoposide, cisplatin) or PVB. Among 244 patients who could be evaluated for response, 74% of those receiving PVB and 83% of those receiving BEP became disease-free. Moreover, there was suggestive evidence that patients with bulky disease defined by the MD Anderson classification as well as the Indiana classification were more likely to achieve a CR after BEP than after PVB. Survival among patients on BEP was also higher ($P=0.05$). The regimens were similar in terms of myelo-suppressive effects and pulmonary toxicity, but the incidence of paraesthesiae, abdominal cramps and myalgia was less with the etoposide regimen. It was concluded that BEP was superior to PVB (Williams et al. 1987) because of diminished neuromuscular toxicity and better efficacy in the patients with bulky disease. Comparable results were achieved in study 30824 of the Urological Group of the EORTC (European Organisation for Research on the Treatment of Cancer) in which patients were stratified for low volume metastases (LVM) and high volume metastases (HVM) (defined as lymph node metastases >5 cm in transverse diameter or lung metastases >2 cm). The patients with HVM were randomised to BEP or to an alternating regimen of PVB and BEP for a total of 4 cycles to investigate whether the alternating regimen would yield a higher CR rate. The preliminary results showed no therapeutic difference between the two regimens with CR rates of 78% and 77%, respectively (Stoter et al. 1986b). As expected, the alternating regimen of PVB/BEP was more toxic with regard to bone marrow function and neuromuscular symptoms.

Patients with LVM were randomised to EP (etoposide, cisplatin) or BEP with the objective of reducing the (lung) toxicity by omitting bleomycin without loss of therapeutic activity. Sixty-four of 67 patients (95.5%) achieved CR on BEP and 59 of 62 patients (95.2%) on EP. Relapses occurred in 1 patient on BEP and 2 on EP. BEP appeared to be more myelotoxic both with regard to leukocytopenia and thrombocytopenia. There was a striking difference in skin toxicity: 34% of patients on BEP had grade 1–3 toxicity in contrast to only 3% grade 1 toxicity among patients on EP. Bleomycin-induced fibrosis on chest X-ray films was observed in 8% of the patients on the BEP arm (Stoter et al. 1987a).

Recently, the results obtained with the VAB-6 program of the Memorial Sloan–Kettering Cancer Center have been published. The VAB-6 protocol included cyclophosphamide, vinblastine, bleomycin, actinomycin-D and cisplatin, with and without maintenance chemotherapy (Bosl et al. 1986). The overall CR rate was 78%, 67% after chemotherapy alone and 11% after chemotherapy and resection of viable residual cancer. There were no treatment-related deaths. Maintenance chemotherapy did not prolong either relapse-free or overall survival in that study.

Bosl et al. (1987) also attempted to improve the treatment results in "poor risk" patients (i.e. bulky and extragonadal germ cell tumours) using the VAB-6 and the EP regimen (etoposide plus cisplatin) alternately for a total of 6 cycles. The rationale for this approach with alternating regimens is based on non-cross-resistance. However, response rate and survival of 39 patients treated with VAB-6 and EP alternately were identical to the results in 29 patients who were treated with VAB-6 alone (Bosl et al. 1987).

With respect to the role of maintenance therapy following CR, 3 studies showed that maintenance therapy is not effective in preventing relapse in well-documented complete responders (Einhorn et al. 1981; Stoter et al. 1986a; Bosl et al. 1986).

Forthcoming Clinical Research

At present, data with regard to prognostic factors are accumulating and permit a more sophisticated approach for the individual patient. The extent of metastatic disease and the serum levels of tumour markers have been shown to be the most important prognostic factors by several investigators, both in the US and in Europe (Bosl et al. 1983; Medical Research Council Working Party 1985; Birch et al. 1986; Stoter et al. 1987b). The EORTC analyses showed that patients with a β-HCG of 10 000 ng/ml or more have a CR rate below 20%. Other studies have indicated that metastases in brain, bone and liver are also associated with a worse prognosis, as are lymph node metastases >10 cm (Pizzocaro 1985a).

The present situation in the treatment of testicular cancer parallels the developments in the treatment of Hodgkin's disease. Once a curative treatment has been established, the next step is to define prognostic variables in order to separate patients with a good prognosis from those in whom it is bad. The objective is to decrease the intensity of treatment in good-risk patients to reduce toxicity while maintaining the therapeutic efficacy. In bad-risk patients, however, the treatment should be intensified to improve the therapeutic results while accepting the increased toxicities.

Combining the results of various analyses, the EORTC has decided to subdivide patients into 3 categories – good risk, intermediate risk and poor risk, defined as follows:

Good prognosis (*all* of the following)
  lymph node metastases <5 cm in diameter
  lung metastases ≤4 in number, ≤3 cm in diameter
  β-HCG <1000 ng/ml
  AFP <1000 ng/ml
Intermediate prognosis (*any* of the following)
  lymph node metastases 5–10 cm in diameter
  lung metastases >3 cm in diameter
  β-HCG 100–9999 ng/ml
  AFP ≥ 1000 ng/ml

Poor prognosis (*any* of the following)
  lymph node metastases >10 cm
  βHCG $\geqslant$ 10 000 ng/ml
  metastatic sites other than lymph nodes and lung (liver, bone, brain, etc.)

For patients with minimal and moderate disease, (according to the Indiana staging system) the Southeastern Cancer Study Group (SECSG) is evaluating the standard 4 cycles of BEP versus 3 cycles (Einhorn 1987). At the Royal Marsden Hospital, the "classical" BEP regimen (bleomycin 30 mg once a week) for 4 cycles is being compared to a "BEP" regimen in which bleomycin is given only once every 3 weeks for 4 cycles. Prelimimary results indicate that the reduced bleomycin regimen is less effective than standard BEP (Brada et al. 1987). With respect to the intermediate risk group, both EORTC and ECOG will randomise this category of patients either to VIP (VP-16, iphosphamide and cisplatin) (Loehrer et al. 1985) or BEP, to evaluate whether iphosphamide is more active than bleomycin. However, VP-16 will be given in a different dose-interval scheme in these studies.

Intensified treatment strategies (e.g. using high dose cisplatin) are now being developed to improve the treatment results in bad-risk patients. At NCI a randomised trial of standard PVB versus a regimen of cisplatin 40 mg/m^2 day 1–5, vinblastine 0.2 mg/kg i.v. day 1, VP-16 100 mg/m^2 day 1–5 and bleomycin 30 mg i.v. once a week, every 21 days, for a total of 3 or 4 cycles has been performed (Ozols et al. 1987).

The randomisation was 2:1 in favour of PVB-VP16. CR was achieved in 26/30 patients (87%) on PVB-VP16, and in 10/16 patients (62%) on PVB. Fatal pulmonary fibrosis occurred in 6% of the patients. There has been only one relapse (4%) in patients randomised to receive PVB-VP16 compared to a 20% relapse rate in patients receiving PVB. Disease-free survival was superior with PVB-VP16 ($P<0.05$). High-dose cisplatin regimens have also been reported by others. Schmoll et al. (1987) reported on 98 patients with bulky disease, 63% of whom became disease-free following high-dose cisplatin-containing chemo-therapy. Similarly, 24 of 40 patients (60%) are alive without evidence of disease following high-dose cisplatin combination chemotherapy in a series from the Finsen Institute in Denmark, at a median follow-up of 18 months (Daugaard et al. 1987).

Short interval cisplatin administration in combination chemotherapy could also be a useful approach for the bad prognosis group. Wettlaufer et al. (1984) treated 29 patients with bulky disease by using vincristine, bleomycin and cisplatin every week for a maximum of 8 weeks, followed by subsequent surgery and consoli-dation therapy, and obtained a CR rate of 93% in this small series. The EORTC has started a pilot study for their poor-prognosis category of patients, evaluating a schedule of 3 courses of vincristine (Oncovin), bleomycin and cisplatin (BOP) at 10 day intervals, followed by 3 courses of VIP at 21-day intervals. High-dose chemotherapy with autologous bone marrow rescue as first-line treatment is under investigation in France, since this approach has given short-term results in pretreated patients (Pico et al. 1986). No results are available yet.

The phase II studies of intensive chemotherapy summarised in this chapter are inconclusive with regard to their therapeutic value. Notably, Pizzocaro has achieved an 82% CR rate in a group of patients with bad prognostic characteris-tics similar to those in the series reported from the Finsen Institute using the standard BEP regimen (Pizzocaro et al. 1985b). The only randomised study from NCI shows a clearcut superiority for PVB-VP16 over PVB, but unfortunately PVB is obsolete and probably less effective than BEP.

Advanced Seminoma

The relapse rate for patients with bulky abdominal disease (stage IIC, lymph nodes ≥5 cm) following radiotherapy is as high as 28% (Gregory and Peckham 1986). Since seminomas are extremely chemosensitive, chemotherapy should be the treatment of choice for patients with stage IIC, as well as for stages III and IV.

There is growing evidence that the spectrum of drug sensitivity is similar to that of non-seminomatous testicular cancer (Hainsworth and Greco 1983). For instance, collected data from Indiana, the Netherlands and Madrid show that 67 of 80 patients with advanced seminoma (stage IIC, III and IV) achieved a CR to PVB (van Oosterom et al. 1985). About half of these patients had received prior radiotherapy or chemotherapy. At the Royal Marsden Hospital, 36 of 39 patients (92%) are disease-free following chemotherapy with BEP at a median follow-up period of 36 months (Peckham et al. 1985). A recent review showed that cisplatin combination chemotherapy has yielded 81% CRs in over 200 patients in various institutions (Loehrer et al. 1987). At present, therefore, the optimal first-line treatment for patients with advanced seminoma is cisplatin combination chemotherapy.

Recently, cisplatin and carboplatin used as single drugs have been reported to have curative potential in advanced seminoma. Oliver reported on 20 patients treated with cisplatin 50 mg/m^2 on days 1 and 2 every 3 weeks for 4 cycles. So far, 17 of those 20 patients are disease-free at a median follow-up of 36 months (Oliver 1984, 1987). Carboplatin has been employed as a single agent in a dose of 400 mg/m^2 for 4–6 cycles in 33 patients, of whom 22 have a follow-up of at least 1 year. Nineteen of 22 (86%) are disease-free (Horwich, personal communication). These results are preliminary and do not permit the omission of cisplatin combination chemotherapy.

References

Birch R, Williams S, Cone A, Einhorn L, Roark P, Turner S, Greco F (1986) Prognostic factors for favorable outcome in disseminated germ cell tumours. J Clin Oncol 4: 400–407

Bosl GJ, Geller NL, Cirrincione C, Vogelzang NJ, Kennedy BJ, Whitmore WFJr, Vugrin D, Scher H, Nisselbaum J, Golbey RB (1983) Multivariate analysis of prognostic variables in patients with metastatic testicular cancer. Cancer Res 43: 3403–3407

Bosl GJ, Gluckman R, Geller, NL, Golbey RB, Whitmore WF, Herr H, Sogani P, Morse M, Martini N, Bains M, McCormack P (1986) VAB–6: an effective chemotherapy regimen for patients with germ cell tumors. J Clin Oncol 4: 1493–1499

Bosl GJ, Geller NL, Vogelzang NJ, Carey R, Auman J, Whitmore WF, Herr H, Morse M, Sogani P, Chan E (1987) Alternating cycles of etoposide plus cisplatin and VAB-6 in the treatment of poor-risk patients with germ cell tumors. J Clin Oncol 5: 436–440

Brada M, Horwich A, Peckham MJ (1987) Treatment of favorable-prognosis nonseminomatous testicular germ cell tumors with etoposide, cisplatin, and reduced dose of bleomycin. Cancer Treat Rep 71: 655–656

Cavalli F, Klepp O, Renard J, Rohrt M, Alberto P (1981) A phase II study of oral VP-16-213 in non-seminomatous testicular cancer. Eur J Cancer 17: 245-249

Cheng E, Cvitkovic E, Wittes RE, Golbey RB (II) (1978) VAB II in metastatic testicular cancer. Cancer 42: 2162-2168

Daugaard G, Hansen HH, Rørth (1987) Management of advanced metastatic germ cell tumours. Int J Androl 10: 319-324

Einhorn LH (1987) Treatment strategies of testicular cancer in the US. Int J Androl 10: 399-405

Einhorn LH, Donohue JP (1977) Cis-diamminedichloroplatinum, vinblastine and bleomycin combination chemotherapy in disseminated testicular cancer. Ann Intern Med 87: 293-298

Einhorn LH, Williams SD (1980) Chemotherapy of disseminated testicular cancer. Cancer 46: 1339-1344

Einhorn LH, Williams SD, Troner M, Birch R, Greco FA (1981) The role of maintenance therapy in disseminated testicular cancer. N Engl J Med 305: 727-731

Gregory C, Peckham MJ (1986) Results of radiotherapy for stage II testicular seminoma. Radiother Oncol 6: 285-292

Hainsworth JD, Greco FA (1983) Testicular germ cell neoplasms. Am J Med 75: 817-832

Higby DJ, Wallace HJ, Albert DJ, Holland JF (1974) Diamminedichloroplatinum: a phase I study showing response in testicular and other tumors. Cancer 33: 1219-1225

Hubbard SM, McDonald JS (1982) An introduction to current controversies in cancer management: stage I testicular cancer – A case in point. Cancer Treat Rep 66: 1-3

Li MC, Whitmore WF, Golbey R, Grabstald H (1960) Effect of combined drug therapy on metastatic cancer of the testis. JAMA 174: 1291-1299

Loehrer PJ, Einhorn LH, Williams SD (1985) Salvage therapy for refractory germ cell tumors (RGCT) with VP-16 plus ifosfamide (IFX) plus cisplatin (DDP). Proc Am Soc Clin Oncol 4: 100

Loehrer PJ, Birch R, Williams SD, Greco FA, Einhorn LH (1987) Chemotherapy of metastatic seminoma: The Southeastern Cancer Study Group Experience. J Clin Oncol 5: 1212-1220

Medical Research Council Working Party on Testicular Tumours (1985) Prognostic factors in advanced non-seminomatous germ-cell testicular tumours: results of a multicentre study. Lancet I: 8-11

Oliver RTD (1984) Surveillance for stage I seminoma and single agent cisplatinum for metastatic seminoma. Proc Am Soc Clin Oncol 3: 162

Oliver RTD (1987) Limitations to the case of surveillance as an option in the management of stage I seminoma. Int J Androl 10: 263-268

Oosterom AT van, Williams SD, Cortes Funes H, ten Bokkel Huinink WW, Vendrik CP, Einhorn LH (1985) Treatment of seminomas with combination chemotherapy. In: Jones WG, Milford Ward A, Anderson CK (eds) Germ cell tumors II. Pergamon Press, Oxford, pp 229-233

Ozols RF (1987) Treatment of poor prognosis germ cell tumors with high dose cisplatin regimens. Int J Androl 10: 291-300

Peckham MJ, Barrett A, McElwain TJ, Hendry WF (1979) Combined management of malignant teratoma of the testis. Lancet II: 267-270

Peckham MJ, Horwich A, Hendry WF (1985) Advanced seminoma: treatment with cisplatinum-based combination chemotherapy or carboplatin (JM8). Br J Cancer 52: 7-13

Pico JL, Droz JP, Couyette A, Beaujean F, Baume D, Amiel J, Hayat M (1986) High dose chemotherapy followed by autologous bone marrow transplantation for poor prognosis non-seminomatous germ cell tumors. Proc Am Soc Clin Oncol 5: 111

Pizzocaro G (1985a) Personal experience in the management of germinal testis tumors. Acta Urologica Belgica 53: 249-258

Pizzocaro G, Luigi P, Salvioni R, Zanoni F, Milani A (1985b) Cisplatin, etoposide, bleomycin first-line therapy and early resection of residual tumor in far-advanced germinal testis cancer. Cancer 56: 2411-2415

Samuels ML, Johnson DE, Holoye PY (1975) Continuous intravenous bleomycin therapy with vinblastine in stage III testicular neoplasia. Cancer Chemother Rep 59: 563-570

Schmoll HJ, Schubert I, Arnold H, Dölken G, Hecht Th, Bergman L, Illiger J, Fink U, Preiss J, Pfreudschuh M, Kaulen H, Bonfert B, Ho AD, Manegold C, Mayr A, Hoffman L, Weiss J, Hecker H (1987) Disseminated testicular cancer with bulky disease: results of a phase-II study with cisplatin ultra high dose/VP-16/bleomycin. Int J Androl 10: 311-317

Stoter G, Sleijfer DTh, Vendrik CP, Schraffordt Koops H, Struyvenberg A, van Oosterom AT, Brouwers TM, Pinedo HM (1979) Combination chemotherapy with cis-diamminedichloroplatinum, vinblastine and bleomycin in advanced testicular nonseminomas. Lancet I: 941-945

Stoter G, Sleijfer DTh, Bokkel Huinink WW ten, Kaye SB, Jones WG, Oosterom AT van, Vendrik CP, Spaander P, Pauw M de, Sylvester R (1986a) High dose versus low dose vinblastine in cisplatin-vinblastine-bleomycin combination chemotherapy of non-seminomatous testicular cancer: a randomized study of the EORTC Genitourinary Tract Cancer Cooperative Group. J Clin Oncol 4: 1199–1206

Stoter G, Kaye S, Sleijfer DTh, Bokkel Huinink WW ten, Jones WG, Oosterom AT van, Splinter T, Pinedo HM, Sylvester R, Keizer J (1986b) Preliminary results of BEP versus an alternating regimen of BEP and PVB in high volume metastatic testicular non-seminomas. An EORTC study. Proc Am Soc Clin Oncol 5: 106

Stoter G, Kaye S, Jones WG, Bokkel Huinink WW ten, Sleijfer DTh, Splinter T, Oosterom AT van, Harris A, Boven E, Pauw M de, Sylvester R (1987a) Cisplatin and VP-16 in good risk patients with disseminated non-seminomatous testicular cancer: a randomized EORTC GU group study. Proc Am Soc Clin Oncol 6: 110

Stoter G, Sylvester R, Sleijfer DTh, Bokkel Huinink WW ten, Kaye SB, Jones WG, Oosterom AT van, Vendrik CP, Spaander P, Pauw M de (1987b) Multivariate analysis of prognostic factors in patients with disseminated non-seminomatous testicular cancer. Cancer Res 47: 2714–2718

Williams S, Birch R, Einhorn L, Irwin L, Greco A, Loehrer PJ (1987) Treatment of disseminated germ cell tumors with cisplatin, bleomycin and either vinblastine or etoposide. New Engl J Med 316: 1435–1440

Wettlaufer JN, Feiner AS, Robinson WA (1984) Vincristine, cisplatin, and bleomycin with surgery in the management of advanced metastatic nonseminomatous testis tumors. Cancer 53: 203–209

Chapter 11

Cancer of the Penis

W.G. Jones

Squamous cell carcinoma of the penis is rare, with an incidence in Western countries of less than one case per 100 000 of the male population. It is a disease which has *not* been exclusively managed by urological surgeons and oncologists. In its early stages it may be seen and treated by such diverse clinicians as venereologists, dermatologists, general surgeons, radiotherapists and general practitioners. Few doctors, indeed few Oncology Centres, have been able to develop an expertise in the treatment of penile cancer because of this diverse and non-centralised approach to management (Sagerman et al. 1984; Stewart Orr et al. 1977). As a result, reports in the medical literature are either small anecdotal series reported by individuals, or bigger series reported from the larger centres with an accrual rate of perhaps only five or six cases per annum and spanning as much as 20 to 30 years. The changes in medical practice over this length of time, differences in philosophy, and possibly of enthusiasm for a particular therapeutic approach (e.g. a particular radiotherapeutic or surgical technique) makes comparison between the reported series virtually impossible (El-Demiry et al. 1984).

The literature is confusing and controversy exists over a number of different aspects of penile cancer. Because of the rarity of the condition, it is unlikely that these controversies will be resolved by randomised controlled studies simply because sufficient numbers of cases will not be available in a relatively short period of time unless highly organised, multi-institutional, indeed multi-national cooperation is possible. Little has been reported on a combination approach to treatment, apart from the obvious combinations of perhaps radiotherapy for the primary lesion and surgery for metastatic inguinal nodes or vice versa, and the use of bleomycin chemotherapy with radiotherapy. Therefore much of this chapter examines the theoretical approach to combination therapy in this disease. As with other forms of cancer, particularly rare forms of malignant disease, a team approach is needed involving the urological surgeon, radiotherapist, oncologist and other specialists such as the radiologist. They must come together to discuss the patient's management determining the best plan of therapy for each individual case, or whether the patients are suitable for clinical studies for which protocols have been written. The patient must also be involved in the management decision and must recognise one member of the team as being in charge of his treatment and easily approachable by him.

The peak incidence of cancer of the penis is in the sixth or seventh decades of life. As many of the treatments have significant morbidity it is important to take account of the patient's biological rather than his chronological age when taking a treatment decision. When curative therapy is considered, one must ask:

1. Is it important that the function of the penis is maintained?
2. What is the minimum therapy likely to achieve a cure?
3. Is it appropriate to attempt to cure at all costs e.g. by radical surgery and adjuvant therapy despite a reasonably high risk of morbidity or failure?
4. Alternatively is palliation the best course of action, knowing that the disease can remain localised to the penis and the immediate node drainage areas for a considerable period of time?

Staging

Two anatomical staging systems have been used. The system devised by Jackson (1966) has been perhaps more widely used because of its clinical applicability but the TNM system (1982) is much more precise and should be used in preference. A comparison of the two systems is shown in Table 11.1. A revision of the TNM system took place in 1987.

Table 11.1. Staging of cancer of the penis: Comparison of Jackson and TNM Systems

Jackson Stage	Description	TMN Stage
Stage I	Tumour on glans penis and/or prepuce only	T_1,T_2,N_0,M_0
Stage II	Tumour spreading onto shaft	$T_1,T_2/N_0,M_0$
Stage III	Tumour with operable involved inguinal nodes	$T_1,T_2,T_3/N_1,N_2,M_0$
Stage IV	Primary tumour spreading off shaft of penis and/or cases with inoperable nodes or distant metastases	$T_1,T_2,T_3,T_4/N_0,N_3,N_4/M_0,M_1$

Management of the Primary Lesion

I once heard penile cancer described as "the stupid man's disease". That unkind description is, I fear, accurate in that far too many men delay in seeking medical advice (Hoppman 1981), not only presenting with a more advanced primary lesion only manageable by a partial or total amputation of the organ but also running an increasing risk of node involvement. Indeed, patients may neglect themselves so much that they present with an auto-amputation (Hasham 1975). However the incidence of penile cancer seems to be falling slowly (Narayana et al. 1982), perhaps due to better personal hygiene (Hess et al. 1983). Increased awareness that such lesions need early attention and increased willingness to seek advice contribute to earlier diagnosis and affect treatment options. The prognosis is related to the size of the primary lesion, the extent of disease and node involvement at presentation, and the histological differentiation of the tumour. It would appear that the age of the patient is also important, younger men having a somewhat worse prognosis, possibly because of more aggressive histologies (Fraley et al. 1985; Merrin 1980).

Far too many men present with advanced disease. The immediate reaction of many surgeons is to perform either a sub-total amputation or a radical amputation with removal of the genitalia and the fashioning of a perineal urethrostomy. Radical surgery thus has a reputation for being relatively simple therapy, which can be performed almost anywhere and except for very advanced cases gives high cure rates. If patients were referred centrally, more might be considered for radiotherapy since organ (and thus function) sparing therapy is to be preferred in the majority of cases where the primary lesion is small enough (Krieg and Luk 1981; Sagerman et al. 1984).

For small tumours (T_1, T_2 and early T_3) with negative inguinal nodes, radiotherapy alone is probably the treatment of choice, with salvage surgery for the 20% to 25% of patients who do not respond completely and for the very small proportion of patients who go on to develop radionecrosis. This is usually seen only when the initial lesion was large and it is also more common if large lesions are treated with an implantation technique which nowadays usually takes the form of an iridium[192] wire implant (Daly et al. 1982; Mazeron et al. 1984).

One combination approach for early lesions has been to use bleomycin chemotherapy with radiotherapy (Edsmyr et al. 1985; Maich 1983). Bleomycin is capable of causing regression of primary lesions when used on its own but longterm control and cure have not been reported (Persky and deKernion 1976). Bleomycin is also toxic. Adminstration of the drug, usually one hour before irradiation, has been thought to be important, but there would appear to be no real evidence that this produces a greater synergistic effect. The scheduling of bleomycin is also a cause for debate. In view of a maximum cumulative tolerable dose in the region of 500 mg/m^2 (perhaps less in the more elderly patient) consideration might be given to the application of much lower than usual doses given every day before radiation therapy.

In patients with T_3 lesions where the patient is desperate to preserve his penis it may be possible to perform studies using a combination of radiotherapy and bleomycin (and possibly other cytotoxic drugs), although it must be argued that in this case radical surgery is probably the safest approach since the longer an active lesion is present in the primary site the greater the risk of metastatic disease taking place. A combination of radiotherapy and chemotherapy might have the potential for down-staging disease thus making surgery feasible, or may have a role in palliation. Useful combinations have still to be discovered.

In conclusion, for the management of the early lesions, it is necessary for the urologist and the radiotherapist to liaise, the radiotherapist offering treatment if indicated and the urologist, in these circumstances, prepared to undertake salvage therapy or the management of radionecrosis if this becomes a problem (Haile and Delclos 1980). For the more advanced lesions the safest approach is probably with surgery alone although studies of preoperative chemotherapy could be performed. This may give valuable information regarding the chemosensitivity of the disease provided that this is ethically justifiable in the situation where the patient might be cured with surgery. My feeling is that this approach would be better left for the very advanced primary lesions where the objective of management is palliation only, particularly since inguinal node involvement is a function of the size of the primary tumour.

The Management of Inguinal Nodes

The management of the inguinal nodes in patients with penile cancer remains controversial because clinical assessment is inaccurate (Catalona 1980; Grabstald 1980; Mukamel and deKernion 1987). Because the primary tumour is commonly infected, many patients have palpable lymph nodes at presentation and it is probably best to give the patient antibiotics while the primary lesion is being treated and to stage the lymph nodes four to six weeks later by clinical means (Stewart Orr et al. 1977). The usefulness of CT scanning has not yet been fully evaluated and is one area where the combined efforts of the treatment team and the radiologist can be put to good use. In the clinically node-negative patient it is possible to watch and wait, performing a dissection if nodes become clinically evident but the best approach is possibly that advocated by Cabanas (1977) who advocates sentinel lymph node biopsy, or a modified approach as advocated by Scappini et al. (1986) using fine needle aspiration biopsy to obviate the need for surgery. However it must be emphasised that a negative aspiration biopsy does not mean the absence of metastatic disease and it is important that the patient is seen by the oncology team at regular intervals, that patient compliance with follow-up is good and that repeated biopsies are performed at regular intervals as and when required.

Those who advocate a prophylactic block dissection even for patients with early tumours of the penis, must accept that only about 20% of the patients will have such metastases and that 80% of the patients will be over-treated and subject to unnecessary and perhaps considerable morbidity. Mukamel and deKernion (1987) find it difficult to justify routine node dissection in early tumours, for this reason; they suggest that superficial node dissection can be done wherever indicated and stress that the patient needs to be carefully followed up after primary therapy.

When nodes are found to be positive, but clinically impalpable, there is a choice between superficial surgical dissection or radiotherapy (with or without chemotherapy). Unfortunately, controlled clinical trials to discover which is the best or indeed whether a combination of preoperative radiotherapy followed by a superficial dissection would be preferable (Persky and deKernion 1976), have not yet been performed. There is however some evidence that the combination of radiotherapy and surgery for patients with more advanced node disease is no more successful than surgery alone; although the criticism is that inadequate radiation fields may have been employed in the past, remembering that many reports span one or more decades and that advances in radiation techniques and equipment have been quite dramatic in the last 20 years. Mukamel and deKernion (1987) have highlighted the controversy which exists, since some authors have shown that deferring dissection until clinical evidence of involvement appears does not affect survival, while others advocate early intervention especially when there is spread into the shaft of the penis (stage II), since they believe chances of cure are compromised.

For more advanced nodal involvement, radical dissection is probably the treatment of choice since radical radiotherapy might cause not only the same degree of lymphoedema but also hinders continued examination of the groin because of subcutaneous fibrosis. If cure is the attempted goal, this may be an acceptable degree of morbidity. On the other hand it must be remembered that surgery may be contraindicated in some patients. Similarly less radical radiotherapy may be capable of controlling locally advanced disease for a considerable length of time if the objective is palliation.

Theoretically, combinations of surgery, radiotherapy and chemotherapy are possible in the management of inguinal nodes and indeed are practised on an individual basis in many centres but without any coordinated plan. At best these cases are reported (if at all) as small numbers of patients doing either particularly well or particularly badly. The only sensible advice that can be offered is that controlled studies should be encouraged despite the limitations discussed earlier.

As with solid tumours at most sites, the results of chemotherapy in penile cancer have been rather discouraging. Only three active agents have been identified, namely bleomycin (Maiche 1983), cisplatinum and methotrexate, although a recent report from Norway (Fosså et al. 1987) suggests that mitomycin-C and 5-fluorouracil may also be active. All these agents are toxic and require special consideration particularly in a rather older age group (Ahmed et al. 1984; Meyers 1983).

Bleomycin can cause fatal lung toxicity; the risk increases with increasing cumulative dose and is much higher above a dose of about 500 mg/m^2, but idiosyncratic reactions can occur at any time.

Methotrexate is toxic particularly to the bone marrow and the kidney and if renal function is reduced, methotrexate levels capable of inducing and perpetuating toxicity in the gastrointestinal tract and in other mucosal surfaces as well as the marrow can remain in the serum for considerable lengths of time. Fortunately methotrexate has a specific antidote (leucovorin) which can either be given empirically 24 hours after the methotrexate or titrated according to the serum levels of methotrexate measured serially from 24 hours onwards. Cisplatinum is particularly toxic to the kidneys and requires forced diuresis for it to be given safely. This agent is probably the most potent inducer of emesis of all the cytotoxic drugs and causes considerable myelosuppression. Despite the toxicities of these agents they can, in specialists' hands, be used in combination and the few reports on this subject and personal experience indicate that this combination of treatment can at least cause partial objective regression in cases of advanced penile cancer. Fosså et al. (1987) report that two T_4 cases were rendered operable by treatment with 5-fluorouracil and Mitomycin-C, or 5-fluorouracil and cisplatinum with subsequent radiotherapy. Therefore the role of chemotherapy must be evaluated further. Certainly chemotherapy, perhaps in combination with local radiotherapy to obvious metastatic sites, is the only therapy capable of modifying the disease when distant metastases are present.

Conclusion

It is difficult to discuss the arguments for and against combination therapy in the management of penile cancer when there is still so much controversy about the standard management of this uncommon disease. Only theoretical applications of combined therapy can be put forward at this stage. The pattern of disease may change in the years to come, and it is important that clinicians should be encouraged to refer all cases to central clinics where a team of specialists cannot only discuss and devise the best management for individual patients but also accumulate expertise and experience by taking part in clinical trials which will necessarily have to be multi-institutional, if not multi-national, in nature.

References

Ahmed T, Sklaroff R, Yagoda A (1984) Sequential trials of methotrexate, cisplatin and bleomycin for penile cancer. J Urol 132: 465–468

Cabanas RM (1977) An approach for the treatment of penile cancer. Cancer 39: 456–466

Catalona WJ (1980) Role of lymphadenectomy in carcinoma of the penis. Urol Clin North Am 7: 785–792

Daly NJ, Douchez J, Combes PF (1982) Treatment of carcinoma of the penis by iridium[192] wire implant. Int J Radiat Oncol Biol Phys 8: 1239–1243

Edsmyr F, Andersson L, Esposti P (1985) Combined bleomycin and radiation therapy in carcinoma of the penis. Cancer 56: 1257–1263

El-Demiry MIM, Oliver RTD, Hope-Stone HF, Blandy JP (1984) Re-appraisal of the role of radiotherapy and surgery in the management of carcinoma of the penis. Br J Urol 56: 724–728

Fosså SD, Sundly Hall K, Johannessen NB, Urnes T, Kaalhus O (1987) Cancer of the penis. Experience at the Norwegian Radium Hospital 1974–1985. Eur Urol 13: 372–377

Fraley EE, Zhang G, Sazama R, Lange PH (1985) Cancer of the penis. Prognosis and treatment plans. Cancer 55: 1618–1624

Grabstald H (1980) Controversies concerning lymph node dissection for cancer of the penis. Urol Clin North Am 7: 793–799

Haile K, Delclos L (1980) The place of radiation therapy in the treatment of carcinoma of the distal end of the penis. Cancer 45: 1980–1984

Hasham AI (1975) Auto-amputation of penis from carcinoma. Urology 5: 244–245

Hess F, Prignitz R, Walthers E (1983) Treatment of penis cancer. Urology 38: 243–246

Hoppmann HJ (1981) Diagnosis and management of tumours and tumour-like genital lesions. Geriatrics 36: 137–142

Jackson SM (1966) The treatment of carcinoma of the penis. Br J Surg 53: 33–35

Krieg RM, Luk KH (1981) Carcinoma of penis. Review of cases treated by surgery and radiation therapy 1960–1977. Urology 18: 149–154

Maiche AG (1983) Adjuvant treatment using bleomycin in squamous cell carcinoma of penis: study of 19 cases. Br J Urol 55: 542–544

Mazeron JJ, Langlois D, Lobo PA, Huart JA, Calitchi E, Lusinchi A et al. (1984) Interstitial radiation therapy for carcinoma of the penis using iridium[192] wires: The Henri Mondor Experience (1970–1979). Int J Radiat Oncol Biol Phys 10: 1891–1895

Merrin CE (1980) Cancer of the penis. Cancer 45: 1973–1979

Meyers FJ (1983) Penile cancer chemotherapy. In: Torti FM (ed) Urologic cancer: chemotherapeutic principles and management. Springer, Berlin, Heidelburg, New York pp 143–147 (Recent results in cancer research, vol 85)

Mukamel E, deKernion JB (1987) Early versus delayed lymph-node dissection versus no lymph-node dissection in carcinoma of the penis. Urol Clin North Am 14: 707–711

Narayana AS, Olney LE, Loening SA, Weimar GW, Culp DA (1982) Carcinoma of the penis. Analysis of 219 cases. Cancer 49: 2185–2191

Persky L, de Kernion J (1976) Carcinoma of the penis. CA 26: 130–142

Sagerman RH, Yu WS, Chung CT, Puranik A (1984) External beam irradiation of carcinoma of the penis. Radiology 152: 183–185

Scappini P, Piscioli F, Pusiol T, Hofstetter A, Rothenberger K, Luciani L (1986) Penile cancer. Aspiration biopsy cytology for staging. Cancer 58: 1526–1533

Stewart Orr P, Habeshaw T, Scott R (1977) Carcinoma of the penis: a review of 42 cases. Br J Urol 49: 733–738

TNM Classification of malignant tumours (1982) Harmer MH (ed) UICC, Geneva, pp 126–128

Chapter 12

Surgical Preservation and Reconstruction

B. Goldwasser, J. Ramon and O. Nativ

Introduction

The goal of treatment of any patient with cancer is cure. To achieve this, patients are frequently subjected to mutilating surgical procedures and quality of life is often compromised by the various modalities used for treatment.

Over previous decades, there has been an increasing trend towards radical surgery. In recent years evidence has been accumulating suggesting that various urological malignancies may be treated with equal success by less aggressive surgical procedures with organ preservation and improved quality of life for the patient.

In this chapter we shall review the various procedures which are currently being used for organ preservation and reconstruction in urological malignancies. Many should be viewed critically as they have been performed only in small select patient populations, for which follow-up is short. However, it is exciting to see that our colleagues around the world are constantly using their ingenuity, imagination and knowledge to improve the results and quality of patient care.

Renal Carcinoma

Renal cortical tumours, by far the most common tumours of the adult kidney, reach a large size before becoming symptomatic. In the past, treatment of such tumours has been predicated by the fact that they commonly have been of large size and often high stage at the time of diagnosis. However, the clinical spectrum of renal tumours coming to the urologist's attention has changed markedly over the past 5 years and gives every promise of showing continued change in the near future. Many are now being detected by new imaging techniques such as ultrasound, computed tomography and magnetic resonance imaging whilst asymptomatic and during diagnostic tests carried out for non-renal disorders. Such tumours are smaller, are generally of lower pathological stage and should be associated with a more favorable prognosis.

The extent of the recent dramatic change in presentation of renal cortical tumours is illustrated by the fact that as many renal carcinomas are now found incidentally by imaging tests performed for correlated symptoms as are seen in patients presenting with haematuria, flank pain or symptoms from metastatic disease (Konnak and Grossman 1985). In contrast, only a decade ago 90% of patients presenting with renal carcinoma were symptomatic (Lieber and Gold-wasser 1988)

This revolutionary change in renal imaging and renal tumour diagnosis has prompted a re-evaluation of the treatment appropriate for renal carcinoma. Simple nephrectomy, often performed through a flank incision, was standard treatment for renal carcinoma until the mid 1950s, but more extensive surgical procedures have become popular in the past 30 years, with radical nephrectomy as the treatment of choice (Robson et al. 1969). However, the recognition that 3% to 5% of tumours previously classified as renal carcinomas are in fact oncocytomas, a distinct clinico-pathological entity which nearly always presents a benign clinical course (Lieber et al. 1981) and the good results attained with renal parenchymal sparing procedures for bilateral renal carcinomas or this type of cancer in a solitary kidney necessitate a critical review of the longstanding urological surgical practice of performing a radical nephrectomy for every solid renal mass lesion of whatever size. A small tumour, particularly if located on one of the poles of the kidney, or superficially on the parenchyma, may be best treated by partial renal resection.

In approximately 2% of patients presenting with renal carcinoma, it occurs bilaterally (Vermillion et al. 1972). Until recently, it was thought that the identification of bilateral renal carcinomas, particularly if synchronous, indicated a very poor prognosis. However, this has changed following the report by Jacobs et al. (1980) who reviewed the world experience of the surgical treatment of these patients. They demonstrated that patients with synchronous bilateral renal cancer treated surgically, often with a radical nephrectomy on one side and a partial nephrectomy on the other (but occasionally by bilateral partial nephrectomies or bilateral total nephrectomies) showed the same prognosis stage for stage as those patients with unilateral disease treated by radical nephrectomy.

More recently, a number of additional reports have documented a good prognosis for patients treated by partial nephrectomy for renal carcinomas in a solitary kidney or for bilateral renal carcinomas. Zincke and associates (1985) compared survival in patients who had renal carcinoma treated by in situ or extracorporeal partial nephrectomy with that of patients treated by radical nephrectomy for unilateral renal cancer in the presence of a contralateral normal kidney. The projected 5-year survival rates for the two groups seen at the Mayo Clinic were 78% and 50%, respectively. When deaths due to cancer were considered, the 5-year survival rates for the two groups were 85% and 93%, respectively. Smith and co-workers (1984), reviewing the UCLA experience with the same type of patients, reported a 5-year survival rate in patients with bilateral renal carcinoma or in a solitary kidney of 72%, if patients dying from non-cancer-related causes were excluded. Similar good results have been reported by other centres (Topley et al. 1984).

All currently published series appear to agree that patients with a low stage lesion in a solitary kidney treated by adequate partial nephrectomy and patients with synchronous bilateral renal tumours treated surgically do about as well as patients treated by radical nephrectomy in the presence of a contralateral normal kidney. Whereas, in some series, patients with asynchronous bilateral renal cancer have done very poorly, in others the prognosis of patients with asynchronous bilateral disease has been similar to that seen for synchronous tumours (Smith et al. 1984; Topley et al. 1984; Marberger et al. 1981).

For those patients with localised tumours who have been candidates for treatment by partial nephrectomy, local recurrence has been surprisingly uncommon. The overall local recurrence rate from a collection of several series of patients with renal cancer in a solitary kidney or bilateral renal cancer treated by partial resection is just 9% (Jacobs et al. 1980; Smith et al. 1984; Topley et al. 1984; Marshall and Walsh 1984; Zincke and Swanson 1982). When these results are considered according to the surgical technique used, namely in situ resection versus extracorporeal partial nephrectomy, the local recurrence rates were 10% and 3%, respectively. Smith and colleagues (1984) were against enucleation of renal carcinoma because microinvasion of the tumour capsule was common in their experience. Novick (1984) reported on 15 patients treated by tumour enucleation. Tumours were 1.8–7.0 cm in diameter and all patients were alive 3 months to 6 years postoperatively. It was claimed that 87% of all non-metastatic renal carcinomas with a diameter less than 7 cm have an unperforated pseudocapsule which provides an ideal plane of cleavage for enucleation. Therefore, Marberger and associates (1981) recommended that tumours up to 7 cm in diameter be enucleated, whereas larger tumours be excised by partial nephrectomy with frozen sections obtained to verify total tumour removal from the margins.

At present, the prognosis for patients with non-surgically-treated renal carcinoma is gloomy. The 5-year survival rates for these patients have been 4% to 30% (deKernion et al. 1978; Marberger 1980; Patel and Lavengood 1978). Wickham (1975) found that of 30 patients with renal cancer in a solitary kidney treated non-surgically, 75% died within a mean follow-up period of 24 months and all 16 patients with bilateral synchronous tumours died within five months. Unilateral nephrectomy for renal carcinoma in solitary kidney or bilateral nephrectomy for bilateral synchronous renal cancer with postoperative haemodialysis is a poor alternative as many of these patients fare poorly: the majority die from dialysis-related complications (Marberger et al. 1981; Jacobs 1984). Nephrectomy followed by renal transplantation is a more attractive alternative, particularly if performed in patients who were on dialysis for over 15 months following nephrectomy (Penn 1977). However, patient survival is still significantly lower than that achieved by partial nephrectomy with contralateral partial or radical nephrectomy.

Urothelial Tumours of the Upper Urinary Tract

Nephroureterectomy with excision of a cuff of bladder has been standard treatment for transitional cell carcinoma of the upper tract for many years. A rate of tumour recurrence of 30% in the bladder (Murphy et al. 1981) and of 15% to 30% in the ureteral cuff (Murphy et al. 1981; Rubenstein et al. 1978; Strong et al. 1976) were reported following nephrectomy alone.

However, it is increasingly recognised that urothelial tumours of the upper urinary tract differ in their biological behaviour in relation to their stage, grade and location. There have been a number of favourable reports recommending conservative treatment for certain ureteral and renal pelvic tumours (Bloom et al. 1970; Carroll 1985; Marshall 1984; Vest 1945; Wallace et al. 1981). Surgical management in these cases may be by pyelotomy with local excision and fulguration, partial nephrectomy, or segmental resection of the ureter. More recently, endourological procedures by the percutaneous route or by ureter-oscopy have been reported with good results achieved in highly selected cases. In complex situations bench surgery and renal autotransplantation may be required for transitional cell tumours of the renal pelvis (Wallace et al. 1981; McLoughlin 1975).

Most authors recommended conservative surgery in patients with pelvic and ureteral tumours of a solitary kidney, in patients with unilateral tumours and renal insufficiency, in those with bilateral upper tract tumours and in patients with Balkan nephropathy. Opinions differ markedly, however, as to the proper management of unilateral low stage low grade renal pelvic and ureteral urothelial tumours in the presence of a contralateral healthy kidney. In a Mayo Clinic study, the success of conservative treatment was related to the location, stage and grade of the tumours (Zincke and Neves 1984). Whereas the tumour recurred in 23 of 37 patients (62%) with renal pelvic tumours, it recurred in only four of 27 patients (15%) with ureteral tumours.

The grade of tumour was related to the success rate of conservative surgery, particularly in patients with ureteral tumours. Only one of 25 (4%) grade 1 and 2 ureteral tumours recurred locally after conservative treatment, but 3 of 6 (50%) tumours of grade 3 or 4 recurred locally. Grade of tumour was not such a significant factor for patients with renal pelvic tumours: even for patients with grade 1 renal pelvic tumours, the local recurrence rate was 50% and this rate was higher for patients with higher grade lesions. Although survival did not depend significantly on the location of the tumours, non-progression did. Patients with ureteral tumours fared better than those with renal pelvic tumours.

For almost all patients with renal pelvic tumours, total nephroureterectomy and excision of a bladder cuff remains the best treatment option. The high rate of recurrence in the ureteral stump when nephroureterectomy is not done, and the low rate (1.5% to 2%) of tumours in the contralateral upper urinary tract convince us that complete nephroureterectomy remains the treatment of choice even for patients with low grade tumours in the renal pelvis. Patients with low grade (grade 1 or 2), low stage (stage I or II) tumours of the distal ureter should be treated with distal ureterectomy, excision of a bladder cuff and ureteroneocys-tostomy. Patients with grade 1 tumour of the mid or upper ureter can be treated with segmental resection and ureteroureterostomy. Grade 1 tumours have a low rate of recurrence (5%) in the ipsilateral ureter (Murphy et al. 1980). Patients with grade 2 tumour of the mid or upper ureter are best treated with nephroure-terectomy to avoid the expected high rate (30%) of recurrence. Segmental resection of a grade 2 tumour in the mid or upper ureter leaves the distal ureter, the most common site of recurrence, in place. Patients with high grade (grade 3 or 4) or high stage (Stage III or IV) ureteral tumours should be treated with complete nephroureterectomy and excision of a bladder cuff.

In a highly selective group of patients with extensive transitional cell tumours of the renal pelvis in whom every attempt at renal preservation must be made, bench surgery for excision of renal pelvis tumours followed by autotransplan-tation can be considered. In such cases excision of all external pelvis and ureter with pyelocystostomy may be performed (Pettersson et al. 1984). This method affords easy follow-up examinations and allows local treatment by fulguration or intravesical chemotherapy to be performed transurethrally.

Another option for patients with an extensive renal pelvic tumour or multiple ureteral tumours is total resection of the ureter and as much as possible of the renal pelvis and replacement by a segment of ileum or colon. In a patient in whom tumour recurrence occurs in the ureter or renal pelvis, after cystectomy and diversion for bladder cancer, particularly if the patient has a solitary kidney, the entire ureter and extra-renal pelvis may be excised and a short segment of ileum or colon may be used to direct the urine from the kidney to the skin. This will allow renal preservation with easy endoscopic follow-up and direct instillation of chemotherapy into the renal collecting system.

The last few years have witnessed tremendous advances in endourological instrumentation of the upper urinary tracts. Reports of conservative treatment of selected cases either by transurethral ureteroscopic or by percutaneous resection of renal pelvic or ureteral tumours (Smith et al. 1987; Woodhouse et al. 1986; Huffman et al. 1985) relate results similar to those achieved with open conserva-tive surgical procedures (Smith et al. 1987). Adequate access to the renal pelvis and resection of the tumour are accomplished better percutaneously than ureteroscopically. However, ureteroscopic resection may obviate the risks of nephrostomy tract tumour implant. The occurrence of extravasation of irrigating fluids during endourologic procedures warrants a word of caution as to the potential hazard of disseminating tumour cells in the retroperitoneum. Although retroperitoneal recurrence has not been described by Smith and colleagues (1987), their follow-up period was short. The results reported in the literature seem to suggest that endourological treatment may be adequate for small well-localised low stage low grade tumours. High stage and/or high grade tumours may not allow adequate extirpation and adequate margins of resection may be difficult to determine percutaneously given the multifocality that appears to be inherent in high grade invasive lesions.

Adaptation of the use of the laser delivered via the ureteroscope or percuta-neously may also increase the applicability of conservative endoscopic manage-ment of these tumours and reduce the need for open partial resection (Smith et al. 1987; Hutschenreiter 1987).

Patients with squamous cell carcinoma and adenocarcinoma of the upper urinary tract usually appear with advanced disease that is unsuitable for conservative therapy. Patients with renal pelvic tumours of these histological types can be treated by nephrectomy alone, because these tumours are not associated with the diffuse urothelial abnormalities that cause recurrence of ureteral tumour (Utz and McDonald 1957; McDonald and Zincke 1987).

Transitional Cell Carcinoma of the Bladder

Bilateral pelvic lymphadenectomy and cystoprostatectomy with or without urethrectomy is the standard form of treatment for invasive transitional cell carcinoma of the bladder. The therapeutic failures with tumour recurrence following surgery alone are thought to reflect the presence of peripheral tumour processes beyond surgical margins, local implantation of tumour cells at the time of surgery, and vascular or lymphatic dissemination of viable tumour cells as a result of surgical manipulation. The development of high-energy external beam irradiation provided a modality to treat transitional cell cancer that theoretically could counter these events that lead to surgical failure. However, planned definitive radiation, even with salvage cystectomy in patients who failed radio-therapy did not improve survival rates over those obtained with surgery alone. Although there seemed to be no discernible difference in the mortality rates between patients who underwent primary cystectomy and those who underwent salvage cystectomy, the latter group suffered a significantly higher morbidity rate.

A major additional attraction of definitive radiation was that it allowed maintenance of voiding and sexual function for those patients in whom it succeeded and who were therefore not subject later to salvage cystectomy.

Advances made in recent years in continent urinary diversions, a nerve sparing radical cystectomy (and prostatectomy), which decreases the rate of post-cystectomy impotence, and our ability to help those patients who are rendered impotent, by self-injection of papaverine or by implantation of a penile prosthesis, increased the compliance of the urologist to recommend and of the patient to accept radical surgery as the primary treatment for invasive bladder cancer.

Partial Cystectomy

Partial cystectomy for the treatment of bladder carcinoma is controversial. Some reports have suggested that the expected survival approaches that achieved with more radical forms of therapy (Utz et al. 1973; Resnick and O'Connor 1973), but the results have been criticised because of patient selection and recent studies have reported high tumour recurrence rates (over 70%) particularly in patients with high grade tumours (Faysal and Freiha 1979; Schoborg et al. 1979). Many of these patients required subsequent total cystectomy. The major reasons for failure of partial cystectomy are inadequate surgical margins, especially when ureters must be reimplanted, and unrecognised multifocal disease away from the tumour for which the partial resection is planned.

The obvious advantage of partial cystectomy is that it preserves normal bladder function. Other advantages include low operative morbidity and mortality, preservation of erectile potency and continence and the fact that there is no need for an external urinary collecting device. Although it may appear to be an adequate alternative to a radical surgical approach, the 70% recurrence rate limits its applicability. This procedure should be used in selected patients such as elderly or poor risk patients whose tumour is located at the dome or the posterior wall of the bladder and in whom an adequate 2-cm margin around the tumour can be achieved. In addition, preoperative random biopsies should reveal no evidence of mucosal atypia or carcinoma in situ elsewhere in the bladder. Only 10% to 15% of bladder tumours are in areas suitable for partial cystectomy. Partial cystectomy may also be appropriate for tumours occurring in a vesical diverticulum as well as for limited invasion of the bladder wall by tumour from other primary sites such as colon, cervix or endometrium.

Partial cystectomy carries the potential hazard of spillage of tumour cells. This may be ameliorated by preoperative radiation therapy or by irrigating the wound with sterile water or thiotepa. Postoperative bladder drainage is provided only by a urethral catheter since suprapubic drainage is contraindicated because of the risk of tumour recurrence in the cystostomy tract of the abdominal wall incision. Frequent postoperative cystoscopic examination should be performed because of the high rate of tumour recurrence after partial cystectomy.

Radical Prostatectomy and Cystoprostatectomy with Preservation of Potency

Impotence is a common complication of radical pelvic surgery. It is estimated that 90% of all patients who undergo radical prostatectomy and virtually all patients who undergo radical cystoprostatectomy are impotent. In 1982 Walsh and Donker suggested that impotence was produced by injury to the pelvic nerve plexus, which provides autonomic innervation to the corpora cavernosa. This nerve plexus consists of parasympathetic nerves (S_{2-4}) which are situated in association with the capsular vessels of the prostate in neurovascular bundles. These neurovascular bundles are located in the leaves of the lateral pelvic fascia adjacent to the prostate, and are susceptible to injury during standard radical prostatectomy or cystoprostatectomy. There are several points during a standard radical prostatectomy in which the neurovascular bundles may be injured inadvertently and unknowingly: (i) during apical dissection of the prostate with transection of the urethra; (ii) during separation of the prostate and urethra from the rectum with transection of the lateral pelvic fascia, and (iii) during division of the lateral pedicle. These portions of the procedure often are performed blindly and bluntly without precise identification of the neurovascular bundles.

Based upon this knowledge, Walsh and associates developed a modification of radical retropubic prostatectomy and radical cystectomy that spares the nerves to the corpora cavernosa that are responsible for erection. During this nerve-sparing technique the apex of the prostate, the urethra, the lateral pelvic fascia which contains the neurovascular bundle and the lateral pedicle of the prostate are visualised clearly. This enables a precise decision to be made, based upon the operative findings, as to whether these structures may be preserved or be resected widely with the specimen. Initially, this modification was developed for radical retropubic prostatectomy performed for prostatic cancer. Because bladder tumours rarely involve the prostate or lateral pelvic fascia, isolation of the prostate and preservation of the neurovascular bundle is much easier in radical cystoprostatectomy.

Walsh and Mostwin (1984) reported the long-term results of postoperative sexual function in 64 patients who underwent radical retropubic prostatectomy and 11 patients following radical cystoprostatectomy using the nerve-sparing technique. All patients were potent preoperatively. In the 64 patients who underwent radical retropubic prostatectomy, 30% to 40% of patients were potent at 3 and 6 months after surgery, 60% at 9 months postoperatively, and after 1 year

86% of patients experienced the return of sexual function. Age had no significant influence although patients less than 50 years of age appeared to regain sexual function earlier than older patients. Clinical and pathological stage had a significant influence on long-term results. After one year patients with low clinical stage disease (A2, B1N, and B1) recovered potency at a rate between 92% and 100%, whereas only 50% of patients with B2 disease were potent. In patients with tumour confined to the prostate 93% were potent at 1 year, compared to 69% in patients with microscopic penetration through the prostatic capsule and only 25% with seminal vesicle invasion. These data suggest that in patients with extraprostatic extension, attempts to excise all tumour resulted in injury to the neurovascular bundles. Of the 11 patients who underwent radical cystoprostatectomy 82% stated that they were having erections and 67% with sexual partners regained potency within 1 year.

The nerve-sparing approach has been criticised because of the possibility of compromising surgical margins. It is well accepted by all surgeons who used the nerve-sparing technique that the primary goal is to remove all tumour and that potency is of secondary concern. Eggleston and Walsh (1985) have evaluated the pathological specimens removed from the first 100 consecutive patients who underwent nerve-sparing radical retropubic prostatectomy. Of these, 41 had established tumour in the soft periprostatic tissue, yet the surgical margins of resection were positive in only 7 patients. In 5 of the 7 there was involvement of the seminal vesicles, and all 7 had positive margins at sites other than the area of the nerve-sparing modification. Catalona and Dresner (1985) evaluated histopathological findings in 52 patients who underwent a nerve-sparing radical retropubic prostatectomy. The overall incidence of positive margins was 40%. The incidence of positive surgical margins in patients with stages A and B1 disease was 18%, and 57% with stage B2 disease. They compared these results to those in patients who underwent a standard radical retropubic prostatectomy by the same surgeon and found no significant difference.

In conclusion, these results suggest that with nerve-sparing radical prostatectomy and radical cystoprostatectomy it is possible to preserve sexual function in the majority of patients witout compromising the adequacy of the cancer operation. Under certain circumstances, it is necessary to excise the lateral pelvic fascia and neurovascular bundle completely. This decision should be based on intraoperative clinical findings such as induration in the lateral pelvic fascia found after the endopelvic fascia had been opened, or fixation of the neurovascular bundle to the prostatic capsule. It is not clear how often patients will be potent if the neurovascular bundle is sacrificed on one side. Walsh and Mostwin (1984) evaluated 3 patients in whom the neurovascular bundle was excised unilaterally; all were potent after 1 year. In patients undergoing radical extirpation of tumours of the sacrum, it has been shown that sacrifice of the sacral nerve roots on one side does not adversely affect sexual performance. If one side is sufficient to induce erections, the nerve-sparing modification may be performed unilaterally, routinely, thus permitting wider extirpation on the side of the tumour. However proof of this concept must await further clinical experience.

Continent Urinary Diversion

The concept of providing the patient following cystoprostatectomy with volitional control of urine expulsion at convenient intervals is not new. Historically, ureterosigmoidostomy is the oldest form of continent urinary diversion. Reports of its long-term results were disappointing and led to popularisation of the stomal conduit diversions. However, disillusionment with their longterm results and a demand for a more socially acceptable solution have prompted the development of various newer techniques for continent urinary diversion.

The outcome of any method employed for continent urinary diversion should functionally resemble the lower urinary tract as closely as possible. The result should be a continent, low pressure internal reservoir to collect and store urine, allow expulsion of urine under voluntary control and at convenient intervals, protect the upper urinary tracts from obstruction and reflux of urine, and avoid significant shifts of water and electrolytes that may result in metabolic disturbances.

A review of the subject of continent urinary diversion has recently been published (Goldwasser and Webster 1985). We shall, therefore, limit our present discussion to those operations which have received popular support and interest among urologists and that are socially and psychologically acceptable to the patients.

Urine must be collected and stored under low pressure to prevent the hazards of upper urinary tract deterioration and incontinence. Urinary continence depends on factors related to the reservoir and to the outlet. High intra-reservoir pressures resulting from reduced compliance or the presence of high pressure contractions may overcome outlet resistance.

Circumventing the problem of high intra-reservoir pressure by augmenting outlet resistance may be hazardous to the upper urinary tracts as a type of reservoir-outlet dyssynergia may be created. Over the years many reports were published which related the urodynamic properties of various bowel segments in different configurations. However, only recently have reports been published by groups who have compared bowel segments of comparable size, in various configurations using identical urodynamic methodology. Goldwasser et al. (1986) compared the cystometric properties of tubular and detubularised right colon and ileum. Sidi et al. (1986) did the same with sigmoid colon. Both groups reported distinct advantages to detubularisation regardless of the bowel segment utilised. Detubularised segments demonstrated a lower incidence of cystoplasty contractions which were lower in amplitude and first appeared at a higher reservoir capacity.

Camey reported that most of his patients were continent during the daytime and that nocturnal continence depended on the patient's willingness to awaken every 2 to 3 hours (Lilien and Camey 1984). However, others have not experienced such high rates of diurnal continence (Allen et al. 1985; Goldwasser et al. 1987). Goldwasser et al. have suggested, based on urodynamic studies in their patients, that diurnal incontinence may result from the high pressure contractions produced by the tubular shaped ileal reservoir overcoming the closing pressure in what remains of the sphincter active urethra following cystoprostatectomy. Camey believes that meticulous dissection of the prostatic apex, thus preserving as much as possible of the distal sphincter mechanism, is responsible for his superior results.

The realisation that an important factor contributing to continence following cystoprostatectomy is our ability to create a low-pressure internal reservoir led a number of groups to develop ingenious techniques for bladder replacement. All have incorporated the use of the principle of bowel detubularisation and ureteral implantation using an antireflux technique. The Mainz pouch (Thuroff et al. 1986), the "Le Bag" (Light and Engelmann 1986) and the Indiana urinary reservoir (Rowland et al. 1985) achieve detubularisation by patching together adjacent loops of ileum and caecum. The technique described by Goldwasser et al. (1986) incorporates the same principles, yet is more easily accomplished (Fig. 12.1). In this operation the entire right colon and the proximal portion of the transverse colon are mobilised on their mesentery following cystoprostatectomy. This is achieved by dividing the posterior peritoneum lateral to the right colon, and by incising the hepatocolic ligament, followed by blunt dissection separating this segment from its retroperitoneal bed.

The ileocolic, right colic, and middle colic arteries are identified by palpation and transillumination. An incision is extended through the colonic mesentery in as avascular a plane as possible to the right of the middle colic artery. An incision is then made through the ileal mesentery; care should be taken to include the ileocolic artery as part of the right colonic segment (Fig. 12.1A). Next, the ileum and right transverse colon are incised, and the right colonic segment is left isolated on its pedicle; intestinal continuity is established by means of an ileocolostomy. The isolated bowel segment is brought through the mesenteric opening to lie lateral to the bowel anastomosis in the right gutter. This procedure facilitates retroperitonealisation of the bladder replacement at a later stage. The isolated bowel segment is irrigated with saline, after which the ileal stump is resected completely (Fig. 12.1B) and the opening at the ileocaecal valve is closed with inverting sutures of 3–0 Vicryl. The large bowel is opened through a tenia on its antimesenteric side, and about 5–8 cm of the caecum is left tubular shaped (Figs. 12.1B and C). The ureters can be reimplanted into the bowel segment (Fig. 12.1C) by use of the Goodwin technique of submucosal tunneling, by split-cuff nipple reimplantation, or by the technique recommended by Camey for reimplanting the ureters into the small bowel. Care should be taken to leave the ureters sufficiently long to allow subsequent mobilisation of this bowel segment down to the pelvic floor. The ureters should be reimplanted in the proximal half of the bowel segment because the distal part will later be folded over to become the anterior wall. The appendix, if present, is removed.

A small hole is created in the most dependent portion of the caecum, which is then anastomosed to the urethral stump (Fig. 12.1D) over a 20-F Foley catheter by using five interrupted sutures of 2–0 chromic catgut. The distal opened bowel segment is folded over, as previously mentioned (Fig. 12.1E). Running 3–0 Vicryl sutures are used to close the new "bladder" in two layers after bringing the ureteral stents and a 20-F Malecot catheter out through the anterior wall of the imposed bowel segment (Fig. 12.1F).

The final steps include retroperitonealisation of the bowel segment used for the bladder replacement and bringing down the omentum when it is available to wrap it around the suture lines of the new bladder. Two suction drains are left in place, one behind and the other anterior to the newly constructed bladder. The abdominal wound is closed with absorbable sutures. The ureteral stents are removed on the 10th–12th postoperative day. The urethral catheter is removed three weeks postoperatively after a cystogram confirms that there are no leaks (Fig. 12.2). The cystostomy is removed a few days later, after determining that the patient can void with only a small residual volume.

In the patients who remain incontinent following bladder replacement, an artificial urinary sphincter may be placed around the bulbar urethra. However, to

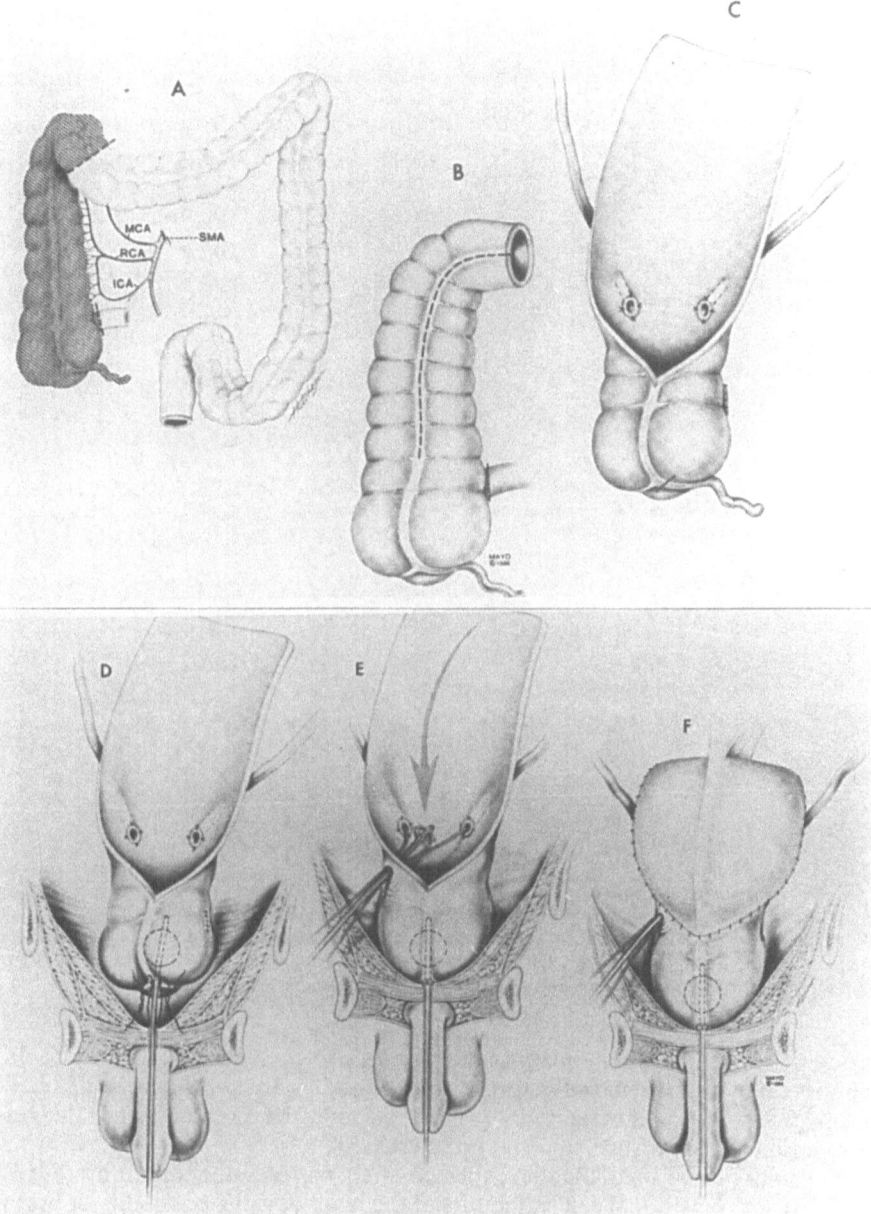

Fig. 12.1. Technique of performing bladder replacement using the detubularised right colon. *A*, the right colon is isolated on a pedicle which incorporates the ileocolic (*ICA*) and right colic arteries (*RCA*). The incision in the colonic mesentery passes to the right of the middle colic artery (*MCA*). *SMA* signifies the superior mesenteric artery. *B*, the ileal stump is removed close to the caecal wall and closed by an inverting running suture. The right colonic segment is opened along the anterior tenia leaving approximately 2–3 in. of proximal caecum tubular shaped. *C*, the ureters are reimplanted using an antireflux technique and the appendix removed. *D*, urethrocaecal anastomosis is performed over a urethral catheter. A suprapubic tube and ureteral stents are passed through the anterior wall of the enterocystoplasty. *E*, the distal opened colonic segment is folded over. *F*, the enterocystoplasty is closed in two layers.

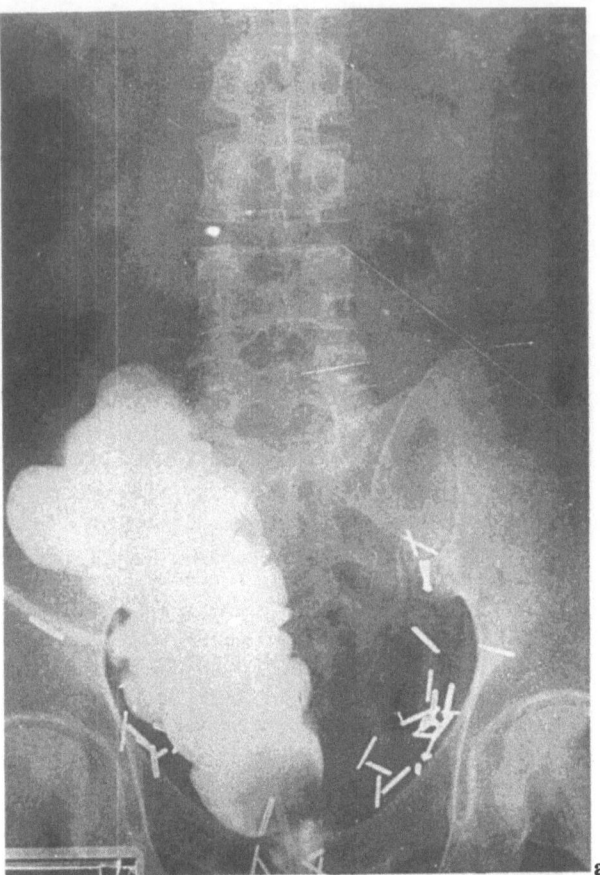

Fig. 12.2a, b. Cystography, three weeks after bladder replacement using a detubularised right colon segment. **a** The bladder filled with 250 ml of contrast dye through the cystostomy tube. **b** Post-void film after urethral catheter was removed and the patient voided per urethra.

attempt to do so when incontinence results from high pressure cystoplasty contractions may be harmful to the upper urinary tracts as a type of bladder artificial urinary sphincter cuff dyssynergia may be created. This danger is minimised if a low pressure reservoir is created.

The major criticism of bladder replacement in patients undergoing cystoprostatectomy for transitional cell carcinoma of the bladder is the possibility of urethral recurrence. Transitional cell carcinoma has a multicentric potential and may involve any portion of the urothelium. This potential for multicentric involvement is frequently separated temporally, and has proved problematic for managing the retained urethra in male patients who have undergone radical cystectomy.

The total incidence of concurrent or subsequent urethral carcinoma is approximately 7%–10% (Raz et al. 1978; Schellhammer and Whitmore 1975). However, if patients with diffuse in situ carcinoma of the bladder, multifocal carcinoma of the bladder, involvement of the prostatic urethra, a history of upper tract

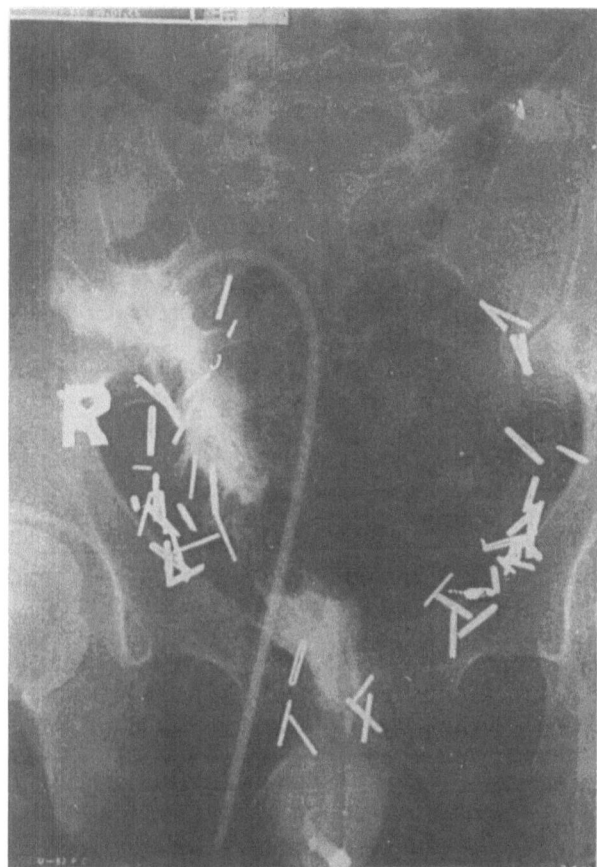

Fig. 12.2b

tumours, and positive margins on frozen section of the transected proximal urethra are excluded, the recurrence rate of carcinoma in the urethra is sufficiently low to justify bladder replacement in these patients.

Continent urinary diversion by creation of an internal reservoir with a continent stoma has a number of distinct advantages over bladder replacement. It may be applied both in males and in females, it can be applied for nearly all aetiologies, and it allows immediate en-bloc cystoprostatectomy and urethrectomy to be performed, thus reducing the risk of urethral recurrence in patients with transitional cell carcinoma of the bladder.

The first technique of external urinary diversion with an attempt to achieve continence was described by Gilchrist and associates in 1950, using the isolated ileocaecal segment. The caecum functioned as a urinary reservoir and the ileum formed the outflow tract and the cutaneous urostoma. They reported complete continence in 68 of their patients (94%). The continence achieved was believed to depend upon the antiperistaltic function of the terminal ileum, the action of the ileocaecal valve, and the small ileal skin stoma. However, others were unable to reproduce these results with this method (Bricker and Eiseman 1950).

Interest in continent urinary stomal diversion was renewed in the 1970s when different groups in Europe began working on various techniques to achieve this goal. Kock and co-workers, who developed the intra-abdominal reservoir (Kock 1969) or continent ileostomy (Kock 1973) for patients undergoing proctocolectomy for ulcerative colitis began considering their technique for continent urinary diversion. Leisinger and associates (1976) described the first successful clinical experience with the continent ileal reservoir and other reports were soon to follow (Madigan 1976; Kock et al. 1978, 1982; Gerber 1983; Skinner et al. 1984). At the same time other workers became interested in the use of the ileocaecal segment for continent urinary diversion (Ashken 1974, 1978; Zingg and Tscholl 1977; Mansson et al. 1984). Various ways of creating a continent valve mechanism were tried, but met with little success (Ashken 1982). The major problems encountered by both those who experimented with the Kock pouch and those who worked on the ileocaecal pouch were related to difficulties with the outlet. Spontaneous dessusception, with resulting incontinence and catheterisation difficulties, were common. After extensive studies in animals, and clinical tests, Kock and co-workers modified the technique for the construction of a nipple valve (Kock et al. 1980). Skinner and co-workers have added their modification which helped decrease the revision rate of the stomas from 58% in the original series of Kock and associates to as low as 6%–25% (Skinner et al. 1984; Boyd et al. 1985).

The major criticism of the Kock pouch is the complexity of the operation and the fact that it is time-consuming. On the other hand, its superior bowel dynamics that allow low pressure collection and storage of urine have helped make it more popular than the caecal reservoir. The development of new techniques (Thuroff et al. 1986; Rowland et al. 1985) based on the concept that detubularisation of the bowel will help create a low pressure reservoir has brought about a renewed interest in the construction of a caecal reservoir. A technique to create a caecoileal continent urinary diversion which has recently been described by Rowland and associates (1985) merits particular interest. Their technique includes detubularisation of the caecal segment to create the low pressure reservoir and plication of 12–15 cm of the terminal ileum leading into the pouch to achieve a continent stoma. This type of outlet seems to be free of the problems of instability inherent in intususcepted valves and makes intermittent catheterisation easier. Their initial results of over 90% continence rate with no revisions make this technique particularly attractive (Rowland et al. 1987).

The ultimate role of continent urinary diversion procedures, and their relative merits with respect to each other and to appliance-dependent conduit diversion must await the results of long-term follow-up of large series. Nonetheless, they are an exciting development with widespread application and the potential to improve the quality of life significantly in patients with diversion.

References

Allen TD, Peters PC, Sagalowsky AI, Roehrborn CP (1985) The Camey Procedure: preliminary results in 11 patients. World J Urol 3: 167–171
Ashken MH (1974) An appliance-free ileocaecal urinary diversion: preliminary communication. Br J Urol 46: 631–637
Ashken MH (1978) Continent ileocaecal urinary reservoir. J Roy Soc Med 71: 357–360

Ashken MH (1982) Urinary reservoirs. In: Ashken MH (ed) Urinary diversion, Springer-Verlag, New York, pp 112–139

Bloom NH, Videne RA, Lytton B (1970) Primary carcinoma of the ureter: a report of 102 new cases. J Urol 103: 590–598

Boyd DS, Skinner DG, Lieskovsky G (1985) Ongoing experience with the Kock continent ileal reservoir for urinary diversion. World J Urol 3: 155–158

Bricker EM, Eiseman B (1950) Bladder reconstruction from caecum and ascending colon following resection of pelvic viscera. Ann Surg 132: 77–84

Carroll G (1985) Bilateral transitional cell carcinoma of the renal pelvis. J Urol 93: 132–135

Catalona WJ (1985) Nerve-sparing radical retropubic prostatectomy. Urol Clin North Am 12: 187–199

Catalona WJ, Dresner SM (1985) Nerve-sparing radical prostatectomy: extraprostatic tumor extension and preservation of erectile function. J Urol 134: 1149–1151

Eggelston JC, Walsh PC (1985) Radical prostatectomy with preservation of sexual function: pathological finding in the first 100 cases. J Urol 134: 1146–1148

Faysal MH, Freiha FS (1979) Evaluation of partial cystectomy for carcinoma of bladder. Urology 14: 352–356

Gerber A (1983) The Kock continent ileal reservoir for supravesical urinary diversion. An early experience. Am J Surg 146: 15–20

Gilchrist RK, Merricks JW, Hamlin MH, Rieger IT (1950) Construction of a substitute bladder and urethra. Surg Gynecol Obst 90: 752–760

Goldwasser B, Lieber MM (1987) Role of partial nephrectomy in management of renal tumors, including surgical technique. In: Skinner DG (ed) Diagnosis and management of genitourinary cancer. W. B. Saunders Co., Philadelphia (In Press)

Goldwasser B, Webster GD (1985) Continent urinary diversion. J Urol 134: 227–236

Goldwasser B, Barrett DM, Kramer DA, Webster GD (1986) Cystometric properties of ileum and right colon in patients following bladder augmentation, substitution and replacement. Proceeding of Third Joint Meeting of the International Continence Society and Urodynamic Society, Boston, p 133

Goldwasser B, Barrett DM, Benson RC (1986) Bladder replacement with use of a detubularized right colonic segment: preliminary report of a new technique. Mayo Clin Proc 61: 615–621

Goldwasser B, Rife CC, Benson RC, Furlow WL, Barrett DM (1987) Urodynamic evaluation of patients after the Camey operation. J Urol 138: 832–835

Huffman JL, Bagley DH, Lyon ES, Morse MJ, Herr HW, Whitmore WF Jr (1985) Endoscopic diagnosis and treatment of upper tract urothelial tumors: a preliminary report. Cancer 55: 1422–1428

Jacobs SC (1984) Role of conservative surgery for patients with bilateral kidney tumors. In: Catalona WJ, Tarliff TL (eds) Urologic oncology. Martinus Nijhoff, Boston

Jacobs SC, Berg SI, Lawson RK (1980) Synchronous bilateral renal cell carcinoma: total surgical excision. Cancer 46: 2341–2345

deKernion JB, Ramming KP, Smith RB (1978) The natural history of metastatic renal cell carcinoma: a computer analysis. J Urol 120: 148–152

Kock NG (1969) Intra-abdominal "Reservoir" in patients with permanent ileostomy. Preliminary observations on a procedure resulting in fecal "continence" in five ileostomy patients. Arch Surg 99: 223–231

Kock NG (1973) Continent ileostomy. Prog Surg 12: 180–201

Kock NG, Nilson AE, Norlen LJ, Sundin T, Trasti H (1978) Urinary diversion via a continent ileum reservoir: clinical experience. Scand J Urol Nephrol [Suppl] 49: 23–31

Kock NG, Myrvold HE, Nilsson LO, Ahren C (1980) Construction of a stable nipple valve for the continent ileostomy. Ann Chir Gynec 69: 132–143

Kock NG, Nilson AE, Nilsson LO, Norlen LJ, Philipson BM (1982) Urinary diversion via a continent ileal reservoir: clinical results in 12 patients. J Urol 128: 469–475

Konnak JW, Grossman HB (1985) Renal cell carcinoma as an incidental finding. J Urol 134: 1094–1096

Leisinger HJ, Sauberli H, Schawwecker T, Mayor G (1976) Continent ileal bladder: first clinical experience. Eur Urol 2: 8–12

Lieber MM, Goldwasser B (1988) Role of partial nephrectomy in management of renal tumors including surgical technique. In: Skinner D, Leiskovsky G (eds) Diagnosis and management of genitourinary cancer. W. B. Saunders Co., Philadelphia, pp 704–720

Lieber MM, Tomera KM, Farron GM (1981) Renal oncocytoma. J Urol 125: 481–483

Light JK, Engelmann UH (1986) Le Bag: total replacement of bladder using ileocolonic pouch. J Urol 136: 27–31

Lilien OM, Camey M (1984) 25-year experience with replacement of the human bladder (Camey procedure). J Urol 132: 886–891

Madigan MR (1976) The continent ileostomy and the isolated ileal bladder. Ann R Coll Surg Engl 58: 62–69

Mansson W, Collen S, Sundin T (1984) Continent caecal reservoir in urinary diversion. Br J Urol 56: 359–365

Marberger M (1980) Organerhallende Chirurgie bein Nierenkarzinom Aktuelle. Urologie 11: 325–334

Marberger M, Pugh RC, Auvert J, Bertermann H, Costantini A, Gammelgaard PA, Petterson S, Wickham JEA (1981) Conservation surgery for renal carcinoma: the EIRSS experience. Br J Urol 53: 528–532

Marshall FF (1984) The in situ surgical management of renal cell carcinoma and transitional cell carcinoma of the kidney. World J Urol 2: 130–135

Marshall FF, Walsh PC (1984) In situ management of renal tumors: renal cell carcinoma and transitional cell carcinoma. J Urol 131: 1045–1049

McDonald MW, Zincke H (1987) Urothelial tumors of the upper urinary tract. In: de Kernion JB, Paulson DF (eds) Genitourinary cancer management. Lea and Febiger, Philadelphia, pp 1–31

McLoughlin MG (1975) The treatment of bilateral synchronous renal pelvic tumors with bench surgery. J Urol 114: 463–465

Murphy DM, Zincke H, Furlow WL (1980) Primary Grade 1 Transitional cell carcinoma of the renal pelvis and ureter. J Urol 123: 629–631

Murphy DM, Zincke H, Furlow WL (1981) Management of high grade transitional cell carcinoma of the upper urinary tract. J Urol 125: 25–29

Novick AC (1984) Editorial comment. In: Catalona WJ, Ratcliff TL (eds) Urologic oncology. Martinus Nijhoff, Boston, p 159

Patel NP, Lavengood RN (1978) Renal cell carcinoma: natural history and results of treatment. J Urol 119: 722–726

Penn I (1977) Transplantation of patients with primary renal malignancies. Transplantation 24: 424–434

Pettersson S, Brynger H, Henriksson C, Jahansson SL, Nilson AE, Ranch T (1984) Treatment of urothelial tumors of the upper urinary tract by nephroureterectomy, renal autotransplantation and pyelocystostomy. Cancer 54: 379–386

Raz S, McLouie G, Johnson S, Skinner DG (1978) Management of the urethra in patients undergoing radical cystectomy for bladder carcinoma. J Urol 120: 298–300

Resnick MI, O'Connor VJ, Jr (1973) Segmental resection for carcinoma of the bladder: review of 102 patients. J Urol 109: 1007–1010

Robson CJ, Churchill BM, Anderson W (1969) The results of radical nephrectomy for renal cell carcinoma. J Urol 101: 297–301

Rowland RG, Mitchell ME, Bihrle R (1985) The cecoileal continent urinary reservoir. World J Urol 3: 185–190

Rowland RG, Mitchell ME, Bihrle R, Kahnoski RJ, Piser JA (1987) Indiana continent urinary reservoir. J Urol 137: 1136–1139

Rubenstein MA, Walz BS, Bucy JG (1978) Transitional cell carcinoma of the kidney: 25 year experience. J Urol 119: 594–597

Schellhammer PF, Whitmore WF, Jr (1975) Transitional cell carcinoma of the urethra in men having cystectomy for bladder cancer. J Urol 115: 56–60

Schoborg TW, Sapolsky JL, Lewis CW, Jr (1979) Carcinoma of the bladder treated by segmental resection. J Urol 122: 473–475

Sidi AA, Reinberg Y, Gonzalez R (1986) Influence of intestinal segment and configuration on the outcome of augmentation enterocystoplasty. J Urol 136: 1201–1204

Skinner DG, Lieskovsky G, Boyd SD (1984) Technique of creation of a continent internal ileal reservoir (Kock pouch) for urinary diversion. Urol Clin North Am 11: 741–749

Skinner DG, Boyd SD, Leiskovsky G (1984) Clinical experience with the Kock continent ileal reservoir for urinary diversion. J Urol 132: 1101–1107

Smith AD, Orihuela E, Crowley AR (1987) Percutaneous management of renal pelvic tumors: treatment option in selected cases. J Urol 137: 852–856

Smith RB, de Kernion JB, Erhlich RM, Skinner DG, Kaufman JJ (1984) Bilateral renal cell carcinoma and renal cell carcinoma in the solitary kidney. J Urol 132: 450–454

Strong DW, Pearse HD, Tank ES, Jr, Hodges CV (1976) The ureteral stump after nephroureterectomy. J Urol 115: 654–655

Thuroff JW, Alken P, Riedmiller H, Engelmann U, Jacobi GH, Hohenfellner R (1986) Mainz pouch (mixed augmentation ileum and cecum) for bladder augmentation and continent urinary diversion J Urol 136: 17–26

Topley M, Novick AC, Montie JE (1984) Long-term results following partial nephrectomy for localized renal adenocarcinoma. J Urol 131: 1050–1052

Utz DC, McDonald JR (1957) Squamous cell carcinoma of the kidney. J Urol 78: 540–552

Utz DC, Schmitz SE, Fulgelso PD, Farrow GM (1973) A clinicopathologic evaluation of partial cystectomy for carcinoma of the urinary bladder. Cancer 32: 1075–1077

Vermillion CD, Skinner DG. Pfister RC (1972) Bilateral renal cell carcinoma. J Urol 108: 219–222

Vest SA (1945) Conservation surgery in certain benign tumors of ureter. J Urol 53: 97–121

Wallace DM, Whitfield HN, Hendry WF, Wickham JEA (1981) The late results of conservative surgery for upper tract urothelial carcinomas. Br J Urol 53: 537–541

Walsh OC, Donker PJ (1982) Impotence following radical prostatectomy: insight into etiology and prevention. J Urol 128: 492–497

Walsh PC, Mostwin JL (1984) Radical prostatectomy and cystoprostatectomy with preservation of potency. Results using a new nerve-sparing technique. Br J Urol 56: 644–697

Walsh PC, Lepor H, Eggleston JC (1983) Radical prostatectomy with preservation of sexual function: anatomical and pathological considerations. Prostate 4: 473–485

Wickham JE (1975) Conservative renal surgery for adenocarcinoma: the place of bench surgery. Br J Urol 47: 25–36

Woodhouse CRJ, Kellett MJ, Bloom HJG (1986) Percutaneous renal surgery and local radiotherapy in the management of renal pelvic transitional cell carcinoma. Br J Urol 58: 245–249

Zincke H, Neves RJ (1984) Feasibility of conservation surgery for transitional cell cancer of the upper urinary tract. Urol Clin North Am 11: 717–724

Zincke H, Swanson SK (1982) Bilateral renal cell carcinoma: influence of synchronous and asynchronous occurrence on patient survival. J Urol 128: 913–915

Zincke H, Engen DE, Henning KM, McDonald MW (1985) Treatment of renal cell carcinoma by in situ partial nephrectomy and extracorporeal operation with autotransplantation. Mayo Clin Proc 60: 651–662

Zingg E, Tscholl R (1977) Continent cecoileal conduit: preliminary report. J Urol 118: 724–728

Chapter 13

Clinical Trials in Genitourinary Oncology: What Have They Achieved?

D. Raghavan and I.F. Tannock

Introduction

When a patient is diagnosed as having urological cancer, a number of factors will influence the treatment that is used. These may include the personal experience of the clinician recommending treatment, his time and place of training, and his awareness of the results of clinical trials which have addressed aspects of management relevant to this particular patient. A recent survey of practice relating to urological cancer has demonstrated very diverse opinions about management (Moore and Tannock, unpublished). Moreover, when presented with the opportunity to enter a hypothetical patient into a randomised clinical trial comparing two treatments (A and B), some respondents refused because their assessment of previous studies indicated treatment A to be vastly superior and B to be inappropriate, while others with equal reputation and experience came to exactly the opposite conclusion. Similar biases led to a reduced rate of entry into a recent controlled, randomised trial of pre-emptive ("neoadjuvant") chemotherapy for invasive bladder cancer (Raghavan 1988). Clinical trials in genitourinary oncology have thus not yet achieved a uniform approach to the management of common clinical problems.

Lack of uniformity in the clinical approach to similar patients does not necessarily reflect a failure of clinical trials to influence practice because, in some instances, they have demonstrated minimal differences in outcome among alternative treatments. This is true, for example, of several which have compared various hormonal manoeuvres to decrease androgen stimulation of metastatic prostate cancer (see Chap. 8). In other situations, the apparent results of clinical trials may rightly be rejected because their design or analysis is flawed, or because patient selection led to differences in the population studied from patients seen commonly in practice. In contrast, clinicians sometimes reject the results of well-conducted clinical trials in favour of personal bias, an approach that we believe to be inappropriate. Anecdotal results from one's own practice often give misleading impressions about therapeutic impact.

It seems unlikely that the outcome for patients with cancer of the bladder, kidney or prostate will improve by quantum leaps. Rather, improved survival and/or decreased morbidity of treatment are likely to result from smaller changes in therapy that will only be demonstrable through the application of well-designed clinical investigations. Thus it behoves all who have an interest in improving patient management to be aware of clinical trials, and to be able to interpret their results after critical evaluation of their design and analysis. In this chapter, we will review the format of various types of clinical trial, comment on factors that may limit their validity, and summarise some of the more important trials relating to the management of genitourinary malignancy.

Scope and Definition of Clinical Trials

Whenever clinicians manage patients who fit defined criteria according to a predetermined plan, and keep records of patient outcome, they are conducting a "clinical trial". This broad definition encompasses investigations that are of varying levels of complexity, and which address a wide variety of questions. One clinical trial may assess a new technique of urinary diversion in 10 suitable patients; another may require randomisation of 300 patients to compare survival when locally advanced bladder cancer is treated by radical cystectomy with or without adjunctive chemotherapy. In general, clinical trials may be classified by the questions they seek to answer, with consequent implications for their design and analysis. The more important features of this classification are outlined below.

Explanatory and Pragmatic Trials

A clinical trial may be assigned to one of two distinct categories, which have been termed "explanatory" and "pragmatic" (Table 13.1; Schwartz and Lellouch 1967). An explanatory trial aims to acquire information; thus it may investigate whether an experimental therapy is feasible or has biological activity, but does not allow conclusions about patient benefit from general use of the therapy. Examples include the feasibility study of a new form of urinary diversion, or the assessment of tumour response in a series of patients treated with an experimental drug. In contrast, a pragmatic trial is concerned with assessment of patient benefit from use of the experimental protocol, so that it can be used as a guide in therapeutic decision-making. An example is provided by the randomised trial of

Table 13.1.   Explanatory and pragmatic clinical trials (Schwartz and Lellouch 1967)

	Explanatory trials	Pragmatic trials
Aim	To acquire information	To make a decision
Design features	Usually require small number of patients	Usually large trials, most often using randomisation between experimental and standard treatment
	Biological endpoints (e.g. tumour shrinkage)	Practical endpoints (e.g. patient survival)
	May analyse only patients receiving full treatment	Should analyse all patients
Examples	Feasibility study of new form of urinary diversion	Randomised trial of cystectomy for muscle invasive bladder cancer with or without neoadjuvant chemotherapy

adjunctive chemotherapy in locally invasive bladder cancer noted above. This classification is important because the goals of each type of trial are quite different, with major implications for their design and analysis (Table 13.1).

An explanatory trial can usually be performed with a small number of patients, and in asking questions about feasibility or biological activity it may be appropriate to report only those patients who could be fully treated according to protocol. For example, in testing for activity of a new drug, it may be legitimate to exclude patients from analysis if they could not tolerate a certain minimal amount of treatment. This practice minimises the chance of rejecting an active agent prematurely but may overestimate the effect of the drug in the patient population. Thus, it does not give information about overall patient benefit, which must be evaluated subsequently in a pragmatic trial.

The goal of a pragmatic trial is to determine the overall benefit of an experimental protocol to all eligible patients. Endpoints should therefore include assessment of both quantity and quality of survival. Also, if the results of the trial are to be relevant to any group of patients who fit the entry criteria, it is important (1) to define those criteria carefully and to record the outcome of eligible patients that are not entered in the trial; and (2) to report the outcome for all patients regardless of the quantity of treatment that they receive.

One example of a pragmatic trial is the evaluation of cystectomy for patients in whom radiological investigations do not reveal extravesical disease. All patients satisfying entry criteria should be evaluated and reported, including those in whom surgery reveals unsuspected nodal disease and patients whose planned operation cannot be completed. Exclusion of such patients from analysis would bias results and overestimate the true benefit of cystectomy to any similar group of clinically and radiologically staged patients (see below).

Many trials are undertaken with the implicit goal of providing patient benefit and are pragmatic in intent, although their results are often analysed by methods more suited to explanatory trials. Thus one finds inappropriate exclusion of patients, and the use of endpoints that do not necessarily reflect benefit to patients (e.g. tumour shrinkage rather than quantity of survival in trials of chemotherapy). This type of faulty design and/or analysis may place severe limitations on the application of their results.

Phase I, II and III Trials

The description of clinical trials as "Phase I, II or III" is used widely in studies of chemotherapy, but has also been adapted to the evaluation of radiotherapy or surgery.

A Phase I trial seeks to evaluate the toxicity of an experimental protocol and, when applied to an experimental drug, may also involve evaluation of pharmacokinetics and the determination of a maximal tolerated dose (MTD). Phase I trials are performed on fully informed volunteer patients who have advanced disease and for whom there is no standard therapy which has a significant probability of favourably influencing their disease. Although possible antitumour activity or therapeutic benefit is recorded, its evaluation is not a major endpoint of a Phase I trial. In fact, the selection of patients with very advanced (and often pretreated) disease makes it unlikely that therapeutic success will be achieved. Phase I trials are explanatory in nature.

Phase II trials are also explanatory and seek to determine whether an experimental protocol shows evidence of anti-tumour activity. They usually involve treatment of a small series of patients with a particular stage and type of malignancy, and use short-term measures of activity. Examples include the assessment of tumour shrinkage in patients with metastatic renal cancer upon treatment with a new drug at the MTD determined from a Phase I trial; or the functional assessment of a new method of continent diversion in patients undergoing cystectomy. As emphasised above, evidence of response in a small, selected series of patients in a Phase II trial does not necessarily imply longterm therapeutic benefit in the broader general population of patients.

Phase III trials attempt to define the role of a new therapeutic strategy in patient management and are pragmatic in intent. They therefore involve a comparison with a standard treatment, and the preferred design involves random allocation ("randomisation") of patients to receive experimental or standard treatment. However, other factors frequently make it difficult to design or execute a randomised trial (see below) and the Phase III trial then involves treatment of a large series of patients with the newer therapy. Assessment of patient benefit relative to standard treatment then requires comparison with historical controls or with a series of patients treated in another institution. Unfortunately, many factors can introduce bias, usually in the direction of making the new therapy appear better than the old (Tonkin and Tannock 1988; Raghavan 1988a). Careful attention to experimental design and complete reporting of the results is then of paramount importance.

Design and Analysis of Clinical Trials

One of the major difficulties in designing and executing clinical trials in genitourinary oncology is to establish and maintain an appropriate balance between statistical validity and the reality of clinical practice. For example, in an ideal setting, a clinical trial in which more than 300 patient with deeply invasive bladder cancer are randomly allocated to undergo radical radiotherapy or radical cystectomy would answer one of the most important questions in the management of this disease. The large number of patients would assure a high statistical probability of defining whether a survival difference actually exists between these two treatment options and would avoid a signficant likelihood of missing a small difference (if it exists). However, several practical problems would flaw the study design:

1. Variation in surgical skill and technique among different participating surgeons
2. A small likelihood that patients today would consent to the loss of their bladders merely on the basis of a randomisation procedure
3. Differences in radiotherapy techniques and equipment among participating institutions, perhaps accentuated by conflicts on what constitutes optimal dose and fractionation of treatment
4. Changes in technology and practice in the diagnosis and management of the disease during the time course of the trial (including the approach to the salvage of treatment failures)
5. The possible loss of enthusiasm of the participants during the lengthy time interval required for such a large study.

All too often, a trial is initiated simply to utilise an established mechanism or clinical trial unit or to maintain the momentum of an established collaborative group. Several major issues must be resolved prior to the development of a clinical trial:

1. Is the question to be asked of sufficient importance to justify the expenditure of resources?
2. Has the question been studied previously in a well-designed trial and has an unequivocal answer been achieved?
3. Will a new result from the planned trial be of significant clinical or scientific benefit?

Once an important question has been identified, it is essential to ensure that the appropriate resources are available to complete the study:

1. Adequate numbers of patients to allow the question to be answered within a reasonable time frame;
2. Statistical support and data management facilities from the time of inception of the study
3. Committed investigators who are prepared to support the trial and to adhere to the protocol requirements and trial design
4. Sufficient technological resources for diagnosis and treatment to fulfil the requirements of the study protocol.

The design requirements vary with the type of clinical trial. For a Phase I study, smaller numbers of patients are required, as the endpoint is to define a maximum tolerated dose. By convention, 3 patients are treated at each dose level to allow adequate assessment of toxicity whilst minimising the number of patients treated at a potentially subtherapeutic (or toxic) dose. Dose escalations are effected on the basis of a pre-defined schedule (Creaven and Mihich 1977; Marsoni and Wittes 1984).

A Phase II trial, is designed to assess whether or not a new therapy has sufficient anti-tumour activity to merit further evaluation to define its true utility. The requirements have been assessed by a variety of statistical methods and have been found to be similar (Staquet and Sylvester 1977; Lee et al. 1979). For example, if a trial is discontinued after 14 patients have been treated without objective response, there is only a 5% probability of rejecting a drug which would yield a true response rate of greater than 20% when tested in a large sample of patients. By contrast, if there has been one objective response among the first 14 cases and the trial is discontinued, there would be a 20% chance of inappropriately rejecting an active drug; hence, an additional number of patients should then be treated to complete the Phase II trial (Lee et al. 1979).

In a Phase III trial, the number of patients required is determined by the anticipated magnitude of the difference in endpoint(s) of the trial and the nature of those differences. If the endpoint is survival, the number of patients required to achieve statistical significance will be influenced by the shape of the survival curves. Furthermore, the nature of these curves will also determine the required duration of follow-up and a reasonable time-frame for patient accrual. However, if the endpoint of the study is quality of life, the trial may require fewer patients, but a greater number of measurements per patient.

When attempting to assess the number of patients required for a clinical trial, it is also necessary to define what is an acceptable level of error from the methodology employed. Error probabilities (designated alpha and beta) have been described to assist in the calculation of requisite sample size and in the assessment of results. The alpha (or Type I) error is made by declaring that there is a difference between two treatments when it does not really exist. The beta (Type II) error represents a failure to recognise a significant difference between samples when it is truly present in an overall population. By setting specific limits for these indices, the requisite number of patients for a specific trial can be determined.

A lack of understanding of these issues is widely manifest in the literature pertaining to the management of genitourinary cancer. For example, randomised trials have been reported at a stage when the small numbers of cases would not have allowed the detection of small but significant differences between the two groups (Horn et al. 1981; Javadpour et al. 1982) or where a large number of patients has been divided into too many treatment subgroups, effectively reducing the likelihood of detecting differences between each group (Blackard et al. 1972; Prout 1976).

An allied problem is the prevalence of early and interim reports of randomised trials, in which the treatment of a small fraction of the proposed patient accrual is described; for example, a consecutive series of reports on the use of hormonal priming for the management of advanced prostate cancer yielded substantially different results, with the most recent actually revealing a survival disadvantage for the experimental protocol (Manni et al. 1985, 1986, 1987). In this situation, the preliminary communication is often erroneously quoted as reflecting the ultimate outcome of the completed trial, as discussed elsewhere (Raghavan 1988b). Although there is often a strong temptation to report statistically-valid interim data from an ongoing trial (Levi et al. 1986), this practice is subject to abuse and should be discouraged.

Sources of Error

Faults in the design of a study can cause substantial errors, or systematic bias, in the results achieved. As discussed above, inadequate numbers of patients can allow sampling errors; when combined with a bias to publish "positive" small studies (Simes 1986), there may be a false impression of benefit from a new treatment. Similarly, exclusion of patients from analysis and reporting can bias the outcome of a study.

The failure to establish uniform criteria for the assessment of efficacy and toxicity (Miller et al. 1981) can cause major confusion in the evaluation of the results of a trial. Thus, substantial apparent variation between the results of two similar studies can be an artefact due simply to differences in the methodology or criteria of assessment or the inaccuracies of clinical measurement (Moertel and Hanley 1976; Warr et al. 1984; Tonkin et al. 1985). This applies, in particular, to the assessment of treatment for advanced prostatic cancer (see below). In some instances, the absence of such criteria can cause intra-group variation, yielding unpredictable and non-uniform results from different investigators participating in a common trial.

As there are many sources of potential error in the execution of a clinical trial, it is desirable to submit the data to external peer review prior to publication. The design and implementation of a study should also be monitored externally, allowing errors to be identified and resolved prospectively. External assessors should review important indices of the trial, including the classification of "reponse" by participating investigators. A variety of mechanisms can be used, such as review of pre- and post-treatment scans and X-rays or chart reviews.

Controls and Their Limitations

In order to assess the relevance of the observations of a clinical trial, it is necessary to compare the data against some form of standard. For example, in the assessment of a new treatment, a comparison will be made with the results obtained using conventional therapy. This can be done implicitly against one's own experience, but such an approach is flawed by the errors and biases discussed above.

Another approach is to use "historical controls", in which the data from a current trial are compared with information gained from previously completed studies. This approach also can lead to major errors, derived from changes in the characteristics of the patient population and from variations in the methods of diagnosis and management over a period of time. For example, an apparent improvement in the results from a new treatment may simply be due to the introduction of a new staging technique, such as computed axial tomographic (CAT) scanning. In this situation, the use of the CAT scan may change the distribution of allocated stage, removing patients with occult metastases from a group with "limited disease" and placing them in a "metastatic" group, albeit with smaller volume metastases ("stage migration" or the "Will Rogers pheno-menon"). In this fashion, the results of treatment for each stage will appear to have improved, although this artefact of improved staging does not reflect a change in overall survival of the group (Batley 1955; Bush 1979; Feinstein et al. 1985). Conversely, when an increase in survival is seen, perhaps after the use of a new cytotoxic drug, this may only reflect improved antibiotic management or the use of more active salvage regimens after first relapse.

Another variant is to compare consecutive series, suggesting (erroneously) that some of the major differences of patient population and management outlined above can be avoided because of the proximity in time of the two series to be compared. While, in theory, this could be possible, it is also likely that major inadvertent biases could be introduced. For example, in the situation in which a particularly aggressive cytotoxic regimen is employed for the management of metastatic prostate cancer, clinicians could defer treatment of elderly unfit patients until the completion of accrual in order to avoid subjecting such patients to undue toxicity – in this fashion, the population undergoing treatment would be heavily biased in favour of the younger more robust patient. Furthermore, when comparing survival curves, the duration of follow-up will differ, as illustrated recently in a comparison of consecutive adjuvant protocols of doxorubicin and mitomycin (Ausfeld et al. 1987). In this situation, an apparent difference in survival curves may simply reflect inadequate time for endpoints (e.g. relapse, death) to occur in the more recently treated cohort.

The currently preferred mechanism for the conduct of clinical trials is to use prospective randomisation, in which patients are allocated to the various treatment arms solely on the basis of chance selection. Using this method, there is less chance of accidentally introducing bias in the selection of patients or the treatment that they receive. A less desirable variant is the use of randomisation by blocks, in which patients in a multi-centre trial are randomised within participating institutions on the basis of small numbers of pre-allocated treatments (see "Clinical Trials in Prostate Cancer" below).

Unfortunately, patients often experience anxiety as a result of their participation in randomised trials; when they receive the details of randomisation and of the uncertainty about the potential differences between the two approaches to treatment, they may lose confidence in their clinicians and often experience high levels of stress and concern (Simes et al. 1986).

Clinical Trials in Bladder Cancer

There are two quite distinct patterns of bladder cancer, based upon natural history, patterns of recurrence and spread, response to treatment and prognosis: superficial and invasive disease (see Chaps. 5 and 6). The dominant histological variant of bladder cancer is transitional cell carcinoma (TCC), which represents more than 90% of cases. As the other histological types (adenocarcinoma, squamous cell carcinoma, sarcoma and other less common patterns) occur infrequently, they have been less prominent as the subjects of clinical trials, apart from an important series of Phase II studies carried out in Egypt (Ghoneim et al. 1979; Gad-el-Mawla et al. 1979).

Superficial Bladder Cancer

For many years, repeated endoscopic resection or transurethral diathermy constituted the hallmarks of management of superficial TCC. Occasionally simple cystectomy was performed for extensive or recurrent tumours. Phase I–II trials have shown that cytotoxic agents can be administered directly into the bladder via a urinary catheter with acceptable toxicity and some anti-tumour activity (Jones and Swinney 1961; Veenema et al. 1962; Riddle and Wallace 1971; Banks et al. 1977; Byar and Blackard 1977; Soloway 1980). This approach, termed "intravesical chemotherapy", has substantially changed the management of superficial bladder cancer. Recently, the efficacy of intravesical chemotherapy as direct therapy, and as prophylaxis after resection of all documented tumour, has been documented in randomised Phase III trials. Data from some of the important studies are summarised in Table 13.2.

Objective response rates of 30%–80% can be achieved by intravesical instillation of drugs such as thiotepa, epodyl, doxorubicin, mitomycin and teniposide (VM-26), or by the use of intravesical Bacille Calmette-Guerin (BCG). Analogous to the use of systemic chemotherapy, response rates are

Table 13.2. Randomised trials of intravesical chemotherapy for superficial bladder cancer

Institution	Number	Design	Result	Reference
EORTC	206	DOX ethoglucid TUR only	Significant benefit for chemotherapy	Kurth et al. 1984
EORTC	308	thiotepa VM26 TUR only	Significant benefit for chemotherapy	Schulman et al. 1982
MRC	417	TTPA stat TTPA monthly Std Rx	No difference	MRC 1985
Tokyo University	575	DOX 1 mg/ml DOX 0.5 mg/ml MMC 0.5 mg/ml std Rx	Significant difference between DOX and standard treatment	Niijima et al. 1983
Mayo Clinic	89	DOX TTPA std Rx	Reduced recurrences with chemotherapy	Zincke et al. 1983
Mayo Clinic	83	TTPA MMC	No difference	Zincke et al. 1985
NBCCGA	93	TTPA std Rx	Longer disease-free interval for TTPA	Koontz et al. 1981
NBCCGA	156	MMC* TTPA*	Benefit for MMC in CR rate	Heney 1985
Tel Aviv University	25	TTPA DOX	No difference but small nos.	Horn et al. 1981
MSKCC	86	BCG std Rx	Benefit for BCG	Pinsky et al. 1985
MSKCC	93	BCG BCG+maint BCG Rx	No difference	Badalament et al. 1987

* therapeutic, not prophylactic, study
Key: DOX, doxorubicin; MMC, mitomycin C; TTPA, thiotepa; BCG, Bacille Calmette-Guerin; maint, maintenance; CR, complete remission; NBCCGA, National Bladder Cancer Collaborative Group A; EORTC, European Organisation for Research and Treatment of Cancer; MRC, Medical Research Council of Great Britain; MSKCC, Memorial Sloan-Kettering Cancer Centre; std Rx, standard treatment; chemo Rx, chemotherapy; VM26, teniposide; TUR only, transurethral resection only; TTPA stat, single, immediate dose of thiotepa.

higher in previously untreated patients. Some of the published trials, which are summarised in Table 13.2, have yielded conflicting results. For example, the NBCCGA showed thiotepa to be an active agent, significantly prolonging the relapse-free interval (Koontz et al. 1981; Prout and Kopp 1984), whereas the EORTC trial, when first analysed, suggested no difference in time to relapse (Schulman et al. 1982). However, subsequent assessment showed a significant reduction in the relative rate of relapse through the use of thiotepa.

One issue that still requires resolution is the difference between statistically significant and clinically relevant information. For stage T_a, grade I TCC, the relapse rate after conventional treatment is low. Although the relapse rate has been shown, in randomised trials, to be further reduced by the use of intravesical chemotherapy, this small clinical benefit may not justify the morbidity of the treatment.

In many of the studies, the doses and schedules have differed, and each trial reflects only the experience with the specific protocols assessed. For BCG therapy, there are substantial differences between the activity of the different strains that are used (Pasteur, Tice, etc.), which may explain the variability in published data.

To date, clinical trials have demonstrated the safety and efficacy of several approaches to intravesical therapy, and have shown that these constitute valid adjuncts and/or alternatives to repeated trans-urethral resection or diathermy or to cystectomy in the management of this disease. However, in 1988, we have still not defined with certainty the optimal schedule, sequencing, or agents for intravesical chemotherapy. This does not represent a failure of clinical trials per se, but rather a reluctance of many clinicians to enter their patients into trials designed to answer these important questions.

Invasive Bladder Cancer

The 5-year survival rate of patients with invasive, clinically non-metastatic bladder cancer is less than 50%, whether the patients are treated by radical cystectomy, radical radiotherapy or a combination of both modalities. The evaluation of the true role of each mode of treatment has been confounded by the biases inherent in each of the published single-arm trials: selection of patients, exclusion from reporting, and the comparison of surgically staged patients (by cystectomy) with clinically staged patients (in radiotherapy series). As discussed previously, the ideal trial to compare the results of radical radiotherapy versus radical surgery for equivalent tumours has not yet been carried out and will probably not be undertaken.

Two important randomised trials have been reported, yielding some insights into the results obtained by these different treatment options. The Clinical Trials Group of the Institute of Urology, London, compared pre-operative pelvic radiotherapy (4000 rads) and elective radical cystectomy with radical radiotherapy (4000 rads plus 2000 rads boost) for deeply invasive bladder cancer (Bloom et al. 1982). A total of 189 patients were randomised, of whom 98 were allocated to pre-operative radiotherapy and surgery and 91 to radical radiotherapy. The details of informed consent and pre-treatment refusal were not reported. The analysis was carried out on the basis of "planned treatment" and "treatment actually received". The following specific 5-year survival figures were obtained:

1. Allocated radiotherapy/cystectomy (n=98): 38%
2. Allocated radical radiotherapy (n=91): 29%   } $P>0.2$
3. Received radiotherapy/cystectomy (n=77): 44%
4. Received radical radiotherapy (n=85): 31%
5. Received radical radiotherapy and salvage cystectomy (n=18): 60%

The major survival benefit from the combined treatment was demonstrated in patients less than 61 years of age. The authors noted that the combined approach allowed a greater opportunity for case selection: the development of metastatic disease during the first phase of treatment or the discovery of inoperability at laparotomy would select a favourably biased group if the analysis was then carried out on the basis of treatment actually received.

At the MD Anderson Hospital, Houston, a smaller randomised, prospective trial compared similar treatment policies to those described above with more marked differences in results – 51% 5-year survival for 35 patients treated by radiotherapy plus cystectomy versus 13% for those treated by radical radio-therapy alone (Miller 1980). This study has been criticised because of the small sample size and doubts regarding the quality of the radiotherapy delivered (in view of the unusually poor survival reported). Notwithstanding these problems, the available data (Table 13.3) appear to support the use of cystectomy, at least in younger patients. Although two of the trials reported no difference in outcome (Blackard et al. 1972; Prout 1976), each was flawed by the inclusion of either too many subgroups or too many randomisation arms.

Table 13.3. Randomised trials of in invasive bladder cancer

Institution	Number	Design	Result	Reference
Institute of Urology, London	189	RT-Cystx RT alone	No significant difference overall[a]	Bloom et al. 1982
MD Anderson Hospital, Houston	67	RT-Cystx RT alone	Survival benefit with surgery	Miller 1980
NBCCGA	475	RT-surgery Surgery	No difference Valid data?	Prout 1976
VA	72	Cystx. RT RT-Cystx	"No difference" ?Validity of data	Blackard et al. 1972
ABCSG	100	cDDP-RT RT alone	Ongoing study	Raghavan 1988a
Birmingham, UK	159	cDDP-RT RT alone	Ongoing study	Wallace et al. unpub.
NCIC	?	RT RT+concurrent cDDP	Ongoing study	Coppin et al. unpub.
Intergroup	?	Cystx MVAC→Cystx	Ongoing study	Einhorn et al. unpub.

Key: NBCCGA: National Bladder Cancer Collaborative Group A; VA: Veterans Administration; ABCSG: Australian Bladder Cancer Study Group; NCIC: National Cancer Institute of Canada; RT: radiotherapy; cDDP: cisplatin; Cystx: cystectomy.
[a] See text.

In many areas, clinical practice does not reflect the results from the above trials. Possible reasons could include concerns about the methodology of these studies, that the data were accrued in patients treated before the introduction of CAT scanning and modern techniques of irradiation, and the impact of the personal biases of individual clinicians (discussed previously).

Recently, the treatment of locally advanced bladder cancer has been complicated by the plethora of attempts to combine first-line ("pre-emptive") cytotoxic chemotherapy with cystectomy and/or radiation in an attempt to improve survival. As discussed in detail elsewhere (Raghavan 1988a), the cautious reports of response rates from single-arm explanatory trials have been over-interpreted to imply that pre-emptive chemotherapy constitutes state-of-the-art medicine. Before the use of this treatment has been validated, a plethora of more toxic combination programmes has now been introduced into clinical practice. Furthermore, at least one ongoing randomised trial (in which pre-emptive chemotherapy plus radiotherapy is compared against radiotherapy alone) has suffered in patient accrual from such clinician biases (Raghavan 1988a). Inclusion of chemotherapy in the treatment of locally invasive bladder cancer should be regarded as investigational, pending the results of the current, incomplete randomised trials.

Recurrent and Metastatic Disease

Extensive data from Phase II clinical trials have shown single agents to give objective response rates of 10%–30% for cisplatin, methotrexate, vinblastine, doxorubicin and mitomycin in the treatment of recurrent and metastatic bladder cancer (see reviews by Yagoda 1980; Ackland and Vogelzang 1988; Tonkin and Tannock 1988; Young and Garnick 1988). Although isolated early reports have suggested a useful role for multiple-agent regimens, such as the combination of cyclophosphamide, doxorubicin and cisplatin (Sternberg et al. 1977), no survival benefit has been demonstrated for a combination regimen over single agent therapy in any randomised clinical trial (Soloway et al. 1983; Khandekar et al. 1985; Hillcoat and Raghavan 1986). Chemotherapy has thus been regarded by many clinicians as an investigational tool, rather than as a well-defined or essential treatment for this disease.

More recently, two important studies, which were initially designed as Phase II trials, have been interpreted to suggest that combination chemotherapy may yield a major improvement in the outcome for patients with advanced bladder cancer. The combination of methotrexate, cisplatin and vinblastine, with or without doxorubicin, the so-called CMV and MVAC regimens, has yielded overall response rates of more than 60%, with a small proportion of complete responses, and a possible prolongation of survival (Harker et al. 1985; Sternberg et al. 1985). These preliminary observations are currently being assessed in a randomised Intergroup clinical trial. Nevertheless, clinicians have already expressed the view that these regimens represent a definite advance (Olsson 1987), ignoring the previously documented discrepancy between the results of Phase II and randomised phase II trials. Uncertainties in our understanding of the true role of chemotherapy do not represent a failure of clinical trials per se, but rather a reluctance of clinicians to await the results of completed trials or, in some cases, to accept the data when available.

Clinical Trials in Prostate Cancer

With the exception of clinical trials evaluating hormonal treatments for metastatic disease, there have been few large randomised trials which have investigated treatment options in prostate cancer. Most have simply recorded the results of treatment for a series of patients, and have tried to judge benefit by comparisons with other series using different types of therapy. Unfortunately, the heterogeneous and often chronic course of this disease increases the potential bias due to selection of patients and other factors, and one can place little confidence in the conclusions derived from such comparisons (Tannock 1985; Eisenberger et al. 1985). The smaller number of randomised trials will therefore be emphasised in the following discussion.

Management of Localised Disease

Randomised clinical trials which have investigated therapeutic options for localised prostate cancer include those conducted by the Veterans' Administration Cooperative Urological Research Group (VACURG) and other trials reported more recently. A summary of the design and outcome of these trials is presented in Tables 13.4 and 13.5.

The results of the VACURG studies in early disease suggest that few of these patients will die from prostate cancer, and that neither radical prostatectomy nor endocrine therapy improve survival. This conclusion has been widely accepted for focal disease found incidentally (stage A1 in the more commonly used American Joint Committee staging system). In contrast, it has been largely rejected for diffuse disease found incidentally (stage A2) or for a palpable nodule confined to the prostate (stage B), and patients with stages A2–B disease usually undergo prostatectomy or radical radiation therapy.

The limited effect of these VACURG trials in influencing clinical practice is due, in part, to criticisms of their design and analysis. Some of these criticisms include:

1. About 20% of the patients with early stage (A–B) disease were not analysed because of protocol violations. However, if their data were analysed on the basis of *intended treatment* only (i.e. not excluding those who sustained protocol violations), the results were not altered.
2. Patient groups were not controlled for subsequent treatment; thus patients randomised to receive placebo may subsequently have undergone hormonal manipulation. This criticism does not seem valid, since the VACURG were testing an *initial* policy of management, and could not have conducted their trials with prescribed treatment for the entire course of disease.
3. The quality of care at that time in Veterans' Administration Hospitals may not have been representative of the standards in the community (perhaps differing from university teaching institutions and from district or community-based hospitals). However, it has not subsequently been shown that the incidence of cancer deaths in the VA Hospitals differed from US national figures.
4. The approach to staging and grading of the tumours may not have been

Table 13.4. Veterans Administration cooperative urological research group (VACURG) trials in prostatic cancer (Byar 1973)

Trial	Stages[a]	No. of patients	Design	Result
VACURG I	I, II	299	Radical Prostatectomy — Placebo / DES 5 mg/d	Early survival favours placebo in Stage I. Otherwise no difference in survival
	III, IV	1903	Placebo Placebo and Orchidectomy DES 5 mg/d DES and Orchidectomy	No difference in overall survival. Increased deaths from cardiovascular causes and decreased deaths from prostate cancer in patients receiving DES
VACURG FOCAL STUDY (Patients unfit for prostatectomy or refusing operation)	I	148	Placebo Placebo and Orchidectomy DES 5 mg/d DES and Orchidectomy	No cancer deaths among first 72 patients who died. No differences in survival
VACURG II	I & II	142	Prostatectomy and placebo Placebo	No difference in survival. Only 14% had disease progression
	III & IV	508	Placebo DES 0.2 mg/d DES 1 mg/d DES 5 mg/d	1 mg/d DES as effective as 5 mg/d in controlling prostate cancer but not associated with increased rate of cardiovascular death

[a] Stage I, incidentally found cancer; Stage II, nodule confined to the prostate; Stage III, extra-prostatic extension; Stage IV, distant metastases and/or raised acid phosphatase.

consistent with modern classifications, perhaps rendering the data less applicable to current practice.

5. The VACURG patients may not have been representative of those seen in the general community. In particular, they may have been older and of lower socio-economic class and performance status, and may have been more prone to intercurrent illness. This criticism is perhaps the most cogent, and may limit the application of the results to other types of practice.

At the very least, however, the VACURG studies suggest that there is no *proven* role for aggressive treatment for early stage prostate cancer. In fact, there would be great merit in repeating some aspects of these initial trials according to modern clinical trials methodology to resolve some of these outstanding issues.

A widely quoted trial, published by the Uro-Oncology Research Group (Table 13.5), purported to show that radical surgery was superior to radiation therapy for the management of stages A2–B prostate cancer (Paulson et al. 1982a, b). However, flaws in the design and analysis of the trial render that conclusion suspect:

Table 13.5. Randomised clinical trials for prostatic cancer that is apparently localised to the pelvis

Eligible patients	Number of patients	Trial design	Results	References
Stages A_2 and B	106 (97 analysed)	Radiation therapy / Radical prostatectomy	Reported to show lower rate of progression with prostatectomy but faulty design renders conclusion suspect	Paulson et al. (1982a)
Extension to pelvic nodes	77	Radiation therapy	Improved survival and decreased progression with radiotherapy	Paulson et al. (1982b)
Stage C without extension to pelvic nodes	73	Initial observation. Orchidectomy or DES on progression	No difference in progression	Paulson et al. (1984)
Stages A_2 or B with extension to pelvic nodes, or Stage C	523 (448 analysed)	Pelvic radiation / Pelvic and para-aortic radiation	No difference in progression or survival	Pilepich et al. (1986)
			Prior TUR appears to convey poorer prognosis	Pilepich et al. (1987)

1. The patients were not adequately randomised. Instead, they were assigned to treatment in blocks of 4 at each participating institution. Thus, after one patient from a centre had been entered, the odds were 2:1 that the next patient would receive the alternative therapy; after 3 patients were entered, it was known with certainty which treatment the next patient would receive. This could have led to major bias in selection of patients for entry (for example, delaying entry of an unfit patient to avoid the need to perform radical surgery on him).

2. Sixteen of the "randomised" patients did not receive their assigned treatment, and were either excluded from analysis, or were analysed with the opposite arm if they happened to receive that treatment. This policy destroyed the validity of any attempt at initial randomisation.

3. The difference between the two groups that were analysed was in the appearance of bony metastases (greater in the radiotherapy-treated group). This endpoint, in isolation, may not be biologically valid as an index of the efficacy of local treatment, and could alternatively reflect a higher initial incidence of occult metastatic disease in the patients who received radiotherapy.

Hormonal Treatment for Metastatic Prostate Cancer

The larger randomised trials which have compared hormonal therapies in metastatic prostate cancer are summarised in Tables 13.4 and 13.6. In the first VACURG study, asymptomatic patients with advanced disease were randomised to receive placebo, placebo plus orchidectomy, DES (5 mg/day), or DES plus orchidectomy; patients randomised to placebo received subsequent hormonal manipulation when symptoms developed. This trial accrued large numbers of patients, but showed no overall survival advantage for any group: thus survival was not compromised by delaying endocrine therapy in asymptomatic patients. However, when patients with stage III disease (extending beyond the prostate) and those with metastases were analysed together, there was a significant increase in deaths due to cardiovascular causes in patients receiving DES, balanced by an overall reduction in cancer deaths (Byar 1973). The subsequent trial showed that DES in a dose of 1 mg/day was equally effective to 5 mg/day in controlling prostatic cancer, but was not associated with excess cardiovascular toxicity, whereas 0.2 mg/day was ineffective. Although the VACURG recommended 1 mg/day as the standard dose, this has not been widely accepted as others have shown that this dose does not lead to uniform suppression of serum testosterone (Shearer et al. 1973).

Table 13.6. Randomised trials comparing hormonal therapies for advanced prostate cancer (see Table 13.2 for VACURG studies

Trial	Number of	Trial design	Result
Henriksson and Edhag (1986)	91	Orchidectomy — Oestrogen	25% major C-V events with oestrogen. None with orchidectomy
Alfthan et al. (1983)	140	Cisobitan — Oestrogen	Similar response rate. Excess C-V events with oestrogen
EORTC 30761 de Voogt et al. (1986) Pavone-Macaluso et al. (1986)	236	DES (3 mg/d) — Cyproterone Acetate — Medroxyprogesterone Acetate	DES and Cyproterone equally effective in controlling disease and superior to Medroxyprogesterone. Greater toxicity with DES
The Leuprolide Study Group (1984)	199	DES (3 mg/d) — Leuprolide	No difference in progression or survival. Greater toxicity with DES
Parmar et al. (1985)	79	Orchidectomy — Long-acting D-TRP-6-LHRH	No major differences
Anderson et al. (1980)	263		No differences in outcome
EORTC 30762 Smith et al. (1986) de Voogt et al. (1986)	248	Estramustine Phosphate — Oestrogen	No differences in time to progression or survival
Benson and Gill (1986)	236		Longer time to progression with estramustine but no difference in survival
NPCP 1300 Murphy et al. (1986)	191		No difference in time to progression or survival

Several of the trials summarised in Table 13.6 have compared oestrogens with other hormonal therapies and have shown that most of these options were equally effective as first-line therapy in controlling prostate cancer, as judged by response to treatment, time to progression and survival. However, medroxyprogesterone acetate was shown to be less effective in one study. In the majority of these trials, oestrogens were used in doses higher than those recommended by the VACURG, and cardiovascular morbidity and mortality were associated with their use.

The results of these studies have had a considerable influence on routine clinical practice. Very elderly patients or those with cardiovascular risk factors are now less often treated with oestrogens. LH-RH agonists and antiandrogens are now offered to many patients as an alternative to castration or oestrogens, although many of the newer agents are more expensive. To date, no trial has demonstrated increased efficiency of any of the new hormonal therapies compared with standard approaches.

Several randomised trials have compared the efficiency and toxicity of oestrogen with that of estramustine phosphate (Table 13.6). The latter drug contains a molecule of oestradiol joined by a carbamate linkage to nitrogen mustard, and may act partly by slow release of oestrogen and partly by direct cytotoxicity. There were only small differences in outcome among the 4 trials, and 3 of them found no difference in time to progression or survival. Cardiovascular side effects were similar, although patients receiving estramustine had increased nausea and diarrhoea. Estramustine is more expensive than DES, and the available trials have not supported its use as routine initial treatment for metastatic prostate cancer.

Chemotherapy for Prostate Cancer

Many trials have sought to evaluate the role of chemotherapy in the treatment of prostate cancer that is no longer responsive to hormonal manipulation. These trials have been reviewed critically elsewhere and many have been shown to be flawed in their design and execution, illustrating many of the problems discussed above (Eisenberger et al. 1985; Tannock 1985). The resulting data have also been difficult to interpret because of the major problems in evaluating tumour response. As noted previously, many of these patients have disease which predominates in the pelvic lymph nodes and bone and it is thus difficult to measure changes in tumour volume. Some trials have been conducted only on the occasional patients with measurable soft-tissue disease, but response to chemotherapy in these patients may not equate with response in bony metastases (Stephens et al. 1984). A broad range of response criteria has been developed, involving a combination of endpoints related to general well-being of the patients (e.g. no weight loss, no decrease in performance status) and to tumour-related factors (changes in bone scan or serum acid phosphatase). Data from the same series of patients may appear to give quite different results when analysed by different criteria of response (Yagoda et al. 1979; Aabo 1987).

A major problem in analysing trials of chemotherapy for prostate cancer is that few patients have definite evidence of tumour shrinkage (5% or less in most trials). Most patients who are classified as "responding" actually fall within the category of "stable disease". It is a fallacy to assume that patients with prostate cancer (which often is a slowly progressive disease) develop stabilisation *because of* treatment (Eisenberger et al. 1985; Tannock 1985). In fact, this category will include tumours that have progressed slowly (and not enough to have been detected as "progressive" over a short time frame) as well as those whose growth has, in fact, been halted or their volume reduced by treatment.

Until recently, the design of the clinical studies of prostate cancer had failed to make this important distinction. For example, some of the most important early trials in the management of hormone-resistant prostate cancer were carried out by the NPCP (Table 13.7). However, their impact has been reduced by systematic flaws in their methodology, including the comparison of survival on the basis of category of response (Anderson et al. 1983) and the use of "stable disease" as an unqualified parameter of objective response. Although non-chemotherapy controls were provided in early studies, the NPCP accepted the higher demonstrable response rate as validation of the role of chemotherapy and has not included such controls in later studies. Despite these problems, the NPCP and other trial groups have made important contributions by attempting to systematise the assessment of response and toxicity following chemotherapy for prostate cancer.

Table 13.7. Summary of reported results of NPCP randomised trials of chemotherapy for patients without extensive prior irradiation who had hormone-resistant stage D prostatic cancer

Protocol	Drugs	No. of patients evaluated	Randomised patients excluded from analysis (%)	Reported responses (%)			Survival (weeks)		Refs
				CR	PR	Stable	Mean	Median	
100	Cyclophosphamide	41		0	7	39	58	NS[a]	Scott
	5-FU	33	12	0	12	24	55	NS	et al.
	Standard treatment	36		0	0	19	57	NS	(1976)
300	Cyclophosphamide	35		0	0	26	NS	26[b]	Schmidt
	DTIC	55	22	0	4	24	NS	40	et al.
	Procarbazine	39		0	0	13	NS	30	(1979)
700	Cyclophosphamide	43		2	5	28	48[c]	42	Loening
	Me-CCNU	27	22	0	4	26	32	22	et al.
	Hydroxyurea	28		4	4	7	27	19	(1981)
1100	Methotrexate	58		2	3	36	46[c]	37	Loening
	Cisplatin	50	16	0	4	32	40	33	et al.
	Estramustine	50		0	2	32	40	43	(1983)

[a] NS, not stated (and data not provided to allow an estimate of mean or median survival for the entire group of patients, regardless of response classification).
[b] Values of median survival estimated by the author from survival curves.
[c] Values of mean survival were stated explicitly but may be updated since the trials were anlaysed before all patients had died.

Some of the larger chemotherapy trials for prostate cancer are reviewed in Table 13.8. While some appear to show a tumour response with quite stringent criteria of evaluation (Paulson et al. 1979; Logothetis et al. 1983), there is no evidence of improved survival as a result of treatment. While chemotherapy appears to have provided palliation of symptoms for some of the responding patients, this may have been offset by toxicity associated with treatment.

In summary, published trials have not yet proved the role of chemotherapy in the management of prostate cancer. New drugs should continue to be evaluated, with an emphasis on the assessment of response in the rarer patient with measurable soft tissue disease, but augmented by an effort to improve the assessment of response in the more common, bone-dominant disease. Promising drugs or combinations should be tested in trials where patients are randomised to

Table 13.8. A summary of some of the larger clinical trials that have sought to evaluate the role of chemotherapy in palliating hormone-resistant chemotherapy

Drugs	Patients	Rate of response (%)	Median survival (weeks)[a]	Comments	References
Cisplatin	45	13/45(29)	NS	Excluded patients receiving <3 doses; poorly defined response criteria included clearance of oedema	Merrin and Beckley (1979)
Melphalan, methotrexate, vincristine, 5-FU, prednisone	88	33/88(38)	NS	Response required a fall in acid or alkaline phosphatase to normal, or weight gain >10%	Paulson et al. (1979)
5-FU v. cyclophosphamide + 5-FU + doxorubicin	101	3/25(12) 7/22(32)	34 25	Responses evaluated for less than half of the patients by >50% decrease in acid phosphatase	Smalley et al. (1981)
Doxorubicin v. 5-FU	147	15/61(25) 3/42(8)	29[b] 24	Response based on patients with measurable disease, includes patients crossing over to alternative drug	De Wys et al. (1983)
Doxorubicin + 5-FU + mitomycin C	62	30/62(48)	NS	Response included >50% fall in acid or alkaline phosphatase on 3 occasions and "improvement" in bone scan	Logothetis et al. (1983)
Doxorubicin	52	2/41(5)	NS	Response based on measurable lesions	Scher et al. (1984)
Hydroxyurea v. doxorubicin + cyclophosphamide	158	1/24(4) 6/19(32)	28 27	Response based on 43 patients with measurable lesions	Stephens et al. (1984)
Doxorubicin + CCNU v. cyclophosphamide + 5-FU	51	12/22(57) 2/25(8)	39 23	PRs by NPCP criteria	Page et al. (1985)

[a] Median survival is for all treated patients: NS, not stated.
[b] Difference in survival between two groups is significant at $P=0.03$. Differences in survival between groups in the other randomised trials are not significant.

receive chemotherapy or standard treatment, in which all patients are analysed, and where the appropriate endpoints are the pragmatic ones of survival and quality of life.

Clinical Trials in Cancer of the Kidney

Informed opinion about treatment for adenocarcinoma of the kidney is perhaps more uniform than for the treatment of other genitourinary tumours. In a patient with a resectable primary tumour and no overt metastases, the treatment of choice is nephrectomy; up to half these patients will be cured (deKernion and Berry 1980; Ritchie and Chisholm 1983). Less clear is the role of aggressive surgery, with radical retroperitoneal lymph node dissection and the resection of metastases.

Two randomised clinical trials have addressed the role of additional treatment in operable disease (Table 13.9). In one, patients were randomised to receive preoperative radiation followed by nephrectomy or nephrectomy alone; in the second, nephrectomy with or without adjuvant medroxyprogesterone acetate for one year. Neither of these studies showed any benefit from the added treatment. Nevertheless, many clinicians still use these added modalities in the hope that they may influence prognosis – a practice that may not be rational or cost-effective, and which does not reflect the results of the available controlled data.

Table 13.9. Randomised clinical trials for patients with operable carcinoma of the kidney without overt metastases

Reference	Number of patients	Trial design	Result
Van der Werf-Messing et al. (1978)	174	Preoperative radiation / Nephrectomy	No difference in 5 yr (~50%) or 10 yr (~45%) survival
Pizzocaro et al. (1986)	136	Nephrectomy + medroxyprogesterone acetate for 1 year / Nephrectomy	No difference in rate of relapse at 3 yr (~25%)

A large number of Phase II trials have been conducted in patients with metastatic disease (Hrushesky and Murphy 1977). All currently available anti-cancer drugs have been tested for activity, as well as many investigational agents, hormones and hormonal antagonists. These trials can be summarised simply by stating that no drug or combination of agents that has been assessed in an adequate number of patients has yielded a consistent rate of tumour response of more than 20%, and for most of them the response rate has been less than 10% (Hrushesky and Murphy 1977). It is clear from these trials, therefore, that neither hormones nor chemotherapy play a role in the standard management of this disease.

The observation that lung metastases from renal cancer may occasionally regress after removal of the primary tumour has suggested the presence of host-mediated factors, and has led to a sustained interest in immunotherapy for this disease. Many recent trials have studied the effect of gamma- or alpha$_2$-interferon on this tumour (Umeda and Niijima 1986; Muss et al. 1987). A review of the results from some of the larger trials indicate that from 5% to 20% of patients may have objective tumour response (i.e. greater than 50% shrinkage in cross-sectional area). Toxicity has been reported to be considerable, and few responses have been sustained after the cessation of treatment. Both the rate of response and the host toxicity appear to be dose-related, suggesting that the interferons may act in part through direct toxic effects, as well as by immune-mediated mechanisms (Queseda et al. 1985). The available data do not suggest that the interferons have a proven role in standard treatment of this disease.

Recently, other immunological manipulations have been tested in small numbers of patients with renal cancer, and there is current interest in the use of interleukin-2 and lymphokine-activated killer (LAK) cells. This treatment may cause disease regression but is very toxic (Rosenberg et al. 1985). It is too early to assess its potential role in routine management. However, the rapid evolution of interest in this approach (augmented by enthusiastic reports in the lay press) may have contributed to a disproportionate level of enthusiasm for its application.

Clinical Trials in Testicular Cancer

The Management of Early Stage Disease

The management of early stage germ cell tumours, including disease limited to the testis (stage I or A) and retroperitoneum (stage II or B) has been controversial (Raghavan 1984). In brief, two treatment policies have traditionally been advocated for stage I non-seminomatous germ cell tumours (NSGCT): retroperitoneal lymph node dissection or radiotherapy. The proponents of each modality have argued on the basis of serial phase II trials, falling into most of the methodological traps outlined previously. To date, no well-designed, randomised trial has been completed to resolve the issue.

On the basis of prognostic factors determined from a series of Phase II trials (Sandeman and Matthews 1979; Raghavan et al. 1982 a, b), a new approach was more recently introduced: the policy of "active surveillance", in which patients with clinical stage I NSGCT are followed according to a strict protocol of non-invasive investigation, including measurement of tumour markers and regular CAT scans (Peckham et al. 1982). To date, the safety and utility of this approach has only been assessed in one randomised trial, completed by the Danish Testicular Cancer Study Group (Rorth et al. 1987). In this study, radiotherapy to the retroperitoneal lymph nodes was compared with a policy of active surveil-lance. Although a higher relapse rate was noted in the latter group, the survival curves were equivalent. However, after nearly 10 years of investigation, it is still not possible to define the optimal protocol for active surveillance, and with the proliferation of small, unregistered trials, it is likely that the answer will not be available for many years (Raghavan et al. 1988b).

Metastatic Germ Cell Tumours

In the past decade, impressive improvements have been achieved in the management of advanced testicular cancer, with an increase in the cure rate of metastatic non-seminomatous germ cell tumours from 20% to more than 80%. This has been largely due to the introduction of effective combination chemotherapy regimens. Several other factors have also played a part including an improved understanding of the biology of the disease, the use of tumour markers in the management of sub-clinical metastases and the identification of prognostic risk factors, advances in imaging technologies, such as the introduction of computed axial tomographic scanning, and improvements in the techniques of retroperitoneal lymph node dissection, thoracotomy for metastatic disease, and the techniques of anaesthesia.

The improvement in the treatment of germ cell tumours clearly illustrates the importance of the balance between statistical validity and clinical common sense. Many of the advances have been achieved through single-arm, non-randomised clinical trials. For example, the introduction of the combination of cisplatin, vinblastine and bleomycin (Einhorn 1981) did not require validation against a "no-treatment" control arm to justify its role. A series of Phase II studies demonstrated a high, reproducible complete response rate which correlated with long-term survival (Einhorn 1981; Peckham et al. 1981; Stoter et al. 1986). Subsequent smaller Phase II trials suggested a possible dose–response relationship for cisplatin (Bosl et al. 1980a, b) and that vinblastine could be replaced by vincristine without major loss of efficacy but with a reduction of toxicity (Wettlaufer et al. 1984). A range of other Phase II studies have demonstrated alternative options for the use of cisplatin-containing chemotherapy regimens, with investigators implying that these are more beneficial than the conventional PVB schedule (Ozols et al. 1983; Bosl et al. 1986).

The implementation of Phase II trials has not been restricted to the assessment of chemotherapy. Several studies have demonstrated the safety and efficacy of post-chemotherapy resection of residual masses (Einhorn 1981; Peckham et al. 1981; Reddel et al. 1983), revealing equal proportions of patients with viable cancer, differentiated teratoma and pure necrosis. Through these studies, the clinical utility of such surgery has been demonstrated, both with regard to the diagnosis of active residual disease and as the final step in achieving cure.

Furthermore, several sets of data from Phase II trials have yielded important prognostic factors for the management of germinal malignancy, including extent of disease, levels of serum tumour markers (alphafetoprotein, human chorionic gonadotrophin and lactic acid dehydrogenase), sites of metastases and performance status (Bosl et al. 1983; MRC 1985; Birch et al. 1986; Levi et al. 1988).

Despite the importance of these investigational studies, many issues were still unresolved. For example, the optimal timing of surgery for abdominal masses was not known after the completion of the Phase II trials outlined above. However, investigators from the National Cancer Institute, Bethesda, demonstrated a trend for improved survival among patients who had chemotherapy first, as compared with those who underwent resection of abdominal masses prior to chemotherapy (Javadpour et al. 1982). However, this study was reported somewhat prematurely and the statistical validity of the data remain somewhat in question.

Several randomised trials have been carried out in an effort to rationalise the use of chemotherapy, increasing cure rates while reducing toxicity and cost. Thus, randomised trials have shown that the addition of doxorubicin to the PVB regimen does not improve survival (Einhorn 1981), that a reduction of vinblastine dosage from 0.4 to 0.3 mg/kg is safe (Einhorn 1981; Stoter et al. 1986), and that there is a dose–response relationship for cisplatin in the management of germinal malignancy (Samson et al. 1984). In an ongoing study in Australia and New Zealand, the feasibility of deleting bleomycin from the PVB schedule for patients with "good risk" disease is being assessed in a prospective, randomised trial (Levi et al. 1986; Raghavan et al. 1989). The issue of prolonging chemotherapy has also been addressed: in a series of randomised trials, the use of vinblastine as maintenance therapy for patients in remission has not been supported (Einhorn 1981; Stoter et al. 1986; Levi et al. 1988).

The management of "bad risk" testicular cancer remains a difficult problem. The reduction in survival rates depends somewhat on the criteria of inclusion in this category of disease. Single arm Phase II trials have suggested improved survival with new regimens (Newlands et al. 1983; Ozols et al. 1983), and the real place of some of these aproaches is now being defined in randomised trials. Thus Ozols et al. (1984) showed a survival benefit from the "PVeBV" regimen, incorporating high dose cisplatin (200 mg/m^2) when compared with the standard PVB regimen. By contrast, not all Phase II trials have been interpreted to show benefit in the managment of "bad risk" disease (Bosl et al. 1987; Raghavan et al. 1989) and thus some of these newer regimens have not been tested against standard therapy. Whether this approach will be validated remains to be seen. One of the most provocative reports has described the use of cycles of cisplatin, vincristine, methotrexate and bleomycin rapidly alternating with actinomycin D, cyclophosphamide and etoposide (the so-called "POMBACE" regimen) (Newlands et al. 1983). This approach has yet to be validated in a controlled trial, despite its use in routine practice for several years.

Summary

There has been substantial progress in the management of genitourinary malignancy in the past 50 years, with the early improvements arising predominantly from innovative, non-randomised clinical trials. It has required the use of well structured clinical trials (both randomised and single arm) to rationalise the use of many of these advances, defining the optimal schedules, doses, and methods of application. Progress has been slower than necessary, usually representing the failure of some clinicians to approach difficult problems in an ordered and rational fashion, rather than due to any inherent deficiency in the tools of the clinical trial. Clinical practice is changing, and there is an increasing need for clinicians to understand and to apply some of the principles outlined in this chapter to the evaluation of clinical trials, and to the application of the results in their own practice. If we are to improve the prognosis for our patients, we must continue to question the methods that we use and the results that we achieve.

References

Aabo K (1987) Prostate cancer: evaluation of response to treatment, response criteria, and the need for standardisation of the reporting of results. Eur J Cancer Clin Oncol 23: 231–236

Ackland SP, Vogelzang NJ (1988) New drugs and old toxicities. In: Raghavan D (ed) The management of bladder cancer. Edward Arnold, London, pp 189–227

Alfthan O, Andersson L, Esposti PH, et al. (1983) Cisobitan in treatment of prostatic cancer. A prospective controlled multicentre study. Scand J Urol Nephrol 17: 37–43

Anderson JR, Cain KC, Gelber RD (1983) Analysis of survival by tumor response. J Clin Oncol 1: 710–719

Andersson L, Berlin T, Boman J et al. (1980) Estramustine versus conventional estrogenic hormones in the initial treatment of highly or moderately differentiated prostatic carcinoma. A randomized study. Scand J Urol Nephrol [Suppl] 55: 143–145

Ausfeld R, Beer M, Muhlethaler JP, Bartlome R, Widmer R, Tscholl R (1987) Adjuvant intravesical chemotherapy of superficial bladder cancer with monthly doxorubicin or intensive mitomycin. Eur Urol 13: 10–14

Badalament RA, Herr HW, Wong GY et al. (1987) A prospective randomized trial of maintenance versus nonmaintenance intravesical Bacillus Calmette-Guerin therapy of superficial bladder cancer. J Clin Oncol 5: 441–449

Banks MD, Pontes JE, Isbicki RM, Pierce JM Jr (1977) Topical instillation of doxorubicin hydrochloride in the treatment of recurring superficial transitional cell carcinoma of the bladder. J Urol 118: 757–760

Batley F (1955) The problem of evaluation of cancer therapy. J Can Assoc Radiol 6: 25–28

Benson RC Jr, Gill GM (1986) Estramustine phosphate compared with diethylstilbestrol. A randomised, double-blind, crossover trial for Stage D prostate cancer. Am J Clin Oncol 9: 341–351

Birch R, Williams S, Cone A et al. (1986) Prognostic factors for favourable outcome in disseminated germ cell tumors. J Clin Oncol 4: 400–407

Blackard DE, Byar DP and the Veterans Administration Cooperative Urological Research Group (1972) Results of a clinical trial of surgery and radiation in stages II and III carcinoma of the bladder. J Urol 108: 875–881

Bloom HJG, Hendry WF, Wallace DM, Skeet RG (1982) Treatment of T3 bladder cancer: Controlled trial of preoperative radiotherapy and radical cystectomy versus radical radiotherapy. Second report and review. Br J Urol 54: 136–151

Bosl GJ (1985) Treatment of germ cell tumors at Memorial Sloan Kettering Cancer Center: 1960 to Present. In: Garnick MB (ed) Genitourinary cancer. Churchill Livingstone, New York, Edinburgh, London and Melbourne, pp 45–59

Bosl GJ, Kwong R, Lange PH, Fraley EE, Kennedy BJ (1980a) Vinblastine, intermittent bleomycin, and single-dose cis-dichlorodiammineplatinum (II) in the management of stage III testicular cancer. Cancer Treat Rep 64: 331–334

Bosl GJ, Lange PH, Fraley EE et al. (1980b) Vinblastine, bleomycin and cis-diamminedichloroplatinum in the treatment of advanced testicular cancer. Possible importance of longer induction and shorter maintenance schedules. Am J Med 68: 492–496

Bosl GJ, Geller N, Cirrincione C et al. (1983) Multivariate analysis of prognostic variables in patients with metastatic testicular cancer. Cancer Res 43: 3403–3407

Bosl GJ, Gluckman R, Geller NL et al. (1986a) VAB-6: An effective chemotherapy regimen for patients with germ cell tumors. J Clin Oncol 4: 1493–1499

Bosl GJ, Bajorin D, Leitner S et al. (1986b) A randomized trial of etoposide (E) plus cisplatin (P) and VAB-6 in the treatment (Rx) of "good risk" patients (Pts) with germ cell tumors (GCT). Proc Am Soc Clin Oncol 5: 104

Bosl GJ, Geller NL, Vogelzang NJ et al. (1987) Alternating cycles of etoposide plus cisplatin and VAB-6 in the treatment of poor-risk patients with germ cell tumors. J Clin Oncol 5: 436–440

Bush RS (1979) Malignancies of the ovary, uterus and cervix. Edward Arnold, London, p 34

Byar DP (1973) The Veterans Administration Cooperative Urological Research Group's Studies of Cancer of the Prostate. Cancer 32: 1126–1130

Byar D, Blackard C (1977) Comparisons of placebo, pyridoxine, and topical thiotepa in preventing recurrence of stage I bladder cancer. Urology 10: 556–560

Creaven PJ, Mihich E (1977) The clinical toxicity of anticancer drugs and its prediction. Semin Oncol 4: 147–163

deKernion JB, Berry D (1980) The diagnosis and treatment of renal cell carcinoma. Cancer 45: 1947–1956

De Voogt HJ, Smith PH, Pavone-Macaluso M et al. (1986) Cardiovascular side effects of diethylstilbestrol, cyproterone acetate, medroxyprogesterone acetate and estramustine phosphate used for the treatment of advanced prostatic cancer: results from European Organization for Research on Treatment of Cancer Trials 30761 and 30762. J Urol 135: 303–307

De Wys WD, Begg CB, Brodovsky H et al. (1983) A comparative clinical trial of Adriamycin and 5-Fluorouracil in advanced prostatic cancer: prognostic factors and response. Prostate 4: 1–11

Einhorn LH (1981) Testicular cancer as a model for a curable neoplasm. Cancer Res 41: 3275–3280

Eisenberger MA, Simon R, O'Dwyer PJ et al. (1985) A reevaluation of non-hormonal cytotoxic chemotherapy in the treatment of prostatic carcinoma. J Clin Oncol 3: 827–841

Feinstein AR, Sosin DM, Wells CK (1985) The Will Rogers phenomenon: Stage migration and new diagnostic techniques as a source of misleading statistics for survival in cancer. New Engl J Med 312: 1604–1608

Gad-El-Mawla NM, Chevlen E, Hamza MR, Ziegler JZ (1979) Phase II trial of c-DDP (II) in cancer of the Bilharzial bladder. Cancer Treat Rep 63: 1577–1578

Ghoneim MA, Ashamallah AG, El-Hammady S, Gaballah MA, Soliman ES (1979) Cystectomy for carcinoma of the Bilharzial bladder: 138 cases, 5 years later. Br J Urol 51: 541–544

Harker WG, Meyers FJ, Freiha FS et al. (1985) Cisplatin, methotrexate and vinblastine (CMV): An effective chemotherapy regimen for metastatic transitional cell carcinoma of the urinary tract. A Northern California Oncology Group Study. J Clin Oncol 3: 1463–1470

Heney NM (1985) First line chemotherapy of superficial bladder cancer: Mitomycin versus thiotepa. Urology 26 [suppl 4]: 27–29

Henriksson P, Edhag O (1986) Orchidectomy versus oestrogen for prostatic cancer: cardiovascular effects. Br Med J 293: 413–415

Hillcoat B, Raghavan D (1986) A randomised comparison of cisplatinum (C) versus cisplatinum and methotrexate (C+M) in advanced bladder cancer. Proc Am Soc Clin Oncol 5: 426

Horn Y, Eidelman A, Walach N, Ilian M (1981) Intravesical chemotherapy in a controlled trial with thio-tepa versus doxorubicin hydrochloride. J Urol 125: 652–654

Hrushesky WJ, Murphy GP (1977) Current status of the therapy of advanced renal carcinoma. J Surg Oncol 9: 277–288

Javadpour N, Ozols RF, Anderson T, Barlock A, Wesley R, Young RC (1982) A randomized trial of cytoreductive surgery followed by chemotherapy versus chemotherapy alone in bulky stage III testicular cancer with poor prognostic features. Cancer 50: 2004–2010

Jones HC, Swinney J (1961) Thio-TEPA in the treatment of tumours of the bladder. Lancet II: 615–618

Khandekar JD, Elson PJ, DeWys WD, Slayton RE, Harris DT (1985) Comparative activity and toxicity of cis-diamminedichloroplatinum (DDP) and a combination of doxorubicin, cyclophosphamide, and DDP in disseminated transitional cell carcinomas of the urinary tract. J Clin Oncol 3: 539–545

Koontz WW Jr, Prout GR Jr, Smith W, Frable WJ, Minnis JE (1981) The use of intravesical thio-tepa in the management of non-invasive carcinoma of the bladder. J Urol 125: 307–312

Kurth KH, Schroder FH, Tunn U et al. (1984) Adjuvant chemotherapy of superficial transitional cell bladder carcinoma: Preliminary results of a European Organisation for Research and Treatment of Cancer randomized trial comparing doxorubicin hydrochloride, ethoglucid and transurethral resection alone. J Urol 132: 258–262

Lee YJ, Staquet M, Simon R, Catane R, Muggia F (1979) Two-stage plans for patient accrual in phase II cancer clinical trials. Cancer Treat Rep 63: 1721–1726

Levi J, Thomson D, Sandeman T et al. (1988) A prospective study of platinum based combination chemotherapy in advanced germ cell malignancy: Role of maintenance and long term follow-up. J Clin Oncol 6: 1154–1160

Levi J, Raghavan D, Harvey V et al. (1986) Deletion of bleomycin from therapy for good prognosis advanced testicular cancer: A prospective, randomized study. Proc Am Soc Clin Oncol 5: 97

Loening SA, Scott WW, De Kernion J et al. (1981) A comparison of hydroxyurea, methylchloroethyl-cyclohexyl-nitrosourea and cyclophosphamide in patients with advanced carcinoma of the prostate. J Urol 125: 812–816

Loening SA, Beckley S, Brady MF et al. (1983) Comparison of estramustine phosphate, methotrexate and cis-platinum in patients with advanced, hormone refractory prostate cancer. J Urol 129: 1001–1006

Logothetis CJ, Samuels ML, Von Eschenbach AC et al. (1983) Doxorubicin, mitomycin C, and 5-fluorouracil (DMF) in the treatment of metastatic hormonal refractory adenocarcinoma of the prostate, with a note on the staging of metastatic prostatic cancer. J Clin Oncol 1: 368–379

Manni A, Santen RJ, Boucher A et al. (1985) Hormone stimulation and chemotherapy in advanced prostate cancer: preliminary results of a prospective controlled clinical trial. Anticancer Res 5: 161–165

Manni A, Santen RJ, Boucher AE et al. (1986) Hormone stimulation and chemotherapy in advanced prostate cancer: interim analysis of an ongoing randomized trial. Anticancer Res 6: 309–314

Manni A, Santen R, Boucher A et al. (1987) Androgen priming and chemotherapy in advanced prostate cancer. Proc Am Soc Clin Oncol 6: 102

Marsoni S, Wittes R (1984) Clinical development of anticancer agents – A National Cancer Institute perspective. Cancer Treat Rep 68: 77–85

Merrin CE, Beckley S (1979) Treatment of estrogen-resistant stage D carcinoma of prostate with cis-Diamminedichloroplatinum. Urology 13: 267–272

Miller AB, Hoogstraten B, Staquet M, Winkler A (1981) Reporting results of cancer treatment. Cancer 47: 207–214

Miller LS (1980) T3 bladder cancer: The case for higher radiation dosage. Cancer 45: 1875–1878

Moertel CG, Hanley JA (1976) The effect of measuring error on the results of therapeutic trials in advanced cancer. Cancer 38: 388–394

MRC Working Party on Testicular Tumours (1985) Prognostic factors in advanced non-seminomatous germ cell testicular tumours: results of a multicentre study. Lancet I: 8–11

MRC Working Party on Urological Cancer (1985) The effect of intravesical thiotepa on the recurrence rate of newly diagnosed superficial bladder cancer. An MRC Study. Br J Urol 57: 680–685

Murphy GP, Beckley S, Brady MF et al. (1983) Treatment of newly diagnosed metastatic prostate cancer patients with chemotherapy agents in combination with hormones versus hormones alone. Cancer 51: 1264–1272

Murphy GP, Huben RP, Priore R and the NPCP (1986) Results of another trial of chemotherapy with and without hormones in patients with newly diagnosed metastatic prostate cancer. Urology 28: 36–40

Muss HB, Constanzi JJ, Leavitt R et al. (1987) Recombinant alfa interferon in renal cell carcinoma: A randomized trial of two routes of administration. J Clin Oncol 5: 286–291

Newlands ES, Begent RHJ, Rustin GJS, Parker D, Bagshawe KD (1983) Further advances in the management of malignant teratomas of the testis and other sites. Lancet I: 948–951

Olsson CA (1987) Management of invasive carcinoma of the bladder. In: De Kernion JB, Paulson DF Genitourinary cancer management. Lea and Febiger, Philadelphia, pp 59–94

Ozols RF, Deisseroth AB, Javadpour N, Barlock A, Messerschmidt GL, Young RC (1983) Treatment of poor prognosis nonseminomatous testicular cancer with a "high dose" platinum combination chemotherapy regimen. Cancer 51: 1803–1807

Ozols RF, Ihde D, Jacob J et al. (1984) Randomized trial of PVeBV [high dose (HD) cisplatin (P), vinblastine (Ve), bleomycin (B), VP-16 (V)] versus PVeB in poor prognosis non-seminomatous testicular cancer (NSTC). Proc Am Soc Clin Oncol 3: 155

Page JP, Levi JA, Woods RL et al. (1985) Randomized trial of combination chemotherapy in hormone-resistant metastatic prostate carcinoma. Cancer Treat Rep 69: 105–107

Parmar H, Phillips RH, Lightman SL et al. (1985) Randomized controlled study of orchidectomy vs long-acting D-TRP-6- LHRH microcapsules in advanced prostatic carcinoma. Lancet II: 1201–1205

Paulson DF, Berry WR, Cox EB et al. (1979) Treatment of metastatic endocrine-unresponsive carcinoma of the prostate gland with multiagent chemotherapy: indicators of response to therapy. J Nat Cancer Inst 63: 615–622

Paulson DF, Cline WA Jr, Koefoot RB Jr et al. (1982a) Extended field radiation therapy versus delayed hormonal therapy in node positive prostatic adenocarcinoma. J Urol 127: 935–937

Paulson DF, Lin GH, Hinshaw W, Sephani S (1982b) Radical surgery versus radiotherapy for adenocarcinoma of the prostate. J Urol 128: 502–504

Paulson DF, Hodge GB Jr, Hinshaw W, The Uro-Oncology Research Group (1984) Radiation therapy versus delayed androgen deprivation for stage C Carcinoma of the Prostate. J Urol 131: 901–902

Pavone-Macaluso M, De Voogt HJ, Viggiano G et al. (1986) Comparison of diethylstilbestrol, cyproterone acetate and medroxyprogesterone acetate in the treatment of advanced prostatic cancer: final analysis of a randomised phase III trial of the European Organization for Research on Treatment of Cancer Urological Group. J Urol 136: 624–631

Peckham MJ, Barrett A, McElwain TJ, Hendry WF, Raghavan D (1981) Non-seminoma germ cell tumours (malignant teratoma) of the testis: results of treatment and an analysis of prognostic factors. Br J Urol 53: 162–172

Peckham MJ, Barrett A, Husband JE et al. (1982) Orchidectomy alone in testicular stage I non-seminomatous germ cell tumours. Lancet II: 678–680

Pilepich MV, Krall JM, Johnson RJ et al. (1986) Extended field (periaortic) irradiation in carcinoma of the prostate – analysis of RTOG 75–06. Int J Radiat Oncol Biol Phys 12: 345–351

Pilepich MV, Krall JM, Hanks GE et al. (1987) Correlation of pre-treatment transurethral resection and prognosis in patients with stage C carcinoma of the prostate treated with definitive radiotherapy – RTOG experience. Int J Radiat Oncol Biol Phys 13: 195–199

Pinsky CM, Camacho FJ, Kerr D et al. (1985) Intravesical administration of Bacillus Calmette-Guerin in patients with recurrent superficial carcinoma of the urinary bladder: report of a prospective, randomized trial. Cancer Treat Rep 69: 47–53

Pizzocaro G, Piva L, Salvioni R et al. (1986) Adjuvant medroxyprogesterone acetate and steroid hormone receptors in category Mo renal cell carcinoma. An interim report of a prospective randomized study. J Urol 135: 18–21

Prout GR Jr (1976) The surgical management of bladder carcinoma. Urol Clin North Am 3: 149–175

Prout GR Jr, Kopp J (1984) Resume of selected studies of the National Bladder Cancer Collaborative Group A and new protocols. Prog Clin Biol Res 162B: 397–427

Quesada JR, Rios A, Swanson D et al. (1985) Antitumor activity of recombinant-derived Interferon Alpha in metastatic renal cell carcinoma. J Clin Oncol 3: 1522–1528

Raghavan D (1984) Expectant therapy for clinical stage A non-seminomatous germ-cell cancers of the testis? A qualified 'yes'. World J Urol 2: 59–63

Raghavan D (1988a) Review: pre-emptive intravenous chemotherapy for invasive bladder cancer. Br J Urol 61: 1–8

Raghavan D (1988b) Non-hormone chemotherapy for prostate cancer: principles of treatment and application to the testing of new drugs. Semin Oncol 15: 371–389

Raghavan D, Peckham MJ, Heyderman E, Tobias JS, Austin DE (1982a) Prognostic factors in clinical stage I non-seminomatous germ-cell tumours of the testis. Br J Cancer 45: 167–173

Raghavan D, Vogelzang NJ, Bosl GJ et al. (1982b) Tumor classification and size in germ-cell testicular cancer. Cancer 50: 1591–1595

Raghavan D, Colls B, Levi J et al. (1988) Surveillance for stage I non-seminoma germ cell tumours of the testis (NSGCT): The optimal protocol has not yet been defined. Br J Urol 61: 522–526

Raghavan D, Levi J, Thomson D et al. (1989) Chemotherapy of advanced germ cell tumors: overview of Australasian Germ Cell Tumor Group studies. In: Von Eschenbach A, Logothetis C, Johnson D (eds) Recent advances in the systemic therapy of genitourinary malignancies. Yearbook Medical Publishers, New York, pp 682–693

Reddel RR, Thompson JF, Raghavan D et al. (1983) Surgery in patients with advanced germ cell malignancy following a clinical partial response to chemotherapy. J Surg Oncol 23: 223–227

Riddle PR, Wallace DM (1971) Intracavitary chemotherapy for multiple non-invasive bladder tumours. Br J Urol 43: 181–184

Ritchie AWS, Chisholm GD (1983) The natural history of renal carcinoma. Semin Oncol 10: 390–400

Rorth M, von der Maase H, Nielsen ES, Pedersen M, Schultz H (1987) Orchidectomy alone versus orchidectomy plus radiotherapy in stage I nonseminomatous testicular cancer: A randomized study by the Danish Testicular Carcinoma Study Group. In: Rorth M, Grigor KM, Daugaard G, Giwercman A, Skakkebaek NE (eds) Carcinoma-in-situ and cancer of the testis: biology and treatment. Blackwell Scientific Publications, Oxford, London, Edinburgh, Melbourne, pp 255–262

Rosenberg SA, Lotze MT, Muul LM et al. (1985) Observations on the systemic administration of autologous lymphokine-activated killer cells and recombinant Interleukin-2 to patients with metastatic cancer. New Engl J Med 313: 1485–1492

Samsen MK, Rivkin SE, Jones SE et al. (1984) Dose-response and dose-survival advantage for high versus low-dose cisplatin combined with vinblastine and bleomycin in disseminated testicular cancer: A SWOG Study. Cancer 53: 1029–1035

Samson MK, Crawford ED, Natale R, Bouroncle, B, Altman S (1986) A randomized comparison of cisplatin, vinblastine (VLB) plus either bleomycin (PVB) or VP-16 (VPV) in patients with advanced testicular cancer. Proc Am Soc Clin Oncol 5: 96

Sandeman TF, Matthews JP (1979) The staging of testicular tumors. Cancer 43: 2514–2525

Scher H, Yagoda A, Watson RC et al. (1984) Phase II trial of Doxorubicin in bidimensionally measureable prostatic adenocarcinoma. J Urol 131: 1099–1102

Schmidt JD, Scott WW, Gibbons RP et al. (1979) Comparison of Procarbazine, Imidazole-Carboxamide and Cyclophosphamide in relapsing patients with advanced carcinoma of the prostate. J Urol 121: 185–189

Schulman C, Kurth KH (1984) Current status of EORTC GU Group protocols for bladder cancer. In: Denis L, Murphy GP, Prout GR Jr, Schroder F (eds) Controlled clinical trials in urological oncology. Raven Press, New York, pp 215–220

Schulman C, Robinson M, Denis L et al. (1982) Prophylactic chemotherapy of superficial bladder carcinoma: An EORTC randomized trial comparing Thiotepa, VM26 and transurethral resection alone. Eur Urol 8: 207–212

Schwartz D, Lellouch J (1967) Explanatory and pragmatic attitudes in therapeutic trials. J Chronic Dis 20: 637–648

Scott WW, Gibbons RP, Johnson DE et al. (1976) The continued evaluation of the effects of chemotherapy in patients with advanced carcinoma of the prostate. J Urol 116: 211–213

Simes RJ (1986) Publication bias: The case for an international registry of clinical trials. J Clin Oncol 4: 1529–1541

Simes RJ, Tattersall MHN, Coates AS, Raghavan D, Solomon HJ, Smartt H (1986) Randomised comparison of procedures for obtaining informed consent in clinical trials of treatment for cancer. Br Med J 293: 1065–1068

Slack NH, Brady MF, Murphy GP et al. (1984) Stable versus partial response in advanced prostate cancer. Prostate 5: 401–415

Smalley RV, Bartolucci AA, Hemstreet G et al. (1981) A phase II evaluation of a 3-drug combination of cyclophosphamide, doxorubicin and 5-fluorouracil in patients with advanced bladder cancer or stage D prostatic carcinoma. J Urol 125: 191–195

Smith PH, Suciu S, Robinson MRG et al. (1986) A comparison of the effect of diethylstilbestrol with low dose estramustine phosphate in the treatment of advanced prostatic cancer: final analysis of a phase III trial of the European Organization for Research on Treatment of Cancer. J Urol 136: 619–623

Soloway MS (1980) Rationale for intensive intravesical chemotherapy for superficial bladder cancer. J Urol 123: 461–466

Soloway MS, Einstein A, Corder MP, Bonney W, Prout GR Jr, Coombs J (1983) A comparison of cisplatin and the combination of cisplatin and cyclophosphamide in advanced urothelial cancer. Cancer 52: 767–772

Shearer RJ, Hendry WF, Sommerville IF, Fergusson JD (1973) Plasma testosterone: an accurate monitor of hormone treatment in prostatic cancer. Br J Urol 45: 668–677

Staquet M, Sylvester R (1977) A decision theory approach to phase II clinical trials. Biomedicine 26: 262–266

Stephens RL, Vaughan C, Lane M et al. (1984) Adriamycin and cyclophosphamide versus hydroxurea in advanced prostatic cancer. A randomized Southwest Oncology Group Study. Cancer 53: 406–410

Sternberg CN, Yagoda A, Scher HI et al. (1985) Preliminary results of M-VAC (methotrexate, vinblastine, doxorubicin and cisplatin) for transitional cell carcinoma of the urothelium. J Urol 133: 403–407

Sternberg JJ, Bracken RB, Handel PB, Johnson DE (1977) Combination chemotherapy (CISCA) for advanced urinary tract carcinoma: A preliminary report. JAMA 238: 2282–2287

Stoter G, Sleyfer DT, Ten Bokkel Huinink WW et al. (1986) High-dose versus low-dose vinblastine in cisplatin-vinblastine-bleomycin combination chemotherapy of non-seminomatous testicular cancer. A randomized study of the EORTC Genitourinary Tract Cancer Cooperative Group. J Clin Oncol 4: 1199–1206

Stoter G, Sylvester R, Sleijfer DT et al. (1987) Multivariate analysis of prognostic variables in patients with disseminated non-seminomatous testicular cancer: Results from an EORTC multi-institutional phase III study. Int J Androl 10: 239–246

Tannock IF (1985) Is there evidence that chemotherapy is of benefit to patients with carcinoma of the prostate? J Clin Oncol 3: 1013–1021

The Leuprolide Study Group (1984) Leuprolide versus Diethylstilbestrol for metastatic prostate cancer. New Engl J Med 311: 1281–1286

Tonkin K, Tannock IF (1988) Evaluation of response and morbidity following treatment of bladder cancer. In: Raghavan D (ed) The management of bladder cancer. Edward Arnold, London, pp 228–244

Tonkin K, Tritchler D, Tannock IF (1985) Criteria of tumor response used in clinical trials of chemotherapy. J Clin Oncol 3: 870–877

Umeda T, Niijima T (1986) Phase II study of alpha interferon on renal cell carcinoma. Summary of three collaborative trials. Cancer 58: 1231–1235

Van der Werf-Messing B, Van der Heul RD, Ledeboer RCh (1978) Renal cell carcinoma trial. Cancer Clin Trials 1: 13–21

Veenema RJ, Dean AL Jr, Roberts M, Fingerhut B, Chowdhury BK, Tarassoly H (1962) Bladder carcinoma treated by direct instillation of thio-tepa. J Urol 88: 60–63

Warr D, McKinney S, Tannock I (1984) Influence of measurement error on assessment of response to anticancer chemotherapy: proposal for new criteria of tumor response. J Clin Oncol 2: 1040–1046

Wettlaufer JN, Feiner AS, Robinson WA (1984) Vincristine, cisplatin, and bleomycin with surgery in the management of advanced metastatic nonseminomatous testis tumors. Cancer 53: 203–209

Yagoda A (1980) Chemotherapy of metastatic bladder cancer. Cancer 45: 1879–1888

Yagoda A, Watson RC, Natale RB et al. (1979) A critical analysis of response criteria in patients with prostatic cancer treatment with cis-diamminedichloride platinum II. Cancer 44: 1553–1562

Young DC, Garnick M (1988) Chemotherapy in bladder cancer: The North American experience. In: Raghavan D (ed) The management of bladder cancer. Edward Arnold, London pp 245–263

Zincke H, Utz DC, Taylor WF, Myers RP, Leary FJ (1983) Influence of thiotepa and doxorubicin instillation at time of transurethral surgical treatment of bladder cancer on tumor recurrence: A prospective, randomized, double-blind, controlled trial. J Urol 129: 505–509

Zincke H, Benson RC Jr, Hilton JF, Taylor WF (1985) Intravesical thiotepa and mitomycin C treatment immediately after transurethral resection and later for superficial (stages Ta and TIS) bladder cancer: A prospective, randomized, stratified study with crossover design. J Urol 134: 1110–1114

Chapter 14

Quality of Life and Palliation Treatment in Urological Cancer

Sophie D. Fosså, N.K. Aaronson and F. Calais da Silva

Introduction

In recent years the assessment of subjective response criteria and of quality of life (QoL) has become a matter of increasing interest in the clinical management of cancer patients (Aaronson 1986; Fayers and Jones 1983; Selby et al. 1984; Orr and Aisner 1986). The individual's physical, functional, psychological and social well-being is recognised as a significant endpoint of cancer treatment. On the one hand, this is due to the awareness that only limited therapeutic improvement has been achieved in the most prevalent malignancies in terms of increased cure rate and prolonged survival. On the other hand, for the curable cancer diseases (i.e. childhood cancer, malignant Hodgkin's disease, testicular cancer), the physician can today choose between several more or less intensive treatment options, with seemingly equivalent therapeutic results but with differing QoL and toxicity effects.

A somewhat arbitrary distinction can be made between subjective response and toxicity criteria (e.g. changes of the performance status, treatment-related side effects) and QoL measures (Aaronson et al. 1988). The former are generally assessed by an external observer (physician, nurse) whereas QoL assessment is most often based on the patient's own description and evaluation of his/her physical and psychosocial health state.

Subjective response criteria, and particularly treatment-induced toxicity, are most often assessed by the WHO grading system (Miller et al. 1981). The WHO system considers the degree of subjective symptoms but not necessarily their frequency or duration. The frequency and duration of symptoms may be of significant importance, however, as in the case of treatment-related nausea and vomiting. For example, many patients may accept severe treatment-related vomiting of short duration, but would not be willing to suffer from more moderate gastrointestinal toxicity lasting for several weeks.

Two main classification systems exist for assessment of performance status: The Karnofsky scale (KPS) (Karnofsky and Burchenal 1949) which employs an 11-step classification system, and the WHO scale which represents a truncated 5-step system (Miller et al. 1981). Though more complicated, the KPS is probably more reliable than the WHO grading system (Aaronson et al. 1988). Additionally, the more refined KPS grading system has the potential for yielding more clinically useful data than the briefer WHO scale (Stanley 1980).

No generally agreed upon evaluation system exists for the assessment of QoL in cancer patients. During recent years many groups have, however, worked out questionnaires for use in patients with specific cancer types (Raghavan et al.1988; Levine et al. 1987; Kaasa et al. 1988). Aaronson et al. (1986) have defined several conditions for QoL assessment in cancer clinical research by questionnaires:

1. Minimal patient burden (i.e. a simple, self-administered questionnaire with a maximum of approximately 40 questions)
2. Use of multiple items for evaluation of each of the 4 domains of QoL (physical, functional, psychological, social)
3. Evaluation of short time periods (e.g. "last week")
4. Use of Likert type response scales
5. Acceptable levels of reliability and validity
6. Feasible and practical data recording and management requirements

Quality of Life Assessment in Patients with Urological Cancer

The literature contains relatively few reports dealing specifically with symptom palliation in patients with urological cancer. Performance status and pain are occasionally considered in patients with advanced cancer. Improvement or worsening of pretreatment micturition problems is less often dealt with. Changes in symptoms during treatment have usually been rated by an external observer. Even less information is available about QoL alterations as a consequence of cancer treatment and malignancy development. Rather, most of the literature deals with treatment-related toxicity and morbidity and the role of subjective symptoms as prognostic parameters, (e.g. performance status and pain) (Fosså et al. 1984; Marcial et al. 1985; Smith et al. 1986).

Cancer of the Prostate

For the localised, theoretically curable stages of prostatic cancer most literature has dealt with treatment-induced toxicity. Radical prostatectomy has historically led to sexual impotence in nearly all patients and to urinary incontinence in 30% (Ackermann and Frohmüller 1983). New operative techniques have decreased these percentages considerably (Eggleston and Walsh 1985), making radical prostatectomy a more acceptable treatment option. The principal side effects following irradiation of the prostate are frequency, dysuria, diarrhoea and abdominal pain, seen in 10%–30% of patients (Dewit et al. 1983; Pilepich et al. 1984; Telhaug et al. 1987). Much of this toxicity can be avoided by the use of CT-based radiation planning, optimal shielding techniques and proper selection of the target dose. Definitive radiation treatment may also lead to decreased sexual function in 20%–30% of the patients (Bergman et al. 1984).

In untreated advanced prostatic cancer bone pain or a decreased performance status are significant parameters associated with poor prognosis (Daponte et al. 1983; Smith et al. 1984). In addition, many patients have urinary symptoms such as frequency and dysuria. Primary androgen-suppressive treatment (medical or surgical castration) reduces these subjective problems in 80% of the patients and increases the performance status for a period lasting between several months and many years (Smith et al. 1986; Pavone-Macaluso et al. 1986; Haapiainen et al. 1986; Presant et al. 1987). Decreased libido and reduced sexual function occur almost universally during androgen-suppressive treatment (Bergman et al. 1984). To date, no clinically significant differences have been shown between the different hormone treatment options regarding the frequency or duration of palliation of these subjective symptoms (Robinson and Hetherington 1986). However, the risk of treatment-related toxicity differs: The risk of oedema, gynaecomastia, thrombo-embolic and cardiovascular side effects must be considered when starting oestrogen treatment (Glashan and Robinson 1981). After surgical castration many patients suffer from hot flushes and emotional instability which sometimes makes continuation of a vocational life difficult. In addition, individual patients may have psychological difficulties in accepting surgical castration (Lunglmayr et al. 1987); the percentage of such patients probably differs from country to country due to variations of the cultural background.

Hormone-resistant prostatic cancer is currently treated with alternative hormone treatment (corticosteroids, medroxyprogesterone acetate, estracyt, aminoglutethimide) or chemotherapy and/or irradiation (Fosså et al. 1985; Rostom et al. 1982; Eisenberger et al. 1985; Logothetis et al. 1982; Benson et al. 1982; Fosså 1987a, 1989b). For these patients improvement of subjective symptoms is a principal treatment aim. Most authors reporting on cytotoxic chemotherapy have, however, concentrated on objective response rates and survival; here treatment-related improvement has been minimal during the last decade (Eisenberger et al. 1985). Some studies have suggested that chemotherapy may occasionally reduce pain and lead to improvement in performance status (Logothetis et al. 1982). Of the patients receiving secondary hormone treatment 20%–30% experience a subjective response (Fosså et al. 1985). Subjective response evaluation has more often been done in radiotherapy studies (i.e. after half-body irradiation, radiotherapy to localised fields) (Benson et al. 1982; Fosså 1987). Pain relief can be expected in 40%–70% of the irradiated patients.

Most of the radiotherapy- and chemotherapy-induced acute subjective toxicity consists of short-lasting nausea, vomiting and diarrhoea. The need for frequent control examinations during intensive chemotherapy should also be viewed as a treatment-related "side effect". Such repeated clinic visits may represent a significant burden for a disabled patient in poor general condition.

Though all these malignancy-related and treatment-induced symptoms have been known for many years, few QoL studies have been performed in patients with prostatic cancer. Currently the Genito-Urinary Group of the European Organisation of Research on the Treatment of Cancer is carrying out two randomised studies in patients with prostatic cancer that include prospective QoL assessments during treatment (Denis 1986; Newling 1986). Such studies will yield more information about the possible superiority of one treatment versus another than can be obtained by evaluation of response and survival rates only, or by simple recording of treatment-induced toxicity or subjective response rate. Further, as the costs of and available resources for the alternative treatment modalities for prostatic cancer differ widely (in spite of similar response and survival rates) QoL studies can provide important information necessary in guiding clinical decision-making.

Bladder Cancer

Subjective symptoms specific to bladder cancer are often the initial signs leading to the diagnosis: haematuria, dysuria, and frequency (Marcial et al. 1985). In other patients such symptoms develop during the course of the disease (Cohen et al. 1986). However, very few reports describe changes in these symptoms during and after treatment. Radiotherapy is reported to palliate tumour-related haematuria, but improvement of other micturition problems seems to be less frequent (Silber et al. 1969; Chan et al. 1979; Culp 1979). Total cystectomy and/or supravesical urinary diversion are sometimes necessary to palliate symptoms of a contracted bladder due to recurrent tumour and/or following radiotherapy (Crawford and Skinner 1980; Montie et al. 1983).

Radiotherapy and radical cystectomy may produce specific problems in bladder cancer patients. The development of a contracted bladder with reduced capacity and long-term gastrointestinal symptoms have been described after irradiation, but are rarely severe (Edsmyr et al. 1978; Quilty and Duncan 1986). Raghavan et al. (1988) performed a QoL investigation of irradiated bladder cancer patients and found that the QoL was good in the majority of relapse-free patients as did Edsmyr et al. (1978). Most of the QoL studies in bladder cancer have concerned patients who have undergone total cystectomy. The conclusions from these reports are that the majority of relapse-free patients adapt sufficiently to the urinary diversion, though leakage problems are significant, particularly during the first months after cystectomy (Jones et al. 1980; Fosså et al. 1987b). Postoperative impotence remains a significant problem and decreases the patient's QoL, particularly if the patient has not been adequately informed about this side effect before the operation (Fosså et al. 1987b). Newer operative techniques of total cystectomy and urinary diversion have now been developed which preserve the erectile function and provide a continent urinary reservoir, independent of urinary bags (Eggleston and Walsh 1985; Montie et al. 1987).

Testicular Cancer

In contrast to prostatic and bladder cancer, testicular cancer is now a highly curable malignancy. Most of these young patients are willing to accept the price of severe, short-lasting, acute subjective toxicity and a transiently reduced QoL for a high probability of being cured. On the other hand, long-lasting chronic toxicity, even if only slight or moderate, may be more difficult to accept.

Each of the three treatment modalities of testicular cancer – surgery, radiotherapy and chemotherapy – has its specific acute side effects. Transient, moderate abdominal pain represents the most common subjective symptom after retroperitoneal lymph node dissection (Fosså et al. 1988). Radiotherapy leads to mild myelosuppression, moderate gastrointestinal side effects and general fatigue (Fosså et al. 1988). These side effects usually settle in the first 2–3 months after the end of treatment. Reversible nausea, vomiting, fatigue and autonomic neuropathy are the most common acute complications during cisplatin-based chemotherapy in testicular cancer (Fosså et al. 1988).

After retroperitoneal surgery "dry" ejaculation and subsequent infertility problems are the principal late toxicities (Fosså et al. 1988). Mild gastrointestinal toxicity is seen in approximately 30% of the patients, even many years after treatment (Hamilton et al. 1986; Fosså et al. 1988) and slight to moderate peripheral neuropathy represents the most frequent late toxicity after cisplatin-based chemotherapy. Both radiotherapy and chemotherapy lead to azoospermia which is reversible in many, but not in all, patients (Fosså et al. 1988).

During recent years increasing attention has been paid to QoL in patients with testicular cancer. Several specific QoL studies have been undertaken dealing with such psychosocial factors as employment, education, family situation, sexuality and emotional status (Schover and von Eschenbach 1984; Rieker et al. 1985). Most have focused on the QoL of cured patients, several years post-treatment. Prospective QoL studies are, however, in progress (Fosså et al. 1988). The overall impression that one gets from these studies is that the QoL of these patients is good. In general, they have a few or no educational or vocational problems and their overall QoL seems comparable to that of age-matched controls. However, individual patients suffer from sexual impairment, residual peripheral neuropathy or gastrointestinal problems (Fosså et al. 1988). Infertility may contribute significantly to a reduced QoL in cured testicular cancer patients (Schover and von Eschenbach 1984; Rieker et al. 1985; Fosså et al. 1988). At the time of diagnosis, 60% of testicular cancer patients consider the ability to father a child after treatment to be of importance for future QoL (Fosså and Aass 1989).

There are currently several treatment options available for testicular cancer patients. Each achieves the goal of cure, and each affects QoL in different ways. Future QoL studies are needed to guide oncologists and urological surgeons in the selection of the most appropriate treatment modality to be offered to the individual patient, considering the stage of the malignancy together with the patient's age and psychosocial status and expected future QoL.

Cancer of the Penis

Though the psychosocial implications of this malignancy and its treatment (partial or total penectomy, radiotherapy to the penis) are obvious, no specifically designed QoL study has been conducted among patients with penile cancer. Future studies are needed to document the psychosocial consequences of penile cancer and, particularly, to compare the relative impact of radical surgery versus radiotherapy on the QoL of these patients. Though this disease is rare, larger cancer centres and/or cooperative research groups should be able to accrue patient series large enough to undertake such investigations.

Cancer of the Kidney

No therapeutic options exist for metastatic renal cell carcinoma that lead to acceptable objective response rates and/or prolongation of survival. Palliation and improvement of QoL are the principal goals of treatment in these patients. Subjective symptoms such as bone pain due to metastases can be greatly reduced by radiotherapy (Fosså et al. 1982; Reddy et al. 1983; Halperin and Harisiadis 1983). In recent years the role of orthopaedic surgery has been emphasised for patients with incapacitating bone metastases (Sherry et al. 1982) and embolisation of the renal artery if haematuria due to the primary tumour represents a problem (Khoury et al. 1983).

Hormone treatment with high doses of medroxyprogesterone acetate leads to an improved performance status in 30% of the patients (deKernion 1983). Chemotherapy and immunotherapy have resulted in an improved general condition in only a minority of patients with metastatic renal cell carcinoma (deKernion 1983; Fosså and De Garris 1987).

Given the lack of favourable therapeutic results of systemic treatment of metastatic renal cell carcinoma, the clinician should be reluctant to apply aggressive chemo- or immunotherapy routinely in these patients. Such therapy will often reduce the patient's QoL without offering an acceptable chance of benefit. However, for some patients with metastatic renal cell carcinoma, the offer of active treatment, even without assurance of improvement in health status, may be preferred to a "no treatment" option.

Conclusion

The lack of reports of prospectively evaluated subjective response rates and of specifically designed QoL studies in patients with urological cancer necessitates increased activity in these areas in the future. QoL studies offer the opportunity for truly interdisciplinary, cooperative research between physicians, researchers from the behavioural sciences and members of the nursing staff. The results of such research activity can exert a significant influence on the selection of the optimal treatment for patients with urological malignancies.

References

Aaronson NK (1986) Methodological issues in psychosocial oncology with special reference to clinical trials. In: Ventrafridda V et al. (eds) Assessment of quality of life and cancer treatment. Elsevier Science Publishers, Amsterdam, pp 29–41
Aaronson NK, Calais da Silva F, Yoshida O, van Dam FSAM, Fosså SD, Miyakawa M, Raghavan H, Riedl H, Robinson MRG, Worden JW (1986) Quality of life assessment in bladder cancer clinical

trials: conceptual methodological and practical issues. In: Denis L et al. (eds) Development in bladder cancer, Alan R Liss, Inc, New York, pp 149–170

Aaronson NK, Calais da Silva F and de Voogt HJ (1988) Subjective response criteria and quality of life. In Denis L et al. (eds) Progress and controversies in oncological urology. Alan R Liss Inc, New York, pp 261–274

Ackermann R, Frohmüller HGW (1983) Complications and morbidity following radical prostatectomy. World J Urol 1: 62–67

Benson RC jr, Hasan SM, Jones AG and Schlise S (1982) External beam radiotherapy for palliation of pain from metastatic carcinoma of the prostate. J Urol 127: 69–71

Bergman B, Damber JE, Littbrand B, Sjögren K, Tomic R (1984) Sexual function in prostatic cancer patients treated with radiotherapy, orchiectomy or oestrogens. Br J Urol 56: 64–69

Chan RC, Bracken RB, Johnson DE (1979) Single dose whole pelvis megavoltage irradiation for palliative control of hematuria or ureteral obstruction. J Urol 122: 750–751

Cohen JM, Persky L, Resnick MI (1986) Pattern of urinary symptoms in patients with metastatic bladder cancer. J Urol 136: 586–588

Crawford ED, Skinner DG (1980) Salvage cystectomy after irradiation failure. J Urol 123: 32–34

Culp DA (1979) Palliative treatment of the patient with disseminated carcinoma of the bladder. Sem Oncol 6: 249–253

Daponte D, Robinson MRG, Smith PH (1983) Prognostic significance of the symptoms associated with prostatic carcinoma. Eur Urol 9: 270–272

Denis L (1986) EORTC protocol 30853: Phase III protocol for a randomized prospective study of the treatment of patients with metastatic prostatic cancer to compare the therapeutic effects of orchiectomy versus LHRH-analogue depot (Zoladex) preparation supplemented by an anti-androgen (Flutamide) Brussels: EORTC Data Center.

Dewit L, Ang KK, van der Schueren E (1983) Acute side effects and late complications after radiotherapy of localized carcinoma of the prostate. Cancer Treat Rev 10: 79–89

Edsmyr F, Esposti PL, Giertz G, Littbrand B (1978) Radiation treatment of urinary bladder carcinoma. Urol Res 6: 229–232

Eggleston JC, Walsh PC (1985) Radical prostatectomy with preservation of sexual function: pathological findings in the first 100 cases. J Urol 134: 1146–1148

Eisenberger MA, Simon R, O'Dwyer PJ, Wittes RE, Friedman MA (1985) A reevaluation of nonhormonal cytotoxic chemotherapy in the treatment of prostatic carcinoma. J Clin Oncol 3: 827–841

Fayers PM, Jones DR (1983) Measuring and analysing quality of life in cancer clinical trials: A review. Stat Med 2: 429–446

Fosså SD (1987) Palliative pelvic radiotherapy in patients with hormone-resistant prostatic cancer. In: Murphy GP, Khoury S, Küss R, Chatelain CL, Denis L (eds) Prostate Cancer Part B: Imaging Techniques, Radiotherapy, Chemotherapy and Management Issues. Alan R. Liss Inc, New York, pp 479–485

Fosså SD (1989) Estramustine phosphate – a clinician's review. In: Current methods in diagnosis and treatment of prostatic cancer. Thieme, Stuttgart (in press).

Fosså SD, Aass N (1989) Fertility and paternity in patients with testicular cancer. In: Proceedings International Conference on Reproduction and Human Cancer. 11–13 May, Washington

Fosså SD, De Garis ST (1987) Further experience with recombinant interferon α-2A with or without vinblastine in metastatic renal cell carcinoma. A progress report. Int J Cancer [Suppl. 1] 36–40

Fosså SD, Kjølseth I, Lund G (1982) Radiotherapy of metastases from renal cancer. Eur J Urol 8: 340–342

Fosså SD, Kaalhus O, Sauer T, Hager B, Lund G (1984) Radiotherapy of T_4 bladder carcinoma. Rad Oncol 1: 291–298

Fosså SD, Jahnsen JU, Karlsen S, Øgreid P, Haveland H, Trovåg A (1985) High-dose medroxyprogesterone acetate versus prednisolone in hormone-resistant prostatic cancer. A pilot study. Eur Urol 11: 11–16

Fosså SD, Reitan JB, Ous S, Kaalhus O (1987) Life with an ileal conduit in cystectomized bladder cancer patients: expectations and experience. Scand J Oncol Nephrol 21: 97–102

Fosså SD, Aass N, Kaalhus O (1988) Testicular cancer in young Norwegians. J Surg Onc 39: 43–63

Glashan RW, Robinson MRG (1981) Cardiovascular complications in the treatment of prostatic carcinoma. Br J Urol 53: 624–627

Haapiainen R, Rannikko S, Alfthan O (1986) Comparison of primary orchiectomy with oestrogen therapy in advanced prostatic cancer. Br J Urol 58: 528–533

Halperin EC, Harisiadis L (1983) The role of radiation therapy in the management of metastatic renal cell carcinoma. Cancer 51: 614–617

Hamilton C, Horwich A, Easton D, Peckham MJ (1986) Radiotherapy for Stage I seminoma testis: Results of treatment and complications. Radiother Oncol 6: 115–120

Jones MA, Breckman B, Hendry WF (1980) Life with an ileal conduit: results of questionnaire surveys of patients and urological surgeons. Br J Urol 52: 21–25

Kaasa S, Mastekaasa A, Stokke I, Naess S (1988) Validation of a quality of life questionnaire for use in clinical trials for treatment of patients with inoperable lung cancer. Eur J Cancer Clin Oncol 24: 691–701

Karnofsky D, Burchenal JH (1949) The clinical evaluation of chemotherapeutic agents in cancer. In: Mcleod CM (ed) Evaluation of chemotherapeutic agents. Columbia University Press, New York, pp 191–205

DeKernion JB (1983) Treatment of advanced renal cell carcinoma – traditional methods and innovative approaches. J Urol 130: 2–7

Khoury S, Richard F, Kuss R (1983) How often is embolization of renal cancer useful nowadays? In: Cancer of the prostate and kidney. Pavone-Macaluso M, Smith PH (eds) Plenum Press, NY, London, pp 659–662

Levine M, Arnold A, Bush H, Abu-Zahra H, DePauw S (1987) Quality of life in Stage II breast cancer. Proceedings of ASCO. 6: 254

Logothetis CJ, von Eschenbach AC, Samuels ML, Trindade A, Johnson DE (1982) Doxorubicin, mitomycin and 5-FU (DMF) in the treatment of hormone-resistant Stage D prostate cancer: A preliminary report. Cancer Treat Rep 66: 57–63

Lunglmayr G, Girsch E, Bieglmayer C (1987) Acceptability of orchiectomy versus GNRH-agonists in the management of advanced cancer of the prostate. J Endocrinol Invest 10 [Suppl 2]: 20

Marcial VA, Amato DA, Brady LW, Johnson RJ, Goodman R, Martz KL, Hanley JA (1985) Split-course radiotherapy of carcinoma of the urinary bladder Stages C and D_1. Am J Clin Oncol 8: 185–199

Miller AB, Hoogstraten B, Staquet M, Winkler A (1981) Reporting results of cancer treatment. Cancer 47: 207–214

Montie JE, Whitmore WF, Grabstald HM, Yagoda A (1983) Unresectable carcinoma of the bladder. Cancer 51: 2351–2355

Montie JE, Pontes E, Smyth EM (1986) Selection of the type of urinary diversion in conjunction with radical cystectomy. J Urol 137: 1154–1155

Newling DWW (1986) EORTC protocol 30865: A randomised phase III study comparing estracyt and mitomycin-c in hormone escaped advanced prostatic cancer. Brussels: EORTC Data Center.

Orr ST, Aisner J (1986) Performance status assessment among oncology patients: A review. Cancer Treat Rep 70: 1423–1429

Pavone-Macaluso M, de Voogt HJ, Viggiano G, Barasolo E, Lardennois B, DePauw M, Sylvester R (1986) Comparison of diethylstilbestrol, cyproterone acetate and medroxyprogesterone acetate in the treatment of advanced prostatic cancer: Final analysis of a randomized phase III trial of the European Organization for Research on Treatment of Cancer Urological Group. J Urol 136: 624–631

Pilepich MV, Krall J, George FW, Asbell SO, Plenk HD, Johnson RJ, Stetz J, Zinninger RN, Ralz BJ (1984) Treatment-related morbidity in phase III, RTOG studies of extended-field irradiation for carcinoma of the prostate. Int J Radiat Oncol Biol Phys 10: 1861–1867

Presant CA, Soloway MS, Klioze SS, Yakabow A, Presant SN, Mendez RG, Kennedy PS, Wyres MR, Naessig VL, Todd B, Wiseman CL, Bouzaglou A, Tanenbaum B, Eventov D (1986) Buserelin treatment of advanced prostatic carcinoma. Cancer 59: 1713–1716

Quilty PM, Duncan W (1986) Primary radical radiotherapy for T3 transitional cell cancer of the bladder: An analysis of survival and control. Int J Rad Oncol Biol Phys 12: 853–860

Raghavan D, Grundy R, Lancaster L (1988) Assessment of quality of life in long-term survivors treated by first-line intravenous cisplatin for invasive bladder cancer. In: Smith PH, Pavone-Macaluso M (eds). Management of advanced cancer of prostate and bladder. EORTC Genitourinary Group Monograph 4. Alan Liss, New York, pp. 625–631

Reddy S, Hendrickson FR, Hoeksema J, Gelber R (1983) The role of radiation therapy in the palliation of metastatic genitourinary tract carcinomas. Cancer 52: 25–29

Rieker PP, Edbril SD, Garnick MB (1985) Curative testis cancer therapy: Psychosocial sequelae. J Clin Oncol 3: 1117–1126

Robinson MRG, Hetherington J (1986) The EORTC studies: is there an optimal endocrine management for M1 prostatic cancer? World J Urol 4: 171–175

Rostom AY, Folkes A, Lord C, Notley RG, Schweitzer FAW, White WF (1982) Aminoglutethimide therapy for advanced carcinoma of the prostate. Br J Urol 54: 552–555

Schover LR, von Eschenbach AC (1984) Sexual and marital counseling with men treated for testicular cancer. J Sex Marital Ther 10: 29–40

Selby PJ, Chapman JAW, Etazadi-Amoli J, Dalley D, Boyd NF (1984) The development of a method for assessing the quality of life of cancer patients. Br J Cancer 50: 13–22

Sherry HS, Levy RN, Siffert RS (1982) Metastatic disease of bone in orthopedic surgery. Clin Orthop Rel Res 169: 44–52

Silber I, Bowles WT, Cordonnier JJ (1969) Palliative treatment of carcinoma of the urinary bladder. Cancer 23: 586–588

Smith PH, Pavone-Macaluso M, Viggiano G, De Voogt H, Lardennois B, Robinson MRG, Richards B, Glashan RW, de Pauw M, Sylvester R and the EORTC Urological Group (1984) EORTC protocols in prostatic cancer. In: Denis L, Murphy PG, Prout GR, Schroder F (eds). Controlled clinical trials in urologic oncology. Raven Press, New York, pp 107–117

Smith PH, Suciu S, Robinson MRG, Richards B, Bastable JRG, Glashan RW, Bouffioux C, Lardennois B, Williams RE, de Pauw M, Sylvester R (1986) A comparison of the effect of diethylstilbestrol with low dose estramustine phosphate in the treatment of advanced prostatic cancer: Final analysis of a phase III trial of the European Organization for Research on Treatment of Cancer. J Urol 136: 619–623

Stanley KE (1980) Prognostic factors for survival in patients with inoperable lung cancer. JNCI 65: 25–32

Telhaug R, Fosså SD, Ous S (1987) Definitive radiotherapy of prostatic cancer: The Norwegian Radium Hospital's experience 1976–1982. Prostate 11: 77–86

Chapter 15

The Cost of Treatment

D.W.W. Newling and J. Hutton

Introduction

Until recent years, it has never been necessary for individual members of the medical profession working in an adequately funded nationalised health service to consider the practice of medicine other than in terms of providing the best treatment possible for an individual patient. In other societies there have, of course, always been constraints brought about by temporary or permanent shortage of resources or by the lack of facilities freely available in other parts of the world.

Nowadays, however, the increasing longevity of the populations in the Western world has resulted in a rapid expansion of services for the elderly within the community and the hospital. Two decades ago such care was merely of a long-term nature in wards which were relatively inexpensive – a form of custodial care – but the demand is now for the provision of adequate acute care as the life expectancy of the ageing population has increased. This requires either an increasing investment in terms of finance and manpower or a reassessment of priorities.

The public expects a comprehensive medical service, the administration expects an efficient service and the medical profession expects a developing service regardless of cost. It seems likely that not all these aims can continue easily to be met. This contribution is designed to highlight some of the economic problems facing the medical profession within the field of urological oncology.

Classification of Costs

There are two main dimensions of cost: the nature of the resources used, e.g., labour, capital, equipment or consumables; and the group on whom the costs fall. In calculating the costs of treating cancer a threefold categorisation of costs is useful – specific hospital costs, general hospital costs, and personal costs to patients and their families. The sum of the three gives the overall social cost of treating a disease. In addition, the costs of attempting to provide any form of screening service which is considered to be desirable should be remembered.

Specific Hospital Costs

These include the cost of diagnostic tests specifically for the patient group under study; the cost of surgical procedures undertaken; and the cost of other treatments, such as radiotherapy or chemotherapy.

General Hospital Costs

This category of costs is common to the treatment of many conditions and often does not vary much between patient groups. It covers the support services provided by the hospital and the costs of providing ward accommodation and out-patient clinics. It is customary in the National Health Service in England to present these in terms of costs per hospital bed-day or per outpatient visit. These are, of course, average cost figures and must be used with caution in calculating additional costs or marginal cost savings.

Personal Costs

These can be out-of-pocket expenses for travel to hospital for treatment or to visit relatives. More serious is the loss of working time, on a temporary or permanent basis, sustained through illness. In many cases, society loses the output of productive members and incurs further costs, often borne by other members of the family as well as the welfare services, in supporting those who are ill. The burden of being ill is a "cost" in itself which must not be ignored but is difficult to measure. Because the emphasis in this chapter is on the costs to the National Health Service of treating cancer the personal costs will not be considered in detail. However, insofar as they may differ between treatment methods they should not be ignored when choosing therapeutic approaches.

Screening Costs

A screening service is not so far routinely provided to detect patients with urological malignant disease but this chapter will consider some of the implications of the development of such services.

Use of Cost Information

Having identified the specific costs of a treatment and estimated the length of hospital stay involved, the total cost can be built up using standard values for each of these items. Some examples of standard values for St. James's Hospital in Leeds are given in Table 15.1.

Table 15.1. Average costs per new referral, subsequent outpatient attendance and inpatient costings, St. James's University Hospital, Leeds, for the year ended March 1986

	Cost in pounds
Outpatient consultation	
New patient	126.00
Follow-up visit	25.00
Inpatient costs	
Per day	75.00
Average per case	725.00

The figures given in Table 15.1 relate to the total cost of providing a diagnostic service for a new patient on an outpatient basis, the average cost of each follow-up visit and the inpatient cost per day. These figures include all services provided by the hospital including medical salaries, catering, the costs of the investigation departments and the upkeep and maintenance of the hospital. There is no allowance for capital investment in building or in certain other major capital items including radiological equipment.

Once the total cost of an individual treatment is known comparison can be made with other therapies, and if information on the relative efficacy of the treatment is available a proper cost-effectiveness comparison can be made. If treatments are considered equally effective then, in the absence of other constraints, the least costly option should be chosen. The generation of good data on effectiveness is difficult because it requires information on patient survival and also on the quality of life during the survival period. This requires the calculation of quality-adjusted life years (QALYs) saved as outlined by Williams (1985). To do this for urological cancer is beyond the scope of this chapter, but in calculating costs to set beside the clinical discussion of the best forms of treatment we hope to move the debate towards this goal.

The following sections outline the principal costs involved in the management of the major urological cancers and discuss the costs of screening for these malignancies. The larger the cost of treatment the greater the potential benefit from preventive health care which reduces the need for it. In this context the cost measures can be used to approximate the resource savings from screening, with the caveat that average costs may over-estimate the savings which may actually accrue.

Costs differ from hospital to hospital and country to country. The figures used in this chapter are based on one hospital and are not necessarily generally applicable. However, they can be used to indicate the significant issues in costing which occur in any situation regardless of the absolute level of the figures. Unless otherwise indicated the cost information used in this chapter is at 1986 prices and totals have been rounded to the nearest pound.

Costs of Diagnosis, Treatment and Follow-up

The initial diagnostic evaluation of tumours of the urinary tract varies but is broadly similar and will include investigations such as full blood count, biochemical profile, chest X-ray, intravenous urogram, ultrasound, computerised tomography, arteriography, lymphography, urine cytology and histological biopsy. An outline of the likely expenditure for the diagnosis of each of the common tumours is shown in Table 15.2.

Table 15.2. Specific cost of diagnostic investigation

Investigation	Cost (£)	Kidney	Bladder	Prostate	Testis
Full blood count	7.00	+	+	+	+
Biochemical profile	3.00	+	+	+	+
Chest X-ray	3.00	+	+	+	+
Intravenous urogram	29.00	+	+	+	+
Ultrasound	6.00	+	−	?	?
CT scan	52.00	+	?	?	+
Arteriography	62.00	?	−	−	−
Cystoscopy	75.00	−	+	−	−
Biopsy	36.00	−	+	+	−
Cytology	15.00	−	+	−	−
Acid Phosphatase	3.00	−	−	+	−
Lymphangiogram	60.00	−	−	−	+
Bone scan	60.00	?	?	+	−
AFP B-HCG	3.00	−	−	−	+
Total (£) (minimal diagnostic evaluation)		100	168	141	157

Treatment costs vary widely from one country to another and also according to the clinical preference of the clinician. Treatment options include surgical excision, radiotherapy, cytotoxic chemotherapy and hormonal treatment. The likely costs of treatment of the different tumours by one or other technique in the United Kingdom is shown in Table 15.3. These costs are very approximate and relate primarily to the length of stay in hospital likely to be required for the treatment to be given. At one end of the scale carcinoma of the kidney can be treated only by radical nephrectomy while lesions of the testis are usually treated initially by orchidectomy and, if advanced, with expensive chemotherapy with or without radiotherapy. The treatment for so-called superficial and invasive bladder cancer and prostatic cancer is very much more variable. The figures given should be regarded only as an outline of the order of costs that may be incurred. Specific costs which may be incurred following the use of intravesical chemotherapy for superficial bladder cancer, and of the different forms of hormonal therapy for prostatic cancer are shown in Tables 15.4 and 15.5

The expenditure on follow-up will be related to the frequency with which the patients are seen, the investigations done on each patient and the duration of survival. These costs are likely to vary widely from hospital to hospital and depend upon the views of the different clinician. Large sums of money can be

Table 15.3. Treatment costs for urological tumours

	Kidney	Bladder	Prostate	Testis
Surgical operation	Radical nephrectomy 10 days £750	Superficial tumours TUR 5 days £375 Invasive tumours radical cystectomy 17 days £1300	TUR 5 days £375	Orchidectomy 4 days £300
Radiotherapy	Rarely applicable	Radical course £2100 (inpatient)	Radical radiotherapy £2100 (inpatient)	Radiotherapy for seminoma £500 (outpatient)
Cytotoxic chemotherapy	Not yet relevant	M-VAC[a] 3 cycles £750	Not yet relevant	BVP[b] 4 cycles £1000
Hormonal treatment	Not relevant	Not relevant	e.g. Stilboestrol 1 mg/day £10/yr or orchidectomy £450 or Estracyt 280 mg/bd £1500/yr	

[a] Methotrexate, Vinblastine, Adriamycin and Cisplatinum
[b] Bleomycin, VP-16, Cisplatinum
Costs of inpatient care for patients receiving cytotoxic chemotherapy including anti-emetics, biochemical and haematological assessment and intravenous fluid are not included.

Table 15.4. Costs of intravesical chemotherapy (up to 15 treatments may be used)

	Per treatment (£)	Total (15 treatments) (£)
Thiotepa 60 mg	18.00	270.00
Epodyl 1.1 g	3.00	45.00
Adriamycin 50 mg	75.00	1125.00
Mitomycin 40 mg	70.00	1050.00

Table 15.5. Annual costs of hormone therapy

	£
Diethylstilboestrol 1 mg/day	10.00
Honovan 100 mg/day	39.00
Megace 160 mg/day	410.00
Anti-androgen, e.g. Cyproterone acetate 300 mg/day	1019.00
LH-RH agonist, e.g. Zoladex, 4 weekly	1492.00
Estracyt 280 mg/bd	1579.00

spent during follow-up by unnecessary frequency of attendance and excessive investigations. The policy should be defined and controlled with great care to minimise the inconvenience for the patient and the expense for the hospital.

Personal Costs

Diagnosis, treatment and follow-up presents the patient with severe and recurrent personal stress. His life is threatened by the diagnosis and treatment and each follow-up visit is a reminder that further problems may lie ahead. The patient's self-esteem, occupation, social life and family are all disturbed. This short section highlights just a few of the problems which may have to be faced.

Adequate surgical excision is followed by temporary disability for all and by permanent disability for some, e.g., radical cystectomy usually leads to impotence in the male and cessation of sexual function in the female, especially if the anterior vaginal wall is removed.

Radiotherapy produces malaise and local irritation for considerable periods of time together with impaired fertility when used in patients with testicular tumours (which may later recover) and a 10% incidence of major complications when used in the pelvis, including fibrosis, bladder irritation, contracture, urethral stricture, irradiation proctitis and stenosis of the sigmoid colon and rectum. The small bowel may also be affected. Although radiotherapy is relatively rarely used in association with primary tumours of the kidney its use is associated with some loss of liver function especially when given to the renal fossa.

Chemotherapy used extensively in patients with testicular tumours causes severe acute problems, is often associated with prolonged sub-fertility or infertility and may lead to the development of second maligancies at some stage in the future.

Hormonal therapy used in prostatic carcinoma mimics castration and results in the cessation of sexual function and other changes including gynaecomastia when oestrogens are used, together with an increased liability to cardiovascular problems.

In addition to these recognised hazards, it is less commonly remembered that the younger patients will need to take considerable periods of time off work for diagnosis, for treatment which will extend over several weeks and, intermittently thereafter, for follow-up. Such patients have to cope with the recognition that their lives are likely to be shortened as a result of the tumour which they have acquired. This leads to psychological disturbance in the short term as the patient grapples with this new, unexpected and unwelcome event in his life and will unsettle the whole family in the medium and longer term since they live in expectation of relapse or the development of disease in some new place. Many patients will find it difficult to continue in the employment which they have chosen, may be forced to retire early and thus suffer financial loss; in addition, they must also face a period of declining capacity as tumour recurrence occurs and further treatment is required or as long-term complications become evident.

The clinical and psychological problems faced by the patient and his advisors determine the intensity and frequency of follow-up. It is important for the professional advisor and for different reasons for the health economist, that it be kept to a minimum with only the essential investigations being carried out on each occasion.

Screening for Urological Malignancies

In most areas of medicine, prevention is often both medically and economically preferable to cure. Screening is not a preventive measure in itself but it may allow earlier treatment which can be more successful. A screening programme can only save resources for the health service if the earlier treatment is less expensive than the later treatment, and the savings made are sufficient to outweigh the cost of the screening programme. These circumstances are unlikely to arise in cancer treatment as early treatment is often quite radical, and late treatment may only be palliative.

If screening programmes are developed for urological malignant disease the most likely benefit will be that of improved health following more successful earlier treatment. The cost of this treatment will, of course, have to be added to the costs of screening. From the health economist's point of view such additional benefits will be related to the additional resource in terms of manpower and finance needed to identify the cases at an appropriately early stage.

In patients with carcinoma of the kidney it would be necessary to carry out routine ultrasound screening, probably in those over 50 years of age (Watanabe et al. 1981). If this were carried out every five years and limited to those particularly at risk, i.e., the male population and smokers, the approximate cost would be as outlined in Table 15.6. Since Hellsten et al. (1981) have already shown that up to one-third of renal tumours never present clinically during the life of the patient such a screening programme would identify a large number of additional tumours for which treatment would be required. Presumably many patients would have an operation which would be unnecessary, while some would benefit from the earlier diagnosis.

Table 15.6. Approximate cost of 5-yearly screening for carcinoma of the kidney by ultrasound from age 50 years (assuming survival to 70 years)

	Cost (£)
Whole population	176 200 000.00
Male population	85 130 000.00
Smokers only	24 000 000.00

Throughout the world screening programmes for bladder cancer have been undertaken in areas where patients follow occupations which make them particularly susceptible to this disease (Cartwright and Glashan 1984). These include the professions allied to the rubber, chemical and dye-stuffs industries. Such a screening programme involves cytological examination of early morning urines during the patient's working life and at regular intervals for 20 years afterwards, since the latent period for the development of bladder cancer may be long. Each cytological examination of three early-morning specimens of urine costs approximately £15. In the absence of symptoms these examinations will probably be carried out annually; in the presence of symptoms they will be undertaken more frequently and it may well be necessary for them to be accompanied by more expensive and time-consuming procedures such as intravenous urography and cystoscopy. Irrespective of the cost such selected programmes are much simpler to justify.

In patients with carcinoma of the prostate screening is still a debatable issue. From comparative work in the UK and US it seems likely that patients may have in situ or very early focal carcinoma of the prostate for many years with no symptoms or signs. When this group of patients become symptomatic they will probably respond as well as those who are treated initially. Screening may well identify a number of patients who will never need treatment for this very early prostate cancer before dying of other diseases (Newling et al. 1985). If screening is carried out by rectal examination, ultrasound, or aspiration cytology, those patients who now present clinically (8000/year in the UK) are likely to be picked up earlier – at extra cost: the implications of this are shown in Table 15.7.

Table 15.7. Cost implications of screening and treatment in patients with carcinoma of the prostate

Technique	Number of patients	Annual cost (£)
Aspiration cytology	8 000 000	120 000 000
Subsequent minimal investigation of positive cases	8 000	560 000
Treatment	2 000	
All by DES		20 000
All by radical operation		6 000 000

Screening for testicular cancer is carried out by the individual patient and by doctors. Intensive programmes are underway to teach testicular self-examination. Already these are achieving some results in that there is an increasing referral of young men with innocent and occasionally suspicious scrotal swellings to urological outpatient clinics. Screening is also carried out by medical staff during the course of insurance or other medical examinations at work.

Such screening does not require money for equipment or special tests. The need is for adequate financial resources to allow for printing of pamphlets and to make educational video programmes for private or television usage. The cost of such ventures is hard to identify but a recent video accompanied by pamphlets on testicular self-examination produced by the testicular subgroup of the Yorkshire Urological Cancer Research Group cost approximately £3000. Treatment of this tumour is so well defined and the possibility of cure (if diagnosed early) so great, that screening for this urological tumour could produce very great health benefits.

Summary

At first sight it may be thought that the most useful and cost-effective innovation for malignant disease of the urinary tract would be the development of appropriate screening programmes for patients at risk in order that effective treatment could be instituted as early as possible. Such screening programmes, however, especially if involving laboratory investigations (e.g., cytology) or imaging studies (e.g., ultrasound) are expensive and, in the context of the majority of patients with urological malignances, are likely to be of doubtful efficiency since treatment, except for those with testicular disease, is not yet guaranteed to be effective.

In patients with cancer of the testis, in whom early investigation and correct primary and secondary therapy commonly saves lives, a screening programme involving testicular self-examination is almost certainly valuable since it will allow an increasing number of patients to be diagnosed before dissemination has occurred.

On the other hand, in carcinoma of the prostate, expensive treatment in many instances is not necessary. In this condition, therefore, it is important to rationalise the management by identifying those patients who need treatment and in whom such treatment will increase survival witout adversely affecting quality of life.

The particular problem posed by patients with carcinoma of the bladder is the identification of that subgroup of patients with superficial disease who will require intensive intravesical chemotherapy; also that subgroup in whom invasive disease will later occur in order that cystectomy may be carried out only when indicated and at such a time that it will be curative.

Carcinoma of the kidney remains the most enigmatic of urological tumours. Although we know a great deal about its pathology we are not yet very good at treating it other than by surgical excision: at least 20% of such patients present with metastatic disease for which we can do virtually nothing.

When new treatment regimens are proposed, they are usually subject to clinical trials and at this stage it may be of some relevance to consider the costs of such trials and their contribution to the management of these disease processes. Over the course of the last 25 years many advances have come, in part as a result of patient clinical trial work by a number of important, dedicated and conscientious groups. Clinical trials in urological oncology are not, however, undertaken without considerable expense and if we are to look at a global sum for the cost of urological malignances, it should be borne in mind that for every patient submitted to a Phase II study of a new agent in urological oncology, the likely annual expense is of the order of £1000. For patients submitted to Phase III studies it is slightly less, and has been quoted at £600. Although much of this expense is borne by research institutions, pharmaceutical companies and a variety of private funds, governments do contribute to organisations such as the European Organisation for Research and Treatment of Cancer (EORTC) and the National Cancer Institute of America (NCI). From all available sources, the cost of running the Data Centre for the EORTC is some $600 000 annually. The total annual budget for the EORTC as a whole is over $2.2 million. The exact proportion that comes from the EEC and individual governments varies from year to year but may well be as much as 50% of this amount.

Although some trials, including those of the Veterans Administrative Cooperative Urological Research Group (VACURG) and the trial of bladder cancer carried out by Wallace and Bloom (1976), have demonstrated certain risk factors including the cardiotoxicity of stilboestrol 5 mg a day in patients with prostatic cancer and the fact that patients over 65 years of age with invasive bladder cancer are probably better treated initially by radiotherapy than by cystectomy, most have either shown no difference between the two proposed treatments or have tended to demonstrate that the newer option is not superior to the established treatment. Many such trials have been started with enthusiasm and if positive would have led to a significant increase in costs since the majority of newer treatments are more expensive than those which they are designed to replace.

The total annual National Health Service budget in the UK, without capital costs of buildings and major equipment, is of the order of 20 billion pounds. In order that the budget for the management of urological malignancies may command a proportion of that amount consistent with the incidence of morbidity and mortality of its constituent tumours the attention of all concerned, from research worker to medical superintendent, must be directed to the examination and practice of cost-effective therapy.

References

Cartwright RA, Glashan RW (1984) The epidemiology and management of occupational bladder cancer. In: Smith PH, Prout GR (eds) Bladder Cancer. Butterworths, London, pp 125–150

Hellsten S, Berge T, Wehlin L (1983) Unrecognised renal cell carcinoma. In: Pavone-Macaluso M, Smith PH (eds) Carcinoma of the Kidney and Prostate. Plenum Press, New York, p. 509

Newling DWW, Hall RR, Richards B, Robinson MRG, Hetherington JW (1985) The natural history of prostatic cancer – the argument for a no-treatment policy. In: Pavone-Macaluso M, Smith PH, Bagshaw MA (eds) Testicular Cancer and other Tumors of the Genitourinary Tract. Plenum Press, New York, pp 443–448

VACURG (1973) The Vacurg studies of cancer of the prostate. Cancer 32: 1126–1130

Wallace DM, Bloom HJG (1976) The management of deeply infiltrating (T3) bladder carcinoma: controlled trial of radical radiotherapy versus preoperative radiotherapy and radical cystectomy (first report) Br J Urol 48: 587–594

Watanabe H, Howles JH, Holm HH, Goldberg BB (1981) Diagnostic Ultrasound in Urology and Nephrology. Igaku-Shon, Tokyo

Williams AH (1985) Economics of coronary artery by-pass grafting. Br Med J (3 August)

Subject Index